AF696231

Immunomodulators in the Rheumatic Diseases

INFLAMMATORY DISEASE AND THERAPY

Series Editor

Daniel E. Furst
University of Medicine and Dentistry
of New Jersey
Robert Wood Johnson Medical School
New Brunswick, New Jersey
and Pharmaceuticals Division
CIBA-GEIGY Corporation
Summit, New Jersey

1. Methotrexate Therapy in Rheumatic Disease, *edited by William S. Wilke*
2. Therapy of Inflammatory Bowel Disease: New Medical and Surgical Approaches, *edited by Mark A. Peppercorn*
3. Platelet-Activating Factor in Endotoxin and Immune Disease, *edited by Dean A. Handley, Robert N. Saunders, William J. Houlihan, and John C. Tomesch*
4. Immunomodulators in the Rheumatic Diseases, *edited by Daniel E. Furst and Michael E. Weinblatt*

Additional Volumes in Preparation

Bradykinin Antagonists: Basic and Clinical Research, *edited by Ronald M. Burch*

Immunomodulators in the Rheumatic Diseases

edited by

Daniel E. Furst

University of Medicine and Dentistry of New Jersey
Robert Wood Johnson Medical School
New Brunswick, New Jersey
CIBA-GEIGY Corporation
Summit, New Jersey

Michael E. Weinblatt

Brigham and Women's Hospital
Harvard Medical School
Boston, Massachusetts

MARCEL DEKKER, INC. New York and Basel

Library of Congress Cataloging-in-Publication Data

Immunomodulators in the rheumatic diseases / edited by Daniel E.
Furst, Michael E. Weinblatt.
p. cm. -- (Inflammatory disease and therapy; 4)
Includes bibliographical references.
Includes index
ISBN 0-8247-8214-3 (alk. paper)
1. Rheumatoid arthritis--Immunotherapy. 2. Rheumatism-
-Immunotherapy. 3. Immunosuppressive agents. I. Furst, Daniel E.,
II. Weinblatt, Michael E. III. Series.
[DNLM: 1. Adjuvants, Immunologic--therapeutic use. 2. Rheumatic
Diseases--immunology. 3. Rheumatic Diseases--therapy. W1 IN41LA
v. 4 / WE 544 I338]
RC933.I43 1990
616.7'23061--dc20
DNLM/DLC
for Library of Congress 90-3297
CIP

This book is printed on acid-free paper.

Copyright © 1990 by MARCEL DEKKER, INC. All Rights Reserved

Neither this book nor any part may be reproduced or transmitted in any form or by any means, electronic or mechanical, including photocopying, microfilming, and recording, or by any information storage and retrieval system, without permission in writing from the publisher.

MARCEL DEKKER, INC.
270 Madison Avenue, New York, New York 10016

Current printing (last digit):
10 9 8 7 6 5 4 3 2 1

PRINTED IN THE UNITED STATES OF AMERICA

Series Introduction

As knowledge of inflammation has flourished over the last decade, understanding of the pathogenesis and therapy of inflammatory diseases has also improved. This has been particularly true in the rheumatic diseases, including infectious rheumatic diseases, those rheumatic diseases associated with gastrointestinal inflammation, immunologically mediated illnesses, various forms of vasculitis, and so forth.

Marcel Dekker, Inc., which specializes in high-quality monographs in a variety of focused medical disciplines, has supplied up-to-date, detailed, and practical information for the practicing physician and research scientist. The Inflammatory Disease and Therapy series addresses a number of carefully chosen topics of interest to practicing physicians, rheumatologists, and research scientists.

Daniel E. Furst

Preface

Inflammatory rheumatic diseases affect more than five million Americans; rheumatoid arthritis alone affects between two and three million. These diseases are chronic and recurrent, leading to lost time at work and school and disruption of family life.

Despite the major health influence of the rheumatic diseases, their treatment is only partially successful. Physical therapy, rest, nonsteroidal anti-inflammatory drugs, so-called disease modifying antirheumatics, corticosteroids, and surgery are frequently used. Unfortunately, they leave many patients' needs unmet and their diseases inadequately controlled.

More recently, as the medical community has begun to dissect the immune system and the underlying pathogenesis of some rheumatic diseases, some new approaches to rheumatic disease therapy have begun to emerge. These exciting developments provided the impetus for this book, a book describing the use of immunomodulation to treat rheumatic disease.

The purpose of this book is to take the reader from the forefront of today's immunomodulatory therapies into the treatments of the next five to ten years. Specifically it will:

- Outline and critically review some of the newest and/or most potent therapies for rheumatoid arthritis and other rheumatic diseases. Thus, methotrexate, azathioprine, alkylating agents, and combination therapy are reviewed in some detail.

- Discuss some experimental therapies for rheumatoid arthritis, including cyclosporine and gamma interferon.
- Consider the use and place of some nonmedicinal immunomodulators in the rheumatic diseases. Apheresis and total lymphoid irradiation are reviewed, and a discussion of their present usefulness and what they teach us about the pathogenesis of the rheumatic diseases is included.
- Review some of the exciting new approaches to rheumatic disease therapy and the directions in which such therapy is likely to go. This applies both to the chapters on cyclosporine and gamma interferon and to the discussion of the retinoids and future trends in the diagnosis and treatment of rheumatoid arthritis.

It is our hope that this book can serve as a well-referenced, critical review of the validity and place of some immunomodulator therapy in the treatment of rheumatoid arthritis and other rheumatic diseases.

We are grateful to our fellow contributors for their cooperation and thoroughness and to Rebecca Bernstein for her assistance in the preparation of this book.

Daniel E. Furst
Michael E. Weinblatt

Contents

Contributors

Thomas F. Bumol Lilly Research Laboratories, Indianapolis, Indiana

Grant W. Cannon Division of Rheumatology, University of Utah and Veterans Administration Medical Center, Salt Lake City, Utah

John H. Carstens, Jr. Department of Neuroendocrinology, Sandoz Research Institute, East Hanover, New Jersey

John W. Coffey Department of Allergy and Inflammation Research, Hoffmann-LaRoche, Inc., Nutley, New Jersey

Clifford W. Colwell, Jr. Division of Orthopedic Surgery, Scripps Clinic and Research Foundation, La Jolla, California

John G. Curd Division of Rheumatology, Scripps Clinic and Research Foundation, La Jolla, California

Douglas V. Faller Harvard Medical School, The Children's Hospital, and Dana Farber Cancer Institute, Boston, Massachusetts

Robert I. Fox Department of Rheumatology and Immunology, Scripps Clinic and Research Foundation, La Jolla, California

Andrea Kowal* Department of Neuroendocrinology, Sandoz Research Institute, East Hanover, New Jersey

---

**Present affiliation*: Department of Dermatology

Joel M. Kremer Division of Rheumatology, Albany Medical College, Albany, New York

Harold E. Paulus Division of Rheumatology, Department of Medicine, UCLA School of Medicine, Los Angeles, California

Charles A. Robinson Division of Rheumatology, Scripps Clinic and Research Foundation. La Jolla, California

John D. Schindler Department of Medical Research, Biogen, Inc., Cambridge, Massachusetts

Thomas J. Schnitzer Section of Rheumatology, Department of Internal Medicine, Rush-Presbyterian-St. Luke's Medical Center, Chicago, Illinois

David E. Trentham Division of Rheumatology, Beth Israel Hospital and Harvard Medical School, Boston, Massachusetts

Steven Weiner Department of Medicine, Olive View Medical Center and UCLA School of Medicine, Los Angeles, California

Gary W. Williams Division of Rheumatology, Scripps Clinic and Research Foundation, La Jolla, California

H. James Williams Division of Rheumatology, Department of Internal Medicine, University of Utah, Salt Lake City, Utah

Thasia G. Woodworth* Department of Allergy and Inflammation Research, Hoffmann-LaRoche, Inc., Nutley, New Jersey

**Present affiliation*: Seragen, Inc., Hopkinton, Massachusetts

Immunomodulators in the Rheumatic Diseases

1

Methotrexate in Rheumatoid Arthritis

Joel M. Kremer
Albany Medical College, Albany, New York

I. INTRODUCTION

Methotrexate (MTX) has become one of the most commonly prescribed drugs for the treatment of rheumatoid arthritis (RA). In spite of this fact, controversies exist concerning its proper role in the treatment of rheumatoid arthritis as well as the true incidence of toxicity associated with the drug. Although the mechanism of action of folate antagonists is well studied on a cellular biochemical level, the target cells for methotrexate in rheumatoid arthritis have not been elucidated. Conflicting evidence abounds of an anti-inflammatory versus an immunomodulating mechanism of action in this disease. We will review these areas along with an overview of the published evidence of clinical efficacy. Lastly, we will speculate on some possible directions of future use of this potent agent.

II. CHEMISTRY AND PHARMACOLOGY

A. Cellular Activity

Folic acid is an essential dietary factor which is metabolized intracellularly to reduced tetrahydrofolate (FH_4) by the enzyme dihydrofolate reductase (DHFR). Tetrahydrofolic acid can then function in several key intracellular synthetic reactions (Fig. 1). These include single-carbon transfer such as the conversion of 2-deoxyuridylate (DUMP) to thymidylate, an essential component of DNA. Reduced FH_4 is converted back to FH_2 as a result of the one-carbon transfer and must again be reduced by DHFR to FH_4 to regain its ability to transfer single carbon atoms (1).

Methotrexate is a folate analog which structurally resembles folic acid (Fig. 2). Methotrexate binds to DHFR, preventing the enzyme from forming metabolically active reduced FH_4. Thus, methotrexate will significantly impair cellular metabolism and reproduction via DHFR inhibition and decreased production of the essential FH_4. Inhibiting one-carbon transfer

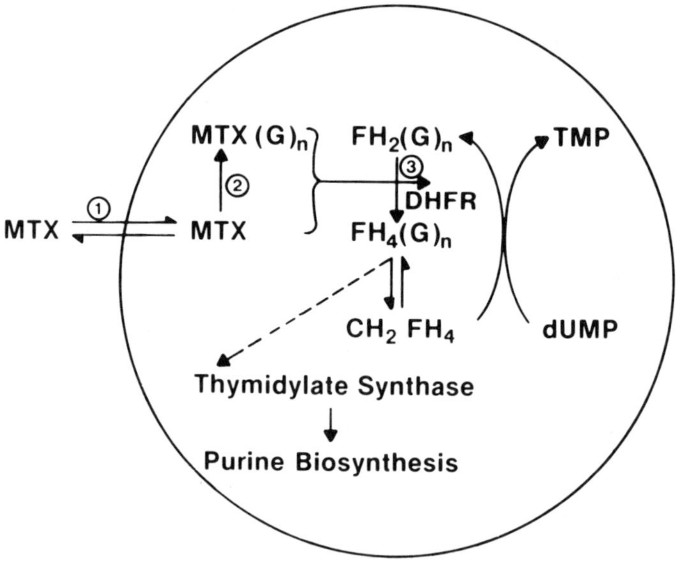

Figure 1 Cellular metabolism of methotrexate. Methotrexate (MTX) is actively transported within the cell (1) where several glutamic acid moieties are added [MTX(G)n] in the process of polyglutamylation (2). MTX(G)n inhibits the conversion of dihydrofolate [FH_2(G)n] to tetrahydrofolic acid [FH_4(G)n] by binding to dihydrofolate reductase (DHFR), the enzyme which catalyzes this reaction (3). The net result of this inhibition is decreased cellular pools of reduced folates [FH_4(G)n], which results in a diminished capacity to transfer methyl groups needed in such key reactions as the conversion of deoxyuridine monophosphate (dUMP) to thymidylate (TMP), essential in purine synthesis, and the production of the amino acid glycine (not shown).

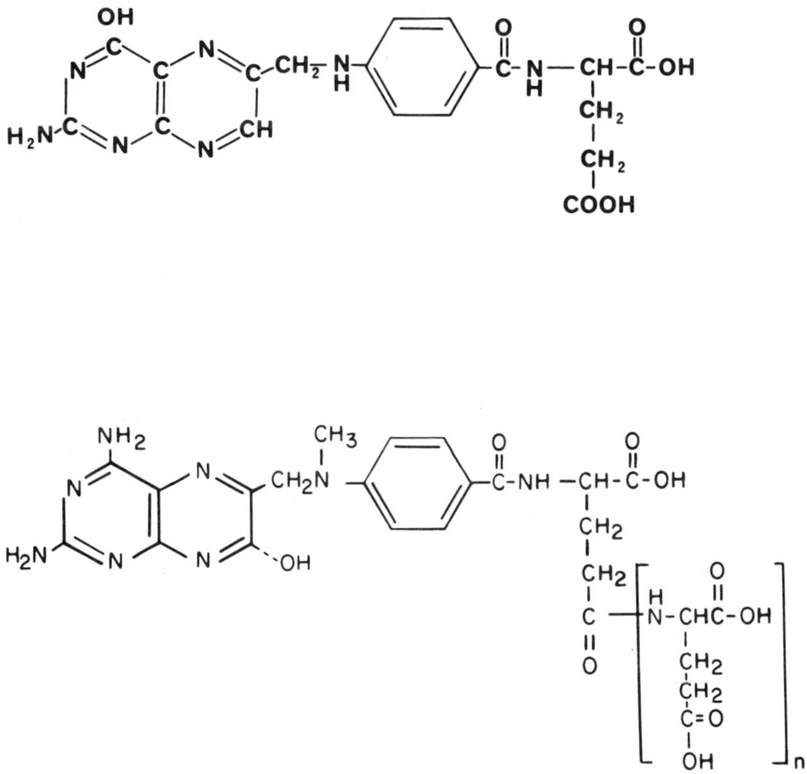

Figure 2 Stucture of folic acid and methotrexate. The similarity in structures between dihydrofolic acid (top) and methotrexate (bottom) is striking. It is easy to see why methotrexate would act to competitively inhibit the binding of folic acid to dihydrofolate reductase (DHFR).

effectively blocks the endogenous synthesis of glycine, thymidylate, and purines (1). Cells grown in tissue culture in a mixture containing these nutrients are indifferent to all methotrexate concentrations.

Methotrexate enters the cell via an active transport system. Once in the cell, glutamyl residues are added in a process termed polyglutamylation (Fig. 1). Methotrexate polyglutamylates have a high affinity for DHFR and are at least as potent inhibitors of this enzyme as methotrexate itself. Methotrexate polyglutamates cross cellular membranes poorly and are trapped within the cell (2). Accumulation of this metabolic product in kidney, liver, and brain is thought to be responsible for chronic toxicity after oncological dosing in these tissues (3). Methotrexate polyglutamate formation, with up to six glutamic acid residues, has been documented in rheumatoid arthritis patients receiving long-term methotrexate therapy (4). The relationship of methotrexate polyglutamate accumulation to chronic hepatotoxicity is currently unclear.

B. Absorption and Excretion

Although oral methotrexate may be well absorbed at doses of 0.1 mg/kg, higher dose ranges may be incompletely absorbed (5). Peak plasma concentrations of 1 μM are achieved 1-2 hr after oral methotrexate ingestion (4). The disappearance from plasma in oncological doses is sometimes triphasic with initial distribution into body fluids taking 45 min followed by a renal clearance phase of 2 hr and a terminal serum half-life of approximately 7 hr (5). This triphasic distribution pattern has not been documented in patients with rheumatoid arthritis.

The major excretory route of methotrexate is renal, involving both glomerular filtration and tubular secretion. Impaired renal function will thus result in delayed methotrexate clearance, increasing the potential for serious toxicity due to prolonged tissue exposure to the drug. After 24 hrs 7-OH-methotrexate appears in the urine (5). It is currently unclear whether this cellular metabolite contributes to efficacy or toxicity in a significant way.

C. Reversal of Cellular Toxicity

A description of methotrexate metabolism is not complete without an understanding of leucovorin's (N^5-formyl FH_4; folic acid) role in the reversal or "rescue" of cells from drug toxicity. Leucovorin is a fully reduced folate coenzyme which enters the cell via a specific carrier-mediated transport system. It is not dependent on reduction by DHFR (the enzyme blocked by methotrexate) and can thus effectively overcome the inhibition of the metabolic steps by the methotrexate-dependent depletion of reduced folates (1).

D. Mechanism of Resistance of Methotrexate

Several mechanisms of acquired cellular resistance to methotrexate have been described in cancer patients (Fig. 1). These include (1) impaired active transport of methotrexate into cells; (2) impaired polyglutamylation of methotrexate; (3) altered DHFR affinity for methotrexate; and (4) gene amplification causing an increased intracellular concentration of DHFR (6). None of these mechanisms has been shown to occur in rheumatoid arthritis patients receiving the drug, although elevated DHFR levels were observed in these patients' peripheral blood mononuclear cells when compared to a control RA population not receiving the drug (7). Increased DHFR levels were uniformly found in the methotrexate-treated patients and did not distinguish poor responders from good responders. The increased levels are thought to be due to a conformational change which renders the enzyme-drug complex less susceptible to proteolysis.

III. CLINICAL EXPERIENCE IN RHEUMATOID ARTHRITIS

A. Early Studies

In the early 1980s there was a proliferation of medical reports which described the clinical experience with methotrexate. These authors were among the first to describe the efficacy and toxicity of methotrexate in rheumatoid arthritis patients. It is largely through these reports, along with word-of-mouth communications among clinicians, that methotrexate became an acceptable alternative in the treatment of refractory disease.

When reviewing this initial clinical experience, one is struck by the lack of uniformity and agreement on such basic questions as how frequently to administer the drug (as well as by what route), how to monitor for toxicity, and what side effects to expect.

Hoffmeister treated 78 patients with methotrexate over a 15-year period (8). All patients failed to improve taking gold or nonsteroidal anti-inflammatory drugs, and most also did not respond to penicillamine or hydroxychloroquine. Methotrexate was administered intramuscularly at 10–15 mg/week, and some patients began oral therapy when maximum benefit was achieved. Hoffmeister found that "complete remission" occurred in 28 patients and that there was "marked improvement" in 45. The drug had "little or no effect" in 14 patients. Of 64 patients, 46 decreased their prednisone dosage because of a beneficial therapeutic effect from methotrexate.

Monitoring for toxicity was done at 2 and 4 weeks initially and on a monthly basis thereafter. Toxicity was limited to occasional stomatitis, headache, and nausea, and only 11 patients had abnormal LFT results. Sixty-seven liver biopsy tests were performed in 34 RA patients, including 24 patients treated for longer than 3 years and seven who had received treatment for between 6 and 15 years. A total of 10 baseline biopsy specimens were obtained. The results of 50 biopsy tests were normal, 17 showed mild to moderate fatty change, and seven showed a mild increase in portal fibrosis.

Hoffmeister concluded that the risk of performing the biopsy tests was not worth the yield and discontinued their use. Of the original 78 patients, 44 discontinued taking the drug.

Willkens and Watson (9) reviewed their experience with 67 patients who were treated with methotrexate for between 3 months and 10 years. Most patients had previously been treated with gold, D-penicillamine, and corticosteroids, and many had received chloroquine and immunosuppressives. Methotrexate was administered orally in three divided doses over 24 hr once a week, for a total dosage of 7.5-22.5 mg/week.

The authors devised criteria for one- and two-step improvement and found that 16 patients had no improvement, 33 had one-step improvement, and 18 had two-step improvement. Thirty-four patients, including five with nausea or dyspepsia and three with liver function abnormalities, had to discontinue methotrexate use. There were also two malignancies that could not be directly attributed to methotrexate use. Five liver biopsy tests were performed, showing mild fatty changes in one patient. The results of the other four tests were normal. The prednisone dosage of 12 of 33 patients was lowered, but the authors did not state whether manipulation of methotrexate dosage contributed to improved safety or efficacy.

In another open study, Steinsson et al. studied 21 patients who had severe RA that was resistant to conventional therapy (10). Patients received 7.5-25 mg of oral or intramuscular methotrexate for a mean of 38 weeks (range 3-114 weeks). Eleven patients had an "unequivocal" response (more than 30% improvement), and five patients had an "equivocal" response (less than 30% improvement). Six (of seven) patients could reduce their prednisone intake. Seven patients had to have the original methotrexate dosage increased to achieve efficacy, while two required a dosage reduction because of toxicity. Patients were monitored every 2-8 weeks; abnormal LFT results were seen in eight patients. The results of two liver biopsy tests were normal. The authors also commented that the size of subcutaneous nodules decreased in several patients.

Groff et al. evaluated their uncontrolled experience with 28 patients with refractory RA who were treated for a mean duration of 12 months (11). Patients received a mean of 8.36 mg of methotrexate orally in a once-a-week, 36-hr regimen. The authors reported tht 14 patients (50%) showed initial subjective improvement over 4-8 weeks. Such improvement had been noted by other investigators. Fourteen patients had a "positive overall response," and eight of 21 were able to lower their prednisone dosage. Patients were monitored every 2 weeks, then monthly; five patients experienced nausea, three had oral ulcerations, three had leukopenia, and two had herpes zoster.

The authors did not state whether the patients who had herpes zoster were taking prednisone. Six liver biopsy tests were performed; one showed minor periportal inflammation. Interestingly, toxicity decreased in 12 of 13 patients when the methotrexate dosage was lowered.

B. Short-Term Controlled Studies

These earlier investigations set the stage for prospective studies to prove that methotrexate was efficacious in the short-term treatment of rheumatoid arthritis. In a 6-week crossover study, Thompson et al. compared 10 mg and 25 mg of weekly intramuscular methotrexate to placebo in 48 patients (12). The authors found that both doses were significantly superior to placebo, but there was no difference in response between the two doses. Anderson et al. also studied intramuscular methotrexate and compared doses between 5 and 25 mg weekly with placebo in a 13-week crossover study (completed by 12 of 16 patients enrolled) (13). The authors found that methotrexate was significantly superior to placebo in most clinical variables measured. Although no significant changes were noted in rheumatoid factor titers, highly significant decreases in concentrations of serum IgG and IgM of 20-30% were observed. Elevated helper/suppressor T-cell ratios in peripheral blood which were noted prior to methotrexate therapy did not change after treatment.

Two short-term prospective controlled investigations established the efficacy of weekly oral methotrexate. Weinblatt et al. reported a 12-week crossover study of 7.5-15.0 mg of methotrexate which was completed by 28/35 patients (14). Methotrexate improved all clinical parameters except grip strength compared to placebo. No significant differences were noted in rheumatoid factor titers, immune complex concentrations, or peripheral blood helper or suppressor T cells. The authors noted transaminase elevation in 21% and nausea in 18% of the patients.

Williams et al. described the experience with 110 patients completing an 18-week double-blind parallel trial of 7.5-15 mg of oral methotrexate versus placebo in rheumatoid arthritis (15). Methotrexate was significantly superior to placebo in all clinical variables measured. One-third of the original 189 patients were withdrawn because they suffered some adverse effect, including transaminase elevation, oral ulceration, and gastrointestinal symptoms. Methotrexate-treated patients did exhibit a significant decrease in mean titer of rheumatoid factor compared to those on placebo.

It is interesting to note that 11/12 of Anderson's subjects, 27/28 of Weinhblatt's, and 38/57 of Williams's patients had to have their starting dose of 7.5 mg of methotrexate increased during these short-term studies in order to achieve a maximum therapeutic effect. These drug-dependent therapeutic effects were also observed for 10 versus 5 mg/M^2 of weekly oral methotrexate (16).

C. Long-Term Prospective Experience in Rheumatoid Arthritis

There are only a few prospective long-term studies, all open, of methotrexate therapy in active rheumatoid arthritis. We will concentrate on our experience with the drug at Albany Medical College (17,18).

It is clear that the long-term experience with methotrexate is different from the short-term in terms of both efficacy and toxicity. An exploration of these differences will give us some useful insights into both the actions of methotrexate and what is actually measured in published long and short-term studies.

All the short-term studies of efficacy comment on the rapid therapeutic benefit of methotrexate. We also found a rapid response which tends to maximize after 6 months of continuous weekly oral methotrexate therapy. After this time patients will generally maintain these gains, although the incremental improvements attained up until 6 months no longer occur. That is, patients reach a "plateau" and most individuals will not be clinically better after 12 months of therapy than they were after 6 months (Fig. 3 and 4). This

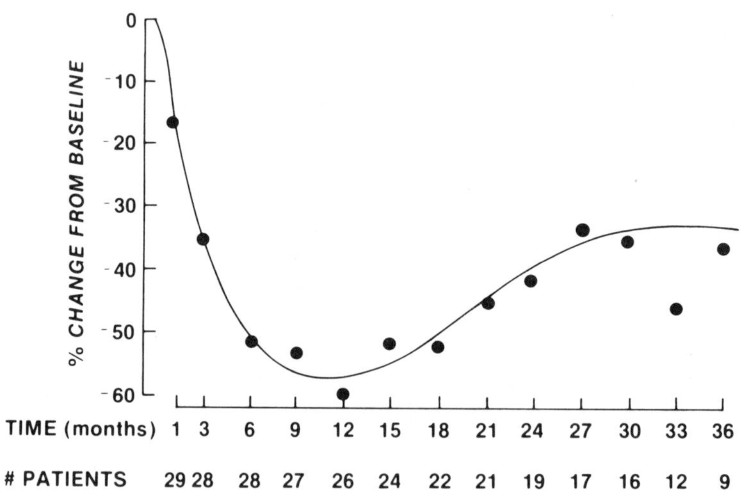

Figure 3 Number of tender joints during long-term methotrexate therapy. Patients achieve their maximal response after 6 months of therapy. After this time plateau in the clinical response is observed.

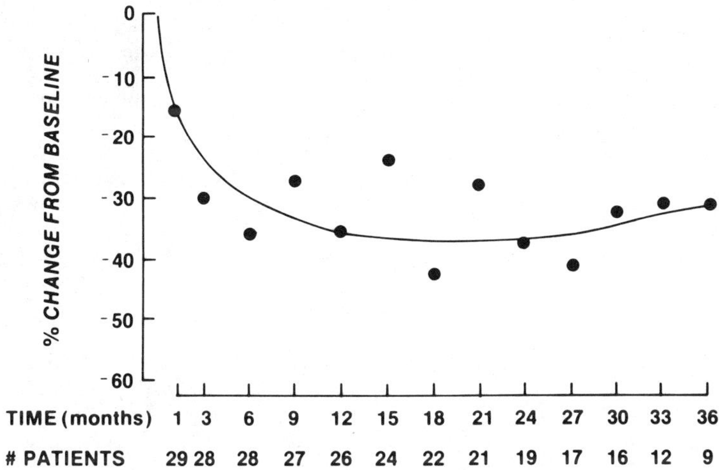

Figure 4 Number of swollen joints during long-term methotrexate therapy. Patients achieve their maximal response after 6 months of therapy. After this time a plateau in the clinical response is achieved.

plateau of clinical efficacy was maintained through 53 months of continuous therapy in our center.

Methotrexate is therefore not a remission-inducing drug; nor is any other drug used in RA regularly remission inducing. Of perhaps more concern are (1) whether the drug can favorably alter a measurable disease outcome such as radiographic progression; (2) whether it will be well tolerated over the long intervals which will be required in a life-long disease such as rheumatoid arthritis; (3) whether it is steroid sparing; and (4) what happens when it is stopped.

1. Radiographic Progression/Long-Term Clinical Response

After 2 years of therapy, we found that seven of 11 patients actually had improvement in erosive disease when examined by a bone radiologist in an open unblinded fashion (16). This effect on radiographic progression has only been reported infrequently after treatment with gold and cyclophosphamide (19-21). We considered this to be encouraging objective evidence that methotrexate could alter the basic course of erosive disease.

We were therefore disappointed to find that the radiographic improvement achieved after 2 years of therapy was not maintained after this time (18) (Fig. 5). In expanded observations of the same study cohort, eight of 22 patients

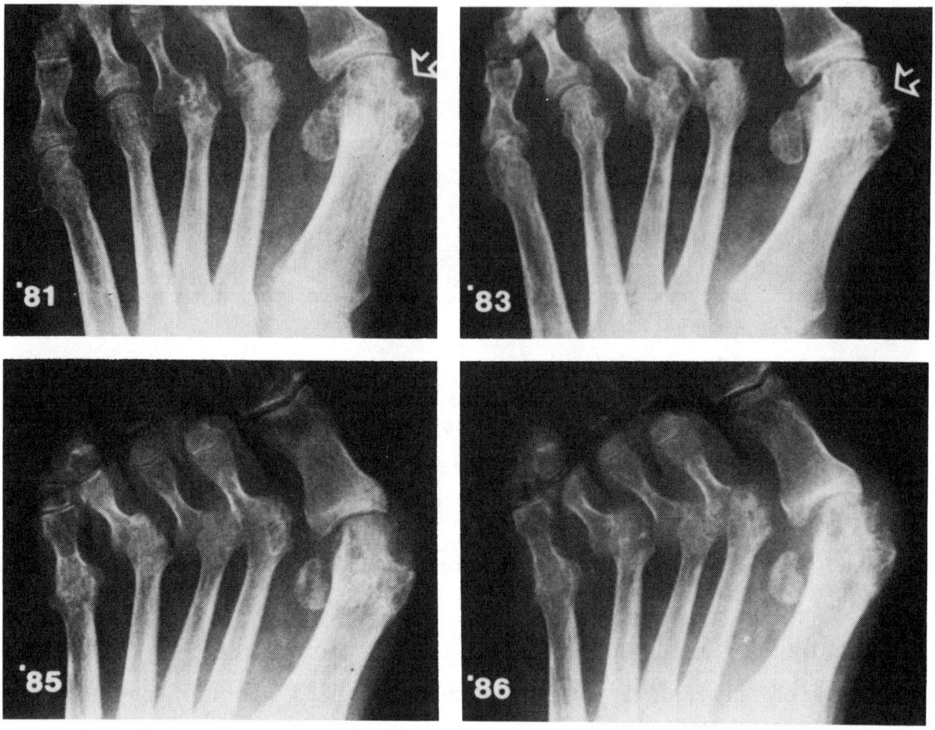

Figure 5 Radiographic changes on methotrexate. Foot radiographs of a patient begun on methotrexate in 1981 (upper left) showed improvement in erosive disease at the 1st metatarsal joint (upper right) in 1983. However, 2 years later (lower left, 1985) there has again been a radiographic deterioration with further worsening in the erosion of the metatarsal head and further destruction of the other metatarsals seen in 1986 (lower right).

exhibited radiographic deterioration in films obtained after 36–60 months of treatment (mean 52.5 months). Some of these individuals had exhibited improvement in erosive disease earlier in their course only to have progression later. Obviously, controlled studies are needed to conclusively decide this important question.

If one examines the slope of the long-term clinical efficacy curve, one observes that there is a noticeable increase in clinical manifestations of disease after 48 months (Fig. 3). The curve represents a mean of the entire study cohort of 25 patients and can thus be influenced if even a small number of patients alter their response to the drug. This in fact seems to be the case as reflected in the eight patients with radiographic deterioration. These same patients also had clinical worsening of disease and have had their weekly methotrexate dose increased to try and regain their original drug response. All of these patients were still improved when compared to their premethotrexate baseline status, yet they are not doing as well as earlier in their course of methotrexate treatment.

It is therefore not possible to extrapolate the efficacy results from short-term studies to long-term therapy. Patients do not continue to have regular incremental improvements and some actually deteriorate clinically while continuing to receive the drug. Possible explanations for this phenomenon lie in altered methotrexate metabolism (discussed in Sec. II) and a change in the underlying disease process. It is well established that rheumatoid arthritis exhibits a cyclical clinical pattern of exacerbations and remissions. It is possible that methotrexate is not potent enough to suppress these cycles. It is even possible that prolonged therapy in certain individuals effects a population of cells which somehow predisposes certain individuals to cyclical exacerbations of disease. In order to understand the mechanism(s) of clinical deterioration, we would undoubtedly be wise to discard our biases until the target cell(s) and mechanism of action of methotrexate in rheumatoid arthritis have been elucidated.

2. Side Effects

For a drug to be considered an appropriate choice for treatment of a chronic life-long disease, it must have an acceptable toxicity profile over long intervals, as will be required in rheumatoid arthritis. Just as it would be a mistake to accept a toxicity profile for insulin derived from a few months of treatment, it would be as significant an error to extrapolate the short-term toxicity data with methotrexate to its long-term use. Rheumatoid arthritis patients treated with methotrexate have life-long disease and the questions of the drug's safety must be formulated in this context.

It is safe to say that almost all patients receiving methotrexate experience some adverse effect, although these are usually rated as only mild to moderate (17,18). The effects are usually transient and can often be avoided entirely with a dosage adjustment. Twenty-six of 29 patients (90%) followed through 29 months experienced toxicity. After a mean of 53 months, 25 of those 29 patients remained on the drug. Of those 25 subjects, 21 experienced some adverse effect by 53 months.

Patients were as likely to experience side effects late in their treatment course as they were during the first year of therapy with the drug (18).

Moreover, the pattern of toxicity remained constant within patients. The patients who reported toxicity within a mean of 30-53 months of therapy also experienced similar adverse experiences during the initial 29 months. Only four patients did not experience toxicity during the mean treatment interval of 30-53 months and three of these four had never experienced an adverse effect during their initial 30 months of methotrexate therapy.

A breakdown of adverse occurrences between 30 and 53 months revealed that 13/25 patients (52%) experienced 34 separate episodes of nausea or gastrointestinal toxicity, 8/25 (32%) experienced 24 separate episodes of mouth soreness, and 9/25 (36%) experienced 18 episodes of headache and/or lightheadedness. This compares with an incidence of adverse experiences through 29 months in a slightly expanded cohort of the same patients of gastrointestinal toxicity in 18/29 patients (62%), oral ulcerations or mouth soreness in 11/29 (38%), and headache or lightheadedness in 6/29 (21%).

Leukopenia was noted in 6/29 patients (21%) through 29 months and 6/25 (24%) through 53 months of therapy. All six patients with depressed white blood cell counts between 30 and 53 months also exhibited transient leukopenia during the first 29 months of therapy. None of the episodes of leukopenia was considered significant; total WBC counts did not go below 2800 mm^3 at any time, nor was there granulocytopenia. All episodes of leukopenia resolved spontaneously without stopping methotrexate, although the dose was temporarily lowered in some cases. Thrombocytopenia has not yet been observed in our patient population, although it has been observed in other studies (D. Furst, pers. commun.).

3. Hepatotoxicity

The experience with methotrexate in psoriatic patients with psoriasis indicates that its use is associated with an incidence of cirrhosis which was as high as 25% in one investigation. Weinstein et al. identified risk factors for the development of hepatotoxicity which were derived from retrospectively collected historical data at the time of liver biopsy in over 500 patients (22). The authors identified alcohol consumption, increasing age, obesity, and the presence of diabetes mellitus to be associated with the development of hepatic fibrosis and cirrhosis.

Biopsy studies of patients with rheumatoid arthritis have not shown an incidence of cirrhosis which approaches that in the psoriasis literature (23-27). Some of these reports suffer from the lack of baseline hepatic histopathology to compare with subsequent biopsies obtained while patients were taking methotrexate. Many of the changes reported in psoriasis studies were also demonstrated in rheumatoid arthritis patients (28-31), although it is not clear whether the observed baseline changes were due to the disease or the drugs used to treat it.

There is therefore a real question as to whether the biopsy results derived from the dermatological experience with psoriasis apply to patients with rheumatoid arthritis. Further, there is a question as to whether the same risk factors for the development of significant hepatic disease will apply in rheumatoid arthritis. Another question arising from the psoriasis experience relates to the utility of routine liver enzyme monitoring, as that experience indicates that there is no correlation of histopathology with these laboratory tests. A careful reading of these studies reveals that the laboratory testing was obtained at the time of the liver biopsy and not in a routine serial fashion while patients continued to receive methotrexate.

We have undertaken a prospective study of liver biopsies in patients with rheumatoid arthritis on long-term methotrexate therapy. All patients underwent baseline biopsies prior to receiving the drug, again after 2 years, and annually thereafter. Clinical status along with monitoring of liver enzymes was performed on a monthly basis. Thus, simultaneously collected longitudinal chemical and laboratory data could be correlated with sequential biopsies which might show the evolution of hepatic changes in the same individual over time.

We found a statistically significant worsening of hepatic histology in the patients between the time of their baseline and last liver biopsy (Table 1) (32). Total cumulative dose and duration of MTX therapy did correlate with fibrotic changes observed at biopsy. These same factors did not correlate with overall histological worsening (i.e., nonfibrotic changes) in the entire study cohort. Enough patients changed their hepatic histological grade earlier on in the trial (second and third year biopsy) to obviate a significant correlation between a change in hepatic histology and the total dose of MTX ingested. The absence of a close correlation between the total dose of MTX and the degree of liver abnormalities has also been reported in psoriatic patients (22, 33-36) and also observed by other investigators in patients with RA (27). Fibrosis appears to be the only uniquely MTX-induced lesion in these patients and thus the finding of a correlation between it and the dose and duration of MTX is potentially meaningful (32).

A statistical analysis performed in order to distinguish which of multiple factors had the most influence on the same outcome (multivariate logistic regression) indicated that only increased body weight was significantly associated with the outcome of fibrosis. Obesity has been reported to correlate with the development of cirrhosis in psoriatic patients receiving MTX (1,3,

Table 1 Hepatic Histological Grade with Time (Mean + SEM)

Time (yr)	Number of patients	Total dose methotrexate mg (mean + SEM)	Mean histological grade (SEM)	p Values	
				Change from previous biopsy	Change from baseline
Baseline	33	0	2.37 + .56	–	–
2	26	1349 + 54	2.54 + .65	.25	–
3	19	2077 + 81	2.63 + .78	.82	12
4	15	2924 + 145	3.07 + .96	.06	.06
5	7	3596 + 121	3.00 + .40	.26	.22
6	1	4500	4.00	–	–

Table 2 Initial Development of Grade IV (Fibrotic) Changes Over Time, in Biopsy Specimens from Patients Receiving Long-Term Methotrexate Therapy for Rheumatoid Arthritis[a]

Time	No. of patients	No. with grade IV (%)
Baseline	27	0
2 yrs.	26	2 (7.7)
3 yrs.	19	3 (15.8)
4 yrs.	15	6 (40.0)
5 yrs.	7	2 (28.6)
6 yrs	1	1 (100)

[a]Fibrosis was seen on trichrome-stained sections only, and is considered early and clinically trivial. See Patients and Methods for explanation of grading system.

22) and has been observed to be a risk factor for hepatic fibrosis in two studies in RA (27,32).

Although 56% of patients exhibited fibrosis (Table 2) it was mild and did not interrupt the hepatic architecture. Whether this degree of change will evolve into clinically significant hepatic fibrosis or cirrhosis will need to be determined with continued observations.

Whether or not patients receiving methotrexate treatment for rheumatoid arthritis should have liver biopsies remains a matter of debate. A pre-MTX biopsy is probably not warranted unless there is a history of liver disease or significant alcohol intake. The issue of whether patients should have subsequent serial liver biopsies is more complex. The risk associated with liver biopsy itself should be less than the risk of persistent fibrosis or cirrhosis. Although we have observed a clear progression of subclinical hepatic architectural worsening, cirrhosis has not yet been reported in any patient with RA. The chances of missing a hypothetical incidence of cirrhosis of 10% with the number of biopsy samples in our study is 0.13 after 3 years and 0.21 after 4 years.

In combined studies of over 211,000 percutaneous liver biopsies for multiple different diagnoses, a mortality rate of between 0.0009 and 0.00017 is reported (37-39), although one survey of the literature listed a mortality of 0.0012 (37). The rate of major complications has been listed as 0.0032 in a review of 10,000 biopsies (37). If we assume an incidence of cirrhosis associated with long-term MTX therapy to be as low as 1% (considerably lower than the 25% incidence reported in some psoriatic studies) (34-36) and use the highester mortality rates for liver biopsy reported in the literature (37), then the relative risk of a liver biopsy is the risk of cirrhosis (0.01) divided by the risk of mortality from a liver biopsy (0.0012), or 8.3. If we use more current references for mortality from liver biopsy (0.0019), then the relative risk increases to over 59, i.e., hypothetically a patient would be 59 times more likely to get cirrhosis than to die from a liver biopsy. Thus, RA patients will have to develop far less hepatotoxicity than that reported in psoriatic patients before liver biopsies in RA patients receiving MTX are unnecessary.

4. Pulmonary Toxicity

Methotrexate pneumonitis has been well described (40–44) in patients receiving the drug for different diagnoses in RA. The acute syndrome may present with a prodrome of headache and malaise followed by a nonproductive cough, dyspnea, and fever (40,41). Tachypnea is common with crepitent rales in one-third and cyanosis in one-half during the clinical course (40). Eosinophilia was reported in 40% in one review (40) but not in another (41). A chest X ray may show linear or reticulonodular infiltrates, but may range from normal to "a widespread alveolar filling process" (40). The syndrome may be steroid-responsive with clinical resolution occurring over 2-4 weeks, although a prolonged pulmonary illness and death have been reported as has resolution when steroids were withheld (40). The syndrome can be distinguished from rheumatoid lung by virtue of its acute onset and short-term course although the clinical and laboratory presentation can be nonspecific (41). Open lung biopsy has shown alveolar damage with prominent epithelial cells as well as a prominent mononuclear cell interstitial infiltrate (which can form nodular aggregates) (41).

In practice the syndrome may be more insidious than the classical syndrome described by Sostman et al. (40). The distinction between methotrexate pneumonitis and rheumatoid lung may be especially difficult in individuals with preexisting interstitial lung disease and baseline functional respiratory impairment. Bronchoalveolar lavage has been espoused to be diagnostically useful in methotrexate pneumonitis (45). In our experience the distinction between the acute hypersensitivity reaction (with a predominance of neutrophils) (46,47) and the pattern seen with stable rheumatoid lung (predominance of lymphocytes on lavage) (46) is difficult and may require repeated samples on an individual patient as the pattern of cellular reactivity seems to be highly variable between individuals (J. K., unpublished data).

The acute pulmonary reaction has been described in the relatively low weekly doses used for rheumatoid arthritis (42-44) (7.5-15 mg/week) and with as little as 165 mg total dose of methotrexate treatment (42). Several patients have had methotrexate reinstituted after recovering from the acute pneumonitis (41) and, although most will not have a recurrence, some severe recurrences and even death have occurred (40). We currently view the presence of documented methotrexate pneumonitis as a contraindication to the continued use of the drug in that individual.

It is currently unclear whether methotrexate benefits preexisting rheumatoid lung disease, or whether preexisting lung disease places that patient at greater risk for developing the pulmonary reaction to methotrexate.

5. Teratogenicity and Carcinogenicity

Methotrexate is a human teratogen which can cause DNA strand breaks and chromatid exchanges (48-50). Thus, it is mandatory that all females of child-bearing potential use an effective birth control method if they are to receive methotrexate (48-50). If the physician is not satisfied that this is the case, it would probably be best not to use the drug in a female with any potential for pregnancy.

The drug has also been shown to transiently effect spermatogenesis (51, 52) and it is probably best that males be counseled about these effects and use effective birth control if their partners are of childbearing potential.

Although there have been a few reports of malignancies in rheumatoid arthritis or psoriatic patients receiving low-dose methotrexate, no increase in malignancies was found in 3522 patient-years of risk in patients receiving methotrexate for treatment of choriocarcinoma (53) or in 245 long-term methotrexate-treated patients with psoriasis (54). At the present time we feel that there is no real evidence that methotrexate is carcinogenic.

6. Mechanism of Action

The mechanism of action of methotrexate in rheumatoid arthritis is unknown (see above). Because it has a relatively rapid onset of action and well-documented steroid-sparing effects, an anti-inflammatory action has been suggested. No effects on the 5-lipooxygenase or cyclooxygenase metabolic pathways were observed in rat adjuvant arthritis (55), although these same studies have not been reported in humans. Effects on rheumatoid factor titers are inconsistent, with most authors reporting no effect (14,15,17), while others showed a definite lowering of titers (13,56).

Reports of effects on helper and suppressor T-cell ratios are also inconsistent. Both increased helper cells (14) and decreased suppressor cells have been reported, along with decreased absolute lymphocyte counts (57). No changes were observed in response to in vitro mitogens in lymphocytes of patients receiving methotrexate (13,14). Methotrexate has been shown to decrease macrophage production of interleukin-1 in rat adjuvant arthritis (58,59), but the significance of this finding in RA is unknown.

Patients receiving methotrexate are not immunocompromised in the same sense as patients receiving azathiopine or cyclophosphamide. There are isolated reports of aspergillosis, histoplasmosis, and herpes zoster (60) in patients on methotrexate, but the exact incidence of these infections is undoubtedly exceedingly low.

IV. FUTURE DIRECTIONS

Although the metabolic activity of methotrexate has been extensively studied and is reasonably well understood, we cannot use this information with precision until the actual site of its activity in rheumatoid arthritis is determined. The situation is actually made easier in oncology where kinetics of neoplastic cell populations are well studied. We need to know more about methotrexate's site of action(s) in the immune and inflammatory (or endothelial cell) systems to optimize its therapeutic effects while minimizing toxicity. For example, perhaps we will be better able to understand the plateau effect of clinical efficacy when some of these mechanistic insights are attained.

Others have speculated on the use of methotrexate earlier in the disease course before the use of more traditional disease-modifying agents. It is possible that methotrexate could be employed simultaneously with these other drugs for limited periods of time so that long-term toxicity problems could be avoided. The clinical flare phenomenon which is marked when methotrexate is discontinued (61) may be more tolerable in the setting of another disease-modifying agent.

A recent review (60) took the position that there are insufficient long-term toxicity data on the use of methotrexate to comfortably recommend it as a first-line agent at the present time. If long-term studies do show an acceptable toxicity profile, we could then support its earlier use. It is also possible that other folate analogs could be employed which would maintain clinical efficacy while reducing toxicity. Further studies of the mechanism of action of methotrexate should allow us to derive meaningful insights about the pathogenesis of rheumatoid arthritis itself.

REFERENCES

1. Chabner B. In: Chabner BA, ed. Methotrexate, pharmacological principles of cancer treatment. Philadelphia: SB Saunders, 1982.
2. Goldman ID. Effects of methotrexate on cellular metabolism: Some critical elements in drug-cell interaction. Cancer Treatment Rep 1977; 61:549–58.
3. Jackson RC, Grindey GB. The biochemical basis of methotrexate cytotoxicity in folate antagonists as therapeutic agents. In: Sirotnak FM, ed. Folate antagnosits as therapeutic agents. Orlando: Academic Press, 1984:280–316.
4. Kremer J, Galivan J, Streckfuss A, Kamen B. Methotrexate metabolism analysis in blood and liver of rheumatoid arthritis patients. Arth Rheum 1986; 29:832–835.
5. Calabresi P, Parks, RE. In: Goodman A, Gilman LS, Rall TW, Murad F, eds. Pharmacological basis for therapeutics. New York: Macmillan 1985.
6. Bertino JR, Rodenhuis S. Methotrexate and drug resistance: Advances in cancer chemotherapy. In Yagoda A, ed. Bladder cancer: future directions for treatment. New York: John Wiley and Sons, 1987.
7. Rodenhuis S, Kremer JM, Bertino JR. Increase of dehydrofolate reductase in peripheral blood lymphocytes of rheumatoid arthritis patients with low dose oral methotrexate. Arth Rheum 30:369–374, 1987.

8. Hoffmeister RT. Methotrexate therapy in rheumatoid arthritis: 15 years experience. Am J Med 1983; 12:69-73.
9. Willkens RF, Watson MA. Methotrexate: a perspective of its use in the treatment of rheumatic diseases. J Lab Clin Med 1982; 100:314-21.
10. Steinsson K, Weinstein A, Korn J, et al. Low dose methotrexate in rheumatoid arthritis. J Rheumatol 1982; 9:860-6.
11. Groff GD, Shenberger KN, Wilke WS, et al. Low dose oral methotrexate in rheumatoid arthritis: an uncontrolled trial and review of the literature. Semin Arth Rheum 1983; 12:333-47.
12. Thompson RN, Watts C, Edelman J, Esdaile J, Russell AS. A controlled two-center trial of parenteral methotrexate therapy for refractory rheumatoid arthritis. J Rheum 1984; 11:6, 760-3.
13. Anderson PA, West SA, O'Dell JR, Via CS, Claypool RG, Kotzin BL. Weekly pulse methotrexate in rheumatoid arthritis. Ann Intern. Med 1985; 103:489-96.
14. Weinblatt ME, Colbyn JS, Fox DA, Holdsworth DE, Glass DN, Trentham, DE. Efficacy of low-dose methotrexate in rheumatoid arthritis. N Engl J Med. 1985; 312:818-22.
15. Williams HJ, Willkens RF, Samuelson CO, Alarcon GS, Guttadauria M, Yarboro C, Polisson RP, Weiner SR, Luggen ME, Billingsley LM, Dahl SL, Egger MJ, Reading JC, Ward JR. Comparison of low-dose oral pulse methotrexate and placebo in the treatment of rheumatoid arthritis. A controlled clinical trial. Arth Rheum 1985; 28:721-30.
16. Furst DE, Burmeister LF, Kohler JA, Koehace R. A dose-response relationship for methotrexate in the treatment of resistant rheumatoid arthritis. Arth Rheum 1987; 30:562 (abstr).
17. Kremer JM, Lee JK. The safety and efficacy of the use of methotrexate in long-term therapy for rheumatoid arthritis. Arth Rheum 1986; 29: 822-31.
18. Kremer JM, Lee JK. A long-term prospective study of the use of methotrexate in rheumatoid arthritis: update after a mean of 53 months. Arth Rheum 1988; 31:577-89.
19. Cooperating Clinics Committee of the American Rheumatism Association: a controlled trial of cyclophosphamide in rheumatoid arthritis. N Engl J Med 1970; 283:883-9.
20. Sigler JW, Gluhm GB, Duncan H, Sharp JT, Ensign DC, McCrum WR. Gold salts in the treatment of rheumatoid arthritis: aA double-blind study. Ann Intern Med 1974; 80:21-6.
21. Cooperating Clinics Committee of the American Rheumatism Association: A controlle dtrial of gold salt therapy in rheumatoid arthritis. Arth Rheum 1973; 16:353-8.
22. Weinstein G, Rocnigk HH, Maiback K, Cosimides J, Halprin K, Millard M. Psoriasis-liver methotrexate interactions. Arch Dermatol 1973; 108:36-42.

23. Aponte J, Petrelli M. Hepatic histology following prolonged treatment of rheumatoid arthritis with bolus methotrexate. Arth Rheum 1985; 28:S37 (abstr).
24. Willkens RF, Clegg DO, Ward JR, Marks CR, Greene ML, Tolman KG, Roth GJ, Jackson-Leonard PA. Liver biopsies in patients on low dose methotrexate for the treatment of rheumatoid arthritis. Arth Rheum 1985; 28:S77 (abst).
25. Rau R, Karger T, Frezel H. Liver biopsy findings in patients with rheumatoid arthritis and psoriatic arthritis on long-term treatment with methotrexate. Arth Rheum 1986; 29:S76 (abstr).
26. Brick JE, Moreland LW, Al-Kiwas F, Chang WWL, Bartolomeo AG. Prospective analysis of pre- and post-methotrexate liver biopsies in rheumatoid arthritis. Arth Rheum 1988; 3:529 (abstr).
27. Shergy W, Polisson R, Rice S, Caldwell D, Allen N. Methotrexate-induced hepatic fibrosis in patients with rheumatoid arthritis. Arth Rheum 1988; 31:529 (abstr).
28. Lefkovits AM, Farrow IJ. Liver in rheumatoid arthritis. Ann Rheum Dis. 1955; 14:162–8.
29. Dietrichson O, From A, Christoffersen P, Juhl E. Morphological changes in liver biopsies from patients with rheumatoid arthritis. Scand J Rheumatol 1976; 5:65–69.
30. Fernandes L, Sullivan S, McFarlane EG, Wojcicka BM, Arues TW, Eddleston ALWF, Hamilton EBD, Williams R. Studies on the frequency and pathogenesis of liver involvement in rheumatoid arthritis. Ann Rheum Dis 1979; 38:501–6.
31. Tolman KG, Kremer JM, Lee RG, Metros F, LeBregue DE, Furst DE. Pretreatment liver histology in rheumatoid arthritis patients treated with low dose methotrexate. Arth Rheum 1986; 29:S18 (abstr).
32. Kremer JM, Tolman KG, Lee RG. Baseline and follow-up liver histology in rheumatoid arthritis patients receiving pulse methotrexate. Arth Rheum 1987; 30:517 (abstr).
33. Roenigk HH, Berfeld WF, St. Jacques R, Owens FJ, Hawk WA. Hepatotoxicity of methotrexate in the treatment of psoriasis. Arch Dermatol 1971; 103:250–61.
34. Nyfors A. Liver biopsies from psoriatics related to methotrexate therapy: Findings in post-methotrexate liver biopsies from 160 psoriatics. Acta Patholog Scand 1977; 85:511–4.
35. Zachariae H, Kragballe K, Sogaard H. Methotrexate-induced liver cirrhosis: Studies including serial liver biopsies during continued treatment. Br J Dermatol 1980; 102:407–12.
36. Robinson JK, Baughman RD, Auerback R, Cimis RJ. Methotrexate hepatotoxicity in psoriasis-consideration of liver biopsies at regular intervals. Arch Dermatol 1980; 116:412–5.

37. Piccinino F, et al. Complications following percutaneous liver biopsy: A multicentre retrospective study on 68,276 biopsies. J Hepatol 1986; 2: 165.
38. Linduer H. Das risiko der perkatanen leberbiopsie. Med Klin 1971; 66: 924.
39. Thaler H. Ueber vorteil und risiko der leberbiopsie methode nach Meughini. Weiu Klin Wschr 1964; 76:533.
40. Sostman HD, Matthay RA, Putman CE. Methotrexate-induced pneumonitis. Medicine 1976; 55:371-88.
41. Carson CW, Cannon GW, Egger MJ, Ward JR, Clegg DO. Pulmonary disease during the treatment of rheumatoid arthritis with low dose pulse methotrexate. Sem Arth Rheum 1987; 21:186-95.
42. Cannon GW, Ward JR, Clegg DO, et al. Acute lung disease associated with low-dose pulse methotrexate therapy in patients with rheumatoid arthritis. Arth Rheum 1983; 26:1269-74.
43. Engelbrecht JA, Calhoon SL, Scherrer JJ. Methotrexate pneumonitis after low-dose therapy for rheumatoid arthritis. Arth Rheum 1983; 26:1275-8.
44. St. Clair EW, Rice JR, Synderman R. Pneumonitis complicating low-dose methotrexate therapy in rheumatoid arthritis. Arch Intern Med 1985; 145:2034-38.
45. Furst DE, Zowala D, Hauser M, Hunninghake G. Pulmonary function testing in rheumatoid arthritis patients on low–dose methotrexate. Arth Rheum 1986; 29:S17 (abstr).
46. Garcia JG, Parhami N, Killam D, Garcia PL, Keogh BA. Bronchoalveolar lavage fluid evaluations in rheumatoid arthritis. Am Rev Resp Dis 1986; 133:450-54.
47. Evans RB, Ettensahn DB, Fawaz-Estrup F, Lally EV, Kaplan SR. Gold lung: recent developments in pathogenesis, diagnosis and therapy. Sem Arth Rheum 1987; 16:196-205.
48. IARC Working Group. Methotrexate. IARC Monogr 1982; 26:282-5.
49. Li JC, Kaminskas E. Accumulation of DNA strand breaks and methotrexate cytotoxicity. Proc Natl Acad Sci USA 1984; 81:5694-8.
50. Lindskov R, Wulf HC, Wantzin GL, Niebuhr E. Sister chromatid exchange in patients treated with methotrexate for psoriasis. J Inv Dermatol 1984; 82:458-9.
51. Grunnet E, Nyfors A, Brogaard-Hansen K. Studies on human semen in topical corticosteroid-treated and in methotrexate psoriatics. Dermatologica 1977; 154:78-84.
52. Sussman S, Leonard JM. Psoriasis, methotrexate and oligospermia. Arch Dermatol 1980; 116:215-7.
53. Rustin GJS, Rustin F, Dent J, Booth M, Salt S, Bagshawe KD. No increase in second tumors after cytotoxic chemotherapy for gestational trophoblastic tumors. N Engl J Med 1983; 308:9,473-6.

54. Nyfors A, Jensen H. Frequency of malignant neoplasms in 248 long-term methotrexate-treated psoriatics. Dermatologica 167:260–261, 1983.
55. Welles WL, Silkworth J, Oronsky AL, Kerwar SS, Galivan J. Studies on the effect of low dose methotrexate on rat adjuvant arthritis. J Rheum 1985; 12:904–6.
56. Olson NJ, Callahan LF, Pincus T. Immunologic studies of rheumatoid arthritis patients treated with methotrexate. Arth Rheum 1987; 30: 481–8.
57. Kremer JM. Lymphocyte subset analysis after long-term methotrexate therapy for rheumatoid arthritis. Arth Rheum 1986; 29:S75 (abstr).
58. Hu SK, Mifeho YL, Oronsky AL, Kerwar SS. Studies on the effect of methotrexate on macrophage function. J Rheum 1988; 15:206–9.
59. Johnson WJ, Di Martino MJ, Mennier KA, Muirhead NH. Methotrexate inhibits macrophage activation as well as vascular and cellular inflammatory events in rat adjuvant arthritis. J Rheum 1988; 15:745–9.
60. Furst DE, Kremer JM. Methotrexate in rheumatoid arthritis. Curr Comm Arth Rheum 31:305–314, 1988.
61. Kremer JM, Rynes RI, Bartholomew LE. Severe flare of rheumatoid arthritis after discontinuation of long-term methotrexate therapy. Double-blind study. Am J Med 1987; 82:781–6.

2

Immunosuppressive Agents: Azathioprine, Alkylating Agents, and Combination Therapy

Grant W. Cannon
University of Utah and Veterans Administration Medical Center, Salt Lake City, Utah

H. James Williams
University of Utah, Salt Lake City, Utah

I. INTRODUCTION

Although patients with rheumatoid arthritis (RA) may respond to a conservative program of rest, physical therapy, and nonsteroidal anti-inflammatory drugs, some RA patients require more aggressive therapy. Other connective tissue diseases frequently have life-threatening manifestations that require chronic corticosteroid therapy. Some patients may not respond to even high-dose steroids and other approaches are necessary.

In an attempt to discover more effective antirheumatic drugs, physicians have begun to evaluate cytotoxic drugs previously developed for the treatment of malignant disease. Use of these agents began in the 1950s with aminopterin (1) and nitrogen mustard (2). The subsequent enthusiasm for corticosteroids overshadowed further cytotoxic study until the hazards of long-term corticosteroids and need for further disease suppression became apparent. While many drugs have been evaluated, those commonly used are azathioprine, chlorambucil, cyclophosphamide, and methotrexate. For a review of methotrexate, please refer to Chap. 1.

II. AZATHIOPRINE

In the early 1960s, 6-mercaptopurine (6-MP) was reported effective in multiple connective tissue disorders including RA (3,4). Efforts to protect 6-MP from rapid metabolism led to the development of azathioprine which is metabolized in vivo to 6-MP (5,6). Early reports described benefit with azathioprine in the treatment of RA (7-11) and systemic lupus erythematosus (SLE) (7,8). Later controlled trials were performed which confirmed the effectiveness of azathioprine in RA (12-14) and long-term follow-up studies demonstrated continued clinical efficacy (15-18). However, the role of azathioprine in SLE (19-27), inflammatory myopathy (28-31), and psoriatic arthritis (12,16) is less well established. The only rheumatic disease for which azathioprine is approved by the Food and Drug Administration (FDA) is RA.

A. Pharmacology

1. Pharmacokinetics

Azathioprine is 6-[(1-methyl-4-nitroimidazol-5-yl)thiol] purine (Fig. 1). Azathioprine is well absorbed orally (6) and approximately 30% of the circulating azathioprine is protein-bound (32). Between 2 and 10% of the drug is excreted unchanged in the urine (32,33). The plasma half-life of azathioprine is 3 hr in subjects with normal renal and hepatic function (32).

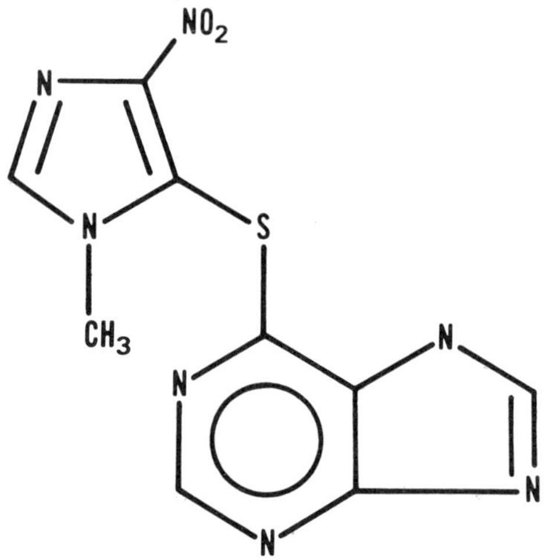

Figure 1 Chemical structure of azathioprine.

Azathioprine is not clinically active but is metabolized to 6-MP by the liver and erythrocytes (34,35). Multiple metabolites of 6-MP have been identified including the cytotoxic compounds 6-thioinosinic acid and 6-thioguanylic acid (5).

Although hepatic metabolism is important, the clinical effects of liver disease on azathioprine metabolism are unclear. Some patients with liver disease may have near-normal azathioprine metabolism (36) while other patients with chronic liver disease appear to be at higher risk for hematological toxicity (37). The half-life of azathioprine may increase to 7.5 hr in renal failure (38), although the effects of renal failure are often not clinically significant. Bach reported no increase in adverse drug reactions for 59 patients who had renal insufficiency treated with azathioprine (33).

Drug interactions with azathioprine are uncommon. Azathioprine and 6-MP are eventually metabolized to 6-thiouric acid by xanthine oxidase. Allopurinol blocks this action and promotes prolonged accumulation of azathioprine metabolites. Although the pharmacokinetics of 6-MP are not significantly altered by allopurinol in some patients (39), the inhibition of azathioprine metabolism by the simultaneous use of allopurinol may result in serious or potentially life-threatening toxicity. If azathioprine and allopurinol are to be used concurrently, the dose of azathioprine must be reduced by 75% and close monitoring performed for toxicity (35). Trimethoprim has been reported to increase the hematological toxicity with azathioprine (40).

2. Proposed Mechanisms of Action

The exact mechanism of action of azathioprine in rheumatic diseases remains unclear. The major effects of azathioprine result from its cleavage in vivo to 6-MP (6). The action of hypoxanthine phosphoribosyltransferase on 6-MP results in 6-thioinosinic acid which suppresses several steps in the synthesis of adenine and guanine by preventing interconversion of purine bases, especially inosinic and guanylic acid. This compound also inhibits production of inosinic acid and thereby inhibits de novo biosynthesis of purines (35). 6-Mercaptopurine may also be incorporated into RNA and DNA as 6-thioguanine (41). These combined effects lead to cell cytotoxicity although the role of cell cytotoxicity remains unclear in the action of these agents in RA.

In addition to cytotoxic effects, it has been suggested that azathioprine suppresses natural killer cell activity (42), antibody production (6), antibody-dependent cellular cytotoxicity (42), and cellular immune assays (43). There may be selective alteration of B cells during treatment with azathioprine (44). No change in adenosine deaminase is seen (45). In general, the immunological variables of patients with rheumatic diseases receiving azathioprine are not grossly altered during treatment (12). Azathioprine suppresses the production of autoantibodies in animal models of SLE (46,47) and has been noted to lower rheumatoid factor in RA patients (48,50), although this is not universally reported (9,13,14,51,52). It is unknown if this alteration of autoantibody level is a primary or secondary effect (46,47).

B. Efficacy

1. Rheumatoid Arthritis

Multiple studies have evaluated the efficacy of azathioprine in RA. Dosages tested have ranged from 1.0 to 4.8 mg/kg/day (16,17) with doses between 1.0 and 2.5 mg/kg/day employed most frequently. Studies comparing 1.25 mg/kg versus 2.5 mg/kg doses did not demonstrate statistically significant differences in clinical outcome (14,53), although the higher dose suggested greater improvement in some measured variables such as an increase in grip strength, a decrease in morning stiffness, and an improvement of disease activity by both physician and patient assessment (53). Adverse drug reactions may have been more common at the higher dose (53). In a large multicenter trial of azathioprine (1.25-1.5 mg/kg/day) compared to penicillamine, 44% of patients on azathioprine experienced "important clinical improvement" defined as improvement of 30% or more in the number of tender joints (54). Comparisons of azathioprine with D-penicillamine (48,52,54,55), gold (50,51), cyclophosphamide (51), chloroquine (50), and levamisole (55) have suggested that azathioprine is equal in efficacy to these agents in the study populations tested. Continued treatment with azathioprine is required to maintain the clinical improvement achieved (15,17).

The disease-modifying effects of azathioprine in RA are unclear. Rheumatoid factor has fallen in some studies but this effect is not universal (13,14, 56). Both progression (15,52) and improvement of bone erosions (55,56) have been reported. An 18-month study comparing gold, cyclophosphamide, and azathioprine suggested that more deterioration developed during gold therapy than during azathioprine and cyclophosphamide therapy (51). Improvement of rheumatoid vasculitis has also been reported during treatment with azathioprine (16).

The recommended initial dose for azathioprine is 1-1.5 mg/kg which may be increased to a maximum dose of 2.5-3 mg/kg in severe cases. Our clinical experience would suggest that the onset of action by azathioprine may be slow (54). A trial of at least 3 months, and preferably 6 months, may be needed to ensure an adequate opportunity for a clinical response. Complete blood counts with platelet counts should be done at baseline and at least every 4 weeks throughout therapy. The role of monitoring hepatic enzymes is unknown. The measurement of liver function tests at baseline would be appropriate with repeat evaluation at one month and then every 3-6 months thereafter. Clinical evaluations should look for gastrointestinal upset, stomatitis, and skin rash. The use of allopurinol should be avoided. If azathioprine and allopurinol are to be used concurrently, the dose of azathioprine must be reduced by 75% (35).

2. Systemic Lupus Erythematosus

The role of azathioprine in SLE is not well defined. Azathioprine doses in studies of SLE patients have ranged from 1.0 to 4.0 mg/kg (19,26) with adjustments for leukopenia. The greatest experience with cytotoxic drugs in SLE is at the National Institutes of Health where a large cohort of SLE patients with nephritis have been followed for several years in randomized protocols (19,24). These studies have been complicated by a general trend toward improvement of SLE outcome over the last decades which makes temporal comparison between the different protocols difficult (57). In general, however, these protocols have shown that cytotoxic drugs, including azathioprine, retard the progression to end-stage renal disease to a greater degree than prednisone alone. The results presently favor cyclophosphamide as the most effective agent, with azathioprine producing some intermediate benefit (19). Other studies have also suggested that azathioprine is much more effective than prednisone alone in SLE renal disease (25,26); however, these studies did not compare azathioprine to cyclophosphamide. Discoid lupus has also been reported to have been successfully treated with azathioprine in an uncontrolled report (27).

3. Inflammatory Muscle Disease

Uncontrolled reports describe improvement of inflammatory myopathy with azathioprine (29,30). A controlled trial evaluating azathioprine and prednisone versus prednisone alone did not show any statistically significant clinical differences in the small groups of patients studied (28). Long-term follow-up of these patients suggested that the group receiving both azathioprine and prednisone may have experienced some greater functional improvement as well as some possible steroid-sparing effects (31). Functional grade improved more significantly in patients receiving azathioprine and prednisone when compared to the prednisone alone group ($p < 0.01$) (31).

4. Psoriatic Arthritis

No controlled trials are available for azathioprine in psoriatic arthritis; however, uncontrolled reports suggest improvement of clinical disease activity (10,12,16) and improvement of skin lesions (10,16).

5. Miscellaneous

Uncontrolled studies have reported success with the use of azathioprine in several vasculitis syndromes. Alkylating agents are often used before azathioprine in severe vasculitides and appear to be more effective (58). However, there are reports of benefit with azathioprine in Wegener's granumomatosis (59), Takayasu's arteritis (60,61), and other necrotizing vasculitis syndromes (62). Weber-Christian disease is also improved by azathioprine in some patients (63). High-dose corticosteroids are often administered with azathioprine in the above diseases.

C. Adverse Drug Effects

Significant adverse drug reactions result in discontinuation of azathioprine in 19-32% of patients treated (51,54). In the majority of instances, these events are rapidly reversed after discontinuing azathioprine. Studies comparing differing doses of azathioprine have suggested a dose-related increase in the frequency of adverse effects (14,53). Often patients experiencing mild toxicity can have azathioprine reinstituted at a lower dose without significant subsequent untoward reaction.

1. Hematologic

Hematological adverse drug reactions are frequently reported occurring in up to 26% of patients (49). Leukopenia (7,10-13,15,16,48,50,51,53,54,64) thrombocytopenia (12,48,55), anemia (11,16,55), pure red cell aplasia (64), and pancytopenia (17) have all been reported in RA patients. Severe leukopenia may lead to serious infections (16).

2. Gastrointestinal

Gastrointestinal complaints occurred in 19% of a worldwide survey and nausea, vomiting (10%), and GI symptoms (6%) were the most frequent complaints in patients receiving azathioprine (7,10,13,15,16,48,50-56). Less frequently, stomatitis (48,55), GI hemorrhage (11), gastric ulcer (16), and diarrhea (48,55) are reported. Pancreatitis has been seen during azathioprine treatment of inflammatory bowel disease and renal transplantation (65-67) but not during the treatment of rheumatic diseases.

3. Hepatic

The incidence of liver disease during azathioprine therapy is unknown. Evaluation of liver disease in renal transplant patients receiving azathioprine suggests that azathioprine is an uncommon cause of hepatic injury in these patients (37). The most common liver abnormality seen with azathioprine is mild elevation of liver enzymes (53). In one study, 5% of 104 patients receiving azathioprine were withdrawn from the drug for abnormal hepatic enzymes (54). However, in the one report of fatal progressive liver failure and cirrhosis with azathioprine, elevated liver enzymes were noted 6 months prior to death (68). It is unknown if the liver disease would have been reversible had the azathioprine been discontinued. There are reports of hepatitis and abnormal liver enzymes which have completely resolved on stopping azathioprine (69) and other reports of fibrosis which has not progressed on serial biopsy during continued azathioprine treatment (70,71). Hepatocellular injury with cholestasis has been seen as well (69-72).

4. Pulmonary

Pulmonary disease is a rare complication during azathioprine therapy and has not been reported during the treatment of rheumatic diseases. Interstitial pneumonitis (73,74) and diffuse alveolar damage have occurred and resulted in death from severe respiratory failure in some renal transplant patients (73).

5. Dermatologic

Maculopapular rashes are reported in most series of azathioprine therapy in RA (10-12,16,48,51,53,54). No major or persistent dermatological complications have been reported in these patients. The rash clears when the drug is discontinued. Psoriasis has improved in some patients with psoriatic arthritis receiving azathioprine (10,12).

6. Reproductive

Azathioprine should not be used in pregnancy, although successful pregnancies have been reported in patients receiving azathioprine during the first trimester and throughout pregnancy (75). However, azathioprine and its metabolites have been shown to cross the placenta (76) and there are reports of significant neonatal complications and chromosomal damage in the offspring of patients receiving azathioprine during pregnancy (77-79).

7. Oncogenesis

Malignancies are increased in renal transplant patients receiving azathioprine and corticosteroids (80). The role of azathioprine in tumor development is unclear. This may represent an increase in malignancies in renal transplant patients independent of immunosuppressive therapy (81), although azathioprine therapy has been associated with chromosome abnormalities with long-term use (15). The possibility of an increase in malignancies in nontransplant patients is still unresolved. Epidemiological studies of malignancies in "non-transplant" patients receiving azathioprine have suggested an increase in malignancies when compared to the baseline malignancy rates (82). During the treatment of RA with azathioprine, leukemias (83,84), lymphomas (84), and solid tumors have been reported (10,16,17,84). A difficulty in evaluating these studies is the conflicting reports of increased malignancies in RA patients independent of antirheumatic therapies (85-87). To truly define the malignancy potential of azathioprine, studies must involve RA control groups without azathioprine therapy.

Symmon reported a retrospective study of malignancy rates in 489 RA patients reviewed for a mean of 12.2 years. Lymphoproliferative malignancies developed in 10 patients (2.2%) (89). Cytotoxic drugs could not be implicated in the pathogenesis of the lymphoproliferative malignancies. A potential increased risk for malignancies in RA patients receiving phenylbutazone and D-penicillamine was suggested but not clearly demonstrated (89). Kinlen reported a prospective study of 1634 nontransplant patients treated with either azathioprine, cyclophosphamide, chlorambucil, or cyclosporine (90). Of these 1634 patients, 643 patients had RA. In this study, a threefold relative risk for malignancies in patients receiving these agents was reported. In RA patients, the relative risk was 1.3 for all malignancies. However, the reported incidence for non-Hodgkin's lymphoma was 13.5 in RA patients. There were no RA controls who did not receive immunosuppressive therapy examined in this study. The malignancy rates in patients were compared to the expected incidence in the normal population. The frequency of malignancies with azathioprine was similar to that seen in patients treated with cyclophosphamide. In a study of 311 patients with RA observed over 11 years, Lewis reported no increased risk for malignancies in the 203 patients treated with azathioprine when they were compared with patients not receiving this agent (91). A recent review discussed these results with the conclusion that "further studies are required to assess the true influence of these drugs on the incidence of tumors in RA" (92). The information to date would suggest that the carcinogenic potential of azathioprine in rheumatic diseases is not well defined.

D. Summary

Azathioprine is an effective second-line agent for the treatment of rheumatoid arthritis. It is approved by the FDA for that use and controlled trials confirm its efficacy. It is similar in efficacy to other second-line agents although controlled studies are few in number. Its utility in other rheumatic diseases is less well established. It is used in lupus nephritis in combination with prednisone, and is more effective than prednisone alone but cannot be considered the drug of choice. Cyclophosphamide would appear to be the superior agent for this condition. Azathioprine may have some benefit as a steroid-sparing agent in patients requiring long-term corticosteroids for rheumatic problems.

Like other second-line agents, azathioprine does have considerable toxicity. Regular monitoring for toxicity is required to prevent serious untoward effects. The oncogenic potential of azathioprine is still being evaluated. While the possibility of tumor induction exists, the risk is probably low.

III. ALKYLATING AGENTS

A. Pharmacology and Pharmacokinetics

1. Cyclophosphamide

Unmodified cyclophophamide (Fig. 2) is an inactive drug. However, the compound is metabolized in vivo by the cytochrome P-450 mixed function oxidase system (93) to form 4-hydroxycyclophosphamide which is in steady state with aldophosphamide. Additional oxidation leads to inactive metabolites (4-ketocyclophosphamide and carobxyphosphamide) and active metabolites (phosphoramide mustard and acrolein) (93). These metabolites are responsible for the clinical actions and adverse effects of cyclophosphamide. Therefore, the activity of the hepatic microsomal enzymes is very important in determining the ultimate effect of this agent. The rate of cyclophosphamide metabolism can be increased by prior exposure to certain drugs like phenobarbitol (94) as well as previous cyclophosphamide therapy (96).

Oral doses of cyclophosphamide are well absorbed (93) and 12-14% of cyclophosphamide is plasma-bound (96). The liver is responsible for the majority of cyclophosphamide metabolism, although there may be some metabolism by the lung and kidney (94). The plasma half-life of

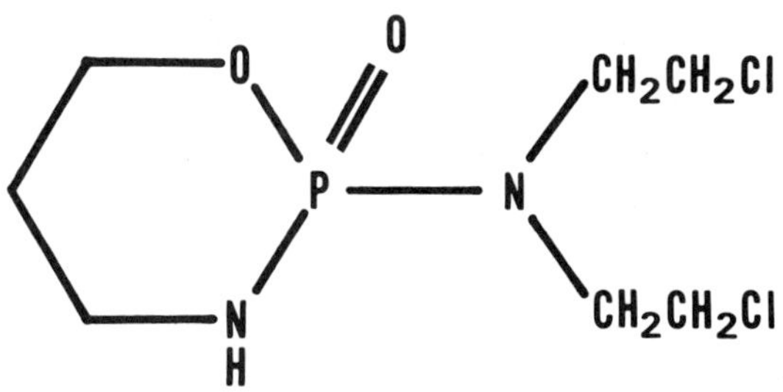

Figure 2 Chemical structure of cyclophosphamide.

cyclophosphamide is 2-10 hr. Less than 20% of cyclophosphamide is excreted unchanged in the urine over the first 24 hr (94).

2. Chlorambucil

Chlorambucil (Fig. 3) pharmacokinetics are not well defined because of the limited number of patients evaluated (94-100). The data available suggest that chlorambucil is rapidly and almost completely absorbed orally. Peak serum concentrations occur after 15-120 min (99,101) with metabolism to phenylacetic acid mustard, and other metabolites with a serum half-life of 1.5-2.6 hr (100,101). The pharmacokinetics are best described by a two-compartment model with an initial distribution phase with a half-life of 0.25-0.85 hr and a terminal phase with half-life of 7.1-20.6 hr (98). Although less than 1% of chlorambucil is excreted unchanged in the urine (99), eventually up to 70% of labeled chlorambucil metabolites are excreted over the first 24 hr. The major metabolism of chlorambucil is through the liver. One of these metabolites, phenylacetic acid mustard, is regarded as having activity equal to that of chlorambucil in vivo (99,100). The induction of cytochrome P-450 by phenobarbital increases the rate of metabolism of chlorambucil in rats (100). The clinical significance of this effect on the cytotoxic effects of this drug are unknown.

3. Drug Interactions

Drug interactions with cyclophosphamide and chlorambucil are rare. The majority of interactions are related to alterations of the metabolism of cyclophosphamide or its metabolites by the liver. Allopurinol may enhance cyclophosphamide toxicity (102) by inhibiting the hepatic microsomal enzyme systems (103). Other agents, such as phenobarbitol, which induce the cytochrome P-450 system may increase cyclophosphamide metabolism (104-109) but appear not to have a clinically significant effect on the antineoplastic effects of cyclophosphamide in animal models. Steroids may also inhibit cyclophosphamide in animal models. Steroids may also inhibit cyclophosphamide metabolism (110). When given to animals chloroquine may inhibit

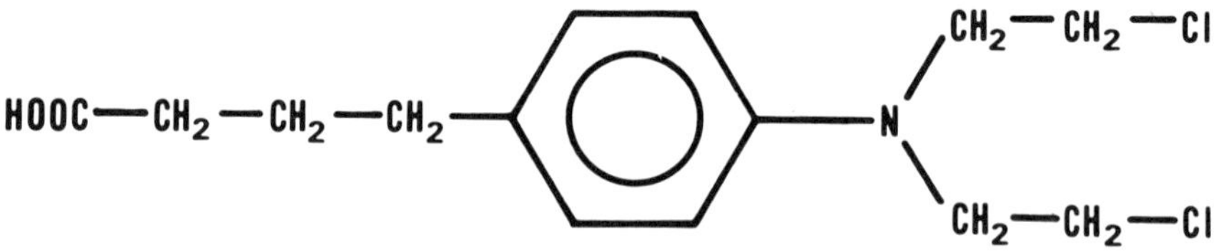

Figure 3 Chemical structure of chlorambucil.

DNA repair enzymes and thus increase cyclophosphamide toxicity (104,105). In the majority of cases, there appears to be little clinical importance of these interactions.

4. Possible Mechanisms of Action for the Alkylating Agents in Rheumatic Disease

The search for the exact antirheumatic action of these drugs has been frustrating. Although many alterations of in vivo and in vitro assays have been reported, it is unclear if these changes are of any significance in the clinical antirheumatic effect of these drugs. The major emphasis in these studies has been to evaluate the cytotoxic and immunological effects of these drugs.

These agents are clearly cytotoxic as a result of alkylation of various cellular constituents. The alkylation of guanine in DNA can lead to miscoding, destruction of the purine ring, and blocked DNA replication through cross-linking (94). These actions appear to be nonspecific, but some cell populations may be protected from alkylating agents by greater amounts of thiols or oxidative enzymes (94). Although a dose-dependent leukopenia has been a consistent observation during treatment with alkylating agents (111), clinical improvement can occur in the absence of leukopenia (112). The cytotoxic effects of these drugs at the site of active inflammation (e.g., synovium in rheumatoid arthritis, kidney in active systemic lupus erythematosus with renal involvement, etc.) is unknown. The local action of these agents may be important but is very difficult to evaluate.

Recently, there has been a significant focus on the effects of alkylating agents on the immune system. Both in vitro and in vivo studies have been undertaken. Although all in vitro evaluation has limitations, this is especially true with alkylating agents. Because cyclophosphamide is itself inactive, its metabolites must be evaluated (113). The exact concentration and proportions of these metabolites which accurately reflect the in vivo status of these drugs are unclear. In addition to these limitations, which must be taken into consideration when evaluating in vitro data, there are also important issues to consider when reviewing in vivo data. The drug dose, duration of therapy, and temporal relationship of drug administration to the immunogen stimulus are all important in determining the effects which will be seen in the immune system. Because many reports, particularly cancer studies, use larger doses of alkylating agents than those used in the treatment of rheumatic diseases, the immunological effects reported may have little bearing on the potential mechanism of action of these drugs at lower doses.

Despite these limitations, there are several observations which may be important. Lymphoid tissues appear to be particularly sensitive to treatment with alkylating agents (114-119). Although a decrease of both T cells and B cells (114-117,120) can occur, the various lymphoid cell populations may not always be equally affected (103,114,116,121-123). B cells may be more sensitive to cyclophosphamide than T cells (114,117). Low-dose cyclophosphamide therapy in children with minimal change nephropathy is associated with a decrease in helper cell subsets (124). These values return to normal after cyclophosphamide was discontinued for 6-12 months (124).

The functional significance of these alterations of cell populations is unclear. Cellular immune function can be both suppressed (115,125-129) and enhanced (130-135) depending on the experimental system utilized. The inhibition of suppressor function may result in an overall enhancement of cellular immune function (134,135) rather than a direct enhancing property. Humoral immunity has generally been depressed (128,136-143), though there are rare examples of increased humoral immunity (144). Although alterations in immune function are frequent during treatment with alkylating agents, many immunological assays may remain unaltered during cyclophosphamide treatment in humans (145). In addition to its immunological effects, the alkylating agents exert anti-inflammatory actions in humans (146).

In summary, the mechanism of action of alkylating agents in the rheumatic diseases remains unknown although data and theories abound. Overall, data would suggest that these compounds act through a nonspecific cytotoxic effect on lymphoid tissue with a resulting alteration of immunological and inflammatory pathways. Although the use of these drugs is associated with change in lymphoid population and immunological assays, the clinical significance of these changes is unclear.

B. Efficacy

1. Historical Perspective

The biological activity of nitrogen mustard was recognized in the late 1800s (94). Alkylating agents were then evaluated in malignancies. Nitrogen mustard was first suggested to be an effective treatment for refractory RA in 1951 (2). Subsequently, cyclophosphamide and chlorambucil were developed and these drugs became the principal agents studied in rheumatic diseases. Cyclophosphamide was the principal agent used by British and American investigators, while chlorambucil was used extensively in France. Initial reports involved their use in RA and SLE with extension to the vasculitides and other rheumatic conditions. Presently, the role of alkylating agents in rheumatic diseases is under reevaluation. They appear to have been proven efficacious in several situations, but uncertainty over the potential long-term toxicity, including the induction of malignancies, is a major concern.

2. General Guidelines

In the United States, the FDA approved the use of cyclophosphamide and chlorambucil only for the treatment of malignancies. There are no alkylating agents which are presently approved for the treatment of rheumatic diseases and it is unlikely that any will be formally approved for this purpose in the future. Thus, the use of alkylating agents in patients with rheumatic diseases must presently be considered experimental. All patients receiving alkylating agents should give informed consent before receiving the drug. An evaluation of the risks and benefits in each patient should determine if potential toxicity from these drugs warrants their use.

3. Rheumatoid Arthritis

Multiple uncontrolled (2,111,147,148) and controlled trials (112,149,150) have documented that cyclophosphamide and chlorambucil are an effective treatment for RA patients. The degree of clinical improvement has varied from 48 to 94% of patients (111). The most widely used dose of cyclophosphamide in RA is 1-2 mg/kg. The optimal dose is unknown. In one trial (112) high-dose cyclophosphamide (150 mg/day) was compared with low-dose cyclophosphamide (75 mg/day) in RA. In this study, both doses of cyclophosphamide were effective. Although there was greater clinical improvement in morning stiffness, grip strength, joint swelling, and joint tenderness in patients taking the higher doses of cyclophosphamide, this difference did not achieve statistical significance. Although there was not a statistically significant difference in toxicity, there was a trend toward greater toxicity in high-dose patients (112).

There are no controlled trials comparing the efficacy and toxicity of different doses of chlorambucil. The doses of chlorambucil used to treat RA have ranged from 0.03 to 0.3 mg/kg/day with the dose frequently adjusted to maintain leukopenia (111).

Reductions in erythrocyte sedimentation rate (151-154), rheumatoid factor (129,152,154), and healing of erosions (155) have all been reported during alkylating agent therapy with both cyclophosphamide and chlorambucil. If a physician decides to use an alkylating agent to treat a rheumatic disease, there must be close clinical and laboratory follow-up. Our protocol is to do clinical monitoring during cyclophosphamide and chlorambucil therapy which includes complete blood counts at least monthly. Patients receiving cyclophosphamide should be instructed to maintain high urine flow to avoid hemorrhagic cystitis. Urinalysis should be performed to detect hematuria suggesting cyclophosphamide bladder toxicity, although recent data from non-Hodgkin's lymphoma patients could not document the predictive value of hemorrhagic cystitis as a predictor of bladder carcinoma (95). This same study showed that use of low-dose, oral cyclophosphamide for 2-4 years was associated with a relative risk of bladder carcinoma of 20.5 confidence interval: 9.8-43.1) (95). Because of this concern over carcinogenicity, alkylating agents are not generally used in RA (94).

4. Systemic Lupus Erythematosus

Most evaluations of cyclophosphamide (19-24) and chlorambucil (156) in SLE have concentrated on lupus nephritis. The NIH studies have been the most extensive. This work has shown that fewer SLE patients progress to end-stage renal disease during treatment with alkylating agents than patients receiving steroids alone (19-24,57). Because of concern over toxicity with continuous oral cyclophosphamide, recent trials have involved pulse cyclophosphamide where regular (1- to 3-month) pulses of intravenous cyclophosphamide (0.5-1.0 g/m^2) (19,57,157) are given with subsequent maintenance therapy at a similar dose. The nadir blood counts 8–12 days after cyclophosphamide treatment must be closely monitored to avoid major hematological complications. The use of cyclophosphamide alone in SLE without steroids has been reported to be ineffective (158).

5. Vasculitis

Treatment of Wegener's granulomatosis, a previously fatal disease, with cyclophosphamide has produced a dramatic change in the outcome of this disease. Long-term remissions are also often seen in many cases and there is better survival than that seen with prednisone alone (159). Fauci reported complete remission in 79 (93%) of 85 patients over Wegener's granulomatosis treated wih cyclophosphamide (159). After mean follow-up of 35.3 months, 23 (27%) of these patients were off all therapy without relapse of their disease. Athough these results are very encouraging, cyclophosphamide treatment failures have been reported (59).

Reports of improvement of polyarteritis nodosa (62), rheumatoid vasculitis (160), Takayasu's arteritis (161), Churg-Strauss syndrome (61), and systemic necrotizing vasculitis (58) during treatment with cyclophosphamide are encouraging. In most of these, high-dose corticosteroids were administered in addition to the alkylating agent.

6. Miscellaneous

In addition to the diseases reported above, there are reports of the use of cyclophosphamide and chlorambucil to treat juvenile RA (162,163), inflammatory muscle disease (159,164), essential mixed cryoglobulinemia (165), Behçet's syndrome (166-168), Goodpasture's syndrome (169), Henoch-Schonlein purpura (167), and scleroderma (171,172).

C. Toxicity

1. Hematological

Hematological complications are common and frequently require an adjustment of dose and/or the discontinuation of the alkylating agent being used in the treatment of rheumatic diseases. Leukopenia (111,112,129,147,151,152, 158,173-181), thrombocytopenia (111,149,152,173,182), anemia (173,180, 181), pancytopenia (180,181,183-185), and eosinophilia (173) have all been reported. The incidence of these complications is not clear. Because many investigators have adjusted the drug dose to produce "mild leukopenia" which is generally in the range of 3000 WBCs/mm^3 (179), many of the reported leukopenias may represent severe leukopenia which is not reversed on dose reduction. In an attempt to more fully define the frequencies of these problems, Deshayes (181) reported the incidence of hematological complications (20%) during chlorambucil treatment including leukopenia (14%), thrombocytopenia (8%), anemia (5%), and pancytopenia (3%). Others have reported an incidence of leukopenia as high as 50% (178). Williams et al. suggested that leukopenia during cyclophosphamide treatment of RA was probably dose-dependent (112). The hematological abnormalities may also be persistent for several months (111). In pulse therapy with alkylating agents the nadir for leukocyte and platelet counts usually occurs 8-12 days after dosing and returns to normal in 2-3 weeks (186).

2. Infections

Significant bacterial and opportunistic infections can occur during treatment with alkylating agents (19,166,173,177,180,181,184). These infections include pneumonia (166,174,177), septic arthritis (184), and sepsis (151, 152,173,177,181,183). Often these infectious events are associated with leukopenia, but they can occur in the absence of peripheral blood abnormalities. Herpes zoster is also frequently reported during treatment of rheumatic disease with cyclophosphamide (19,148-150) and chlorambucil (151,152, 173-175,179,181,183,184).

3. Urological

Cyclophosphamide is metabolized to acrolein, which is excreted in the urine and is probably responsible for the toxicity of this drug on the urinary tract. Urological complications have not been reported with chlorambucil. Cyclophosphamide treatment is often complicated by hemorrhagic cystitis (19,112, 147-150), chronic cystitis (187-189), and carcinoma of the bladder (190, 192). The use of low-dose cyclophosphamide in non-Hodgkin's lymphoma patients was associated with a relative risk of 20.5 for bladder carcinoma, when accounting for the long latency for the development of this tumor (at least 65 months) (95). Efforts to reduce bladder exposure to these toxic agents include vigorous hydration and potentially the use of agents with sulfhydryl groups which may protect against cyclophosphamide bladder toxicity (193).

4. Reproductive

Male infertility involves both toxicity to the germinal epithelium in the seminiferous tubules (194-196) and Leydig cell dysfunction (197,198). Some patients will be permanently sterile (194); however, patients receiving cyclophosphamide have subsequently fathered normal children (199,200). Ovarian failure and amenorrhea is a well-documented complication of cyclophosphamide (147-149,158) and chlorambucil (173-175,181) treatment with ovarian fibrosis and follicular destruction. The use of pulse cyclophosphamide may produce less ovarian failure than daily oral treatment. In a study of 107 patients with systemic lupus erythematosus, 71% of patients receiving oral cyclophosphamide developed premature ovarian failure. The frequency of ovarian failure was higher than that seen in similar patients receiving prednisone alone (8%), azathioprine alone (18%), combined azathioprine and cyclophosphamide (53%), and intravenous cyclophosphamide (45%) (19). The difference was only statistically significantly different in comparing prednisone and azathioprine groups with oral cyclophosphamide, combined oral azathioprine and cyclophosphamide, and intravenous cyclophosphamide groups.

All possible efforts should be made to avoid conception in a woman receiving an alkylating agent. Because pregnancies are generally avoided after alkylating agent treatment, the teratogenic effects of cyclophosphamide and chlorambucil are not well defined. Chromosomal damage has been seen in RA patients receiving cyclophosphamide (171). Fetal abnormalities have been reported in humans after cyclophosphamide (201-203) and chlorambucil (204) treatment, although there are reports of normal pregnancies after cyclophosphamide treatment (205).

5. Pulmonary

Case reports of pulmonary fibrosis and pneumonitis in patients receiving cyclophosphamide have appeared in the literature (206), most often as a component of combination chemotherapy. There is concern that agents or the underlying conditions may have been responsible for the pulmonary disease.

6. Gastrointestinal

During treatment with alkylating agents, gastrointestinal upset (112,147,148, 150,158,175,177,181), stomatitis (112,150), diarrhea (112,149), and rare hepatotoxicity with cholestasis are reported (207).

7. Dermatological

Although infrequent, maculopapular rashes which are severe enough to require discontinuing cyclophosphamide (148) and chlorambucil (173-175,177,181) are described. Hair loss (174-177,184,208) and urticaria (209) are also reported.

8. Potential for Malignancies

Increasing evidence is documenting the potential for alkylating agents to produce malignancies. There have been multiple reports of leukemia (111, 163,180,182,210-218), lymphomas (206,217,219,220), solid tumors (180, 210,220), and chromosomal damage (171,221) in patients receiving alkylating agents. Renier reported 38 deaths with 15 malignancies (seven lymphomas and leukemias) in 131 RA patients receiving chlorambucil between 1965 and 1973 (180). The prevalence of leukemia in 1612 RA patients receiving chlorambucil has been estimated at 0.74% (211).

In addition to these uncontrolled reviews, Baltus reported a controlled evaluation of the prevalence of malignancies in RA patients receiving cyclophosphamide compared to a similar population not receiving cyclophosphamide (220), and noted an increase in malignancies in patients receiving cyclophosphamide. In this study, 81 RA patients who had received cyclophosphamide were compared to 81 control RA patients with similar disease activity who had not received cyclophosphamide. Malignancies occurred in 15 RA patients treated with cyclophosphamide and in four control patients for a relative risk of 4.1. The total dose and duration of cyclophosphamide therapy in patients who developed malignancies were compared to the total dose and duration of cyclophosphamide therapy in patients who did not develop malignancies. Although the differences were not statistically significant, this analysis showed that patients who developed cancer had received a larger total dose of cyclophosphamide ($p = 0.054$) and had received the cyclophosphamide for a longer duration ($p = 0.229$) than patients who did not develop malignancies.

Other reports have suggested increased malignancies following cyclophosphamide and chlorambucil therapy in RA (111,222). These results strongly suggest that cyclophosphamide and chlorambucil increase the risk for malignancy in these patients. The potential risk of malignancy should be discussed with all patients before using alkylating agents.

9. Miscellaneous

Rare complications include water retention (223), cardiotoxicity (186,224), anaphylaxis with fever (225), and acute oropharyngeal dysesthesias (226).

D. Summary

Cyclophosphamide and chlorambucil are potent cytotoxic drugs which are effective in suppressing disease activity in RA, SLE, vasculitis, and other rheumatic conditions. Toxic reactions are commonly dose-related and will usually resolve after the drug is discontinued. The potential carcinogenicity of these agents is a significant concern and has dampened the original enthusiasm for their use in the rheumatic diseases. Wegener's granulomatosis, severe SLE, and aggressive necrotizing vasculitis represent diseases where the potential benefit offered by alkylating agents may justify their use. The decision to use an alklylating agent to treat a patient with a rheumatic disease must involve a complete review of the risks and benefits, a definition of defined outcomes which will be used to determine if the drug should be continued for long-term therapy, and close follow-up for toxicity.

IV. COMBINATION THERAPY

Treatment of rheumatoid arthritis gives an unpredictable response. Some patients require aggressive therapy and second-line agents have been of help to many patients resistant to the basic therapeutic program. However, there are a small number of patients who are refractory to all standard therapy and whose disease has continued to progress. The persistent nature of the RA in these patients is frustrating to both patient and physician.

Combination chemotherapy was first used in malignant disease in an attempt to combine drugs with different mechanisms of action and different toxicities to increase tumor reduction with an acceptable toxicity. Treatment of malignant disease has been improved by the use of combinations of cytotoxic and immunosuppressive drugs.

Some have described RA as a form of "localized malignancy" (227). The use of multiple second-line agents in RA is gaining increasing acceptability. Combination therapy was first reported by Sievers and Hurri in 1963 when they used a combination of gold and chloroquine (228). Chloroquine in a daily dose of 400-500 mg for 2-4 weeks was followed by a maintenance program of 200-400 mg daily. Parenteral gold was used in combination with chloroquine in a dose of 50 mg weekly for at least 12 weeks. Hydroxychloroquine was substituted for chloroquine in some patients at equivalent doses. Two hundred forty-eight patients were treated for 3-6 weeks with the combination and "major improvement or remission" was seen in 43% of the combination patients compared to 36% of 240 patients on chloroquine alone or 31% of 239 patients on parenteral gold alone.

Young and Scherbel used combination therapy in this country for several decades but neither reported the results (227). Apparently many patients achieved satisfactory results.

Recent interest in combination therapy in RA was stimulated in 1982 when McCarty and Carrera (229) described 17 patients with progressive, erosive RA that was refractory to conventional therapy but improved with combination therapy. Each patient had failed gold injections and each was taking hydroxychloroquine in a dose of 200-400 mg daily. Either cyclophosphamide or azathioprine in an oral dose of 25 mg/day was added to the treatment program. After 2-3 weeks the alternate drug was added to the regimen. The dose of either cytotoxic drug was increased alternately at 2- to 3-week intervals until a white blood cell count of 3000-4000 cells/mm^3 was obtained. The mean daily dose of cyclophosphamide was 39 mg and of azathioprine was 55 mg. The patients were followed for a mean of 27 months (5-60 months). Disease suppression was seen in 14 of the 17 patients. Five patients went into remission with no signs or symptoms of disease activity and two patients had only monoarticular disease. Seven patients had partial improvement. Only three patients had no response. Prednisone dosage was decreased or stopped in nine of 10 patients. Radiographs demonstrated recortication of erosions in nine patients. Four patients discontinued the combination therapy for "severe side effects" which were not detailed. All but five patients had some untoward reaction. Herpes zoster was seen in two patients, cystitis in five, infections in seven, and leukopenia in at least one patient.

This initial report had a follow-up in 1986 (230). Thirty-one patients were reported in this second paper. Previous therapy was variable but the treatment regimen studied was the same as in the preliminary report although two patients did not receive hydroxychloroquine because of previous retinal toxicity. All patients had been followed on the combination therapy for at least a year with the mean duration of therapy being 43 months. The mean maximum daily dose of cyclophosphamide was 54 mg, azathioprine 95 mg, and hydroxychloroquine 310 mg.

Disease suppression was defined as a decrease in morning stiffness of at least 1 hr, increase in grip strength of at least 10%, and a decrease in proximal interphalangeal joint circumfrence of at least 5 mm. Disease suppression was seen as early as 3 months and as late as 24 months with a mean of 9 months. All three patients who had been unresponsive in the first report responded to continued therapy. Sixteen patients achieved complete remission (no swelling or tenderness of any joint) and an additional seven patients reached "near remission" with residual swelling and tenderness in only one joint. Seven patients obtained a partial response and only one patient failed to respond. The nonresponder had to discontinue both cyclophosphamide and azathioprine. Patients in remission required continued drug therapy to remain in remission.

Adverse drug reactions were common and occurred in 25 of the patients although only five patients were withdrawn for untoward drug effects such as thrombocytopenia, diarrhea, stomatitis, pneumonia, and leg ulcers. Four patients developed malignancies and three of them died. It was concluded that the combined use of these agents may be of use in the treatment of refractory progressive RA but it was recommended that cyclophosphamide be replaced with a nonalkylating agent.

Other reports have also evaluated combination second-line therapy. Bunch et al. (231) combined hydroxychloroquine and penicillamine and compared the combination to each drug given alone in a 2-year controlled, double-blind trial. Hydroxychloroquine was given in a dose of 2.2 mg/kg/day and penicillamine was given in a dose of 7 mg/kg/day. While the study had small numbers of participants, penicillamine alone gave more improvement than the combination. Penicillamine alone also had more toxicity than the combination.

Bitter (232) reported on open prospective 5-year trial of five combinations of second-line drugs in 71 patients. Patients who had received gold therapy were randomly assigned gold therapy alone or gold in combination with penicillamine, levamisole, or chlorambucil. Patients who had not responded to penicillamine therapy were randomly assigned penicillamine alone or in combination with levamisole or chlorambucil. Patients were followed for 18 months and patients withdrawn were replaced with other patients. Toleration of the treatments was "surprisingly good." There were two withdrawals for toxicity within 6 months and nine withdrawals for toxicity after 6 months for patients on gold alone or in combination. For the penicillamine groups, there was one withdrawal for toxicity before 6 months of therapy and three withdrawals for untoward reactions after 6 months of treatment. The author concluded that the combination of gold and penicillamine was the most promising but that the overall therapeutic effect was disappointing.

A recent study compared sulfasalazine alone and in combination with penicillamine in a 6-month unblinded study of 30 patients (233). Significant improvement was seen in both treatment groups although 60% of the combination group responded compared to 40% of the sulfasalazine group. The authors concluded that the combination was more effective but less well tolerated.

Butler and Tiliakos (234) conducted a small 6-month study in patients with intractable RA comparing methotrexate, cyclophosphamide, and hydroxychloroquine to methotrexate alone. Both groups improved and recortication of erosions was reported for five patients on combination therapy. The combination therapy was well tolerated.

Biro et al. (235) treated 20 patients who had failed hydroxycholorquine and either methotrexate or azathioprine with a combination of methotrexate and azathioprine. After a mean of 12 months treatment, joint counts fell from a mean of 11 to a mean of 3. One patient was withdrawn for drug toxicity.

Summary

The remarkable results of McCarty and coworkers with combination therapy in patients with intractable RA has led to increased interest in various combinations of second-line agents. Most of the studies are open and uncontrolled. In the only controlled trial (231), a single agent outperformed the combination group. It has been postulated that combinations of second-line drugs in lower dose will give improved efficacy with less toxicity. In the uncontrolled studies reported, both efficacy and toxicity have been acceptable with the exception of the four malignancies reported by Csuka et al. (230). Whether these malignancies developed from the drug treatment or not is unknown. Both cyclophosphamide (220) and azathioprine (92) have been implicated in tumor induction and it is possible that the therapy played some role in the development of cancer in these patients. However, it is known that patients with RA are at a higher risk for development of lymphoproliferative malignancies (85) although the risk for solid tumors is not clear but does not seem to be increased.

Combination therapy holds some promise for the treatment of refractory connective tissue diseases but large, controlled, double-blind comparison studies need to be done before combination therapy can be considered as more than experimental therapy.

ACKNOWLEDGMENT

We acknowledge the excellent assistance of Wanda Moore and Teresa Tanner in preparing this manuscript. The preparation of this chapter was sponsored in part by the Veterans Administration Medical Research Program and Nora Eccles Treadwell Foundation.

REFERENCES

1. Gubner R, August S, Ginsberg V. Therapeutic suppression of tissue reactivity. II. Effect of aminopterin in rheumatoid arthritis and psoriasis. Am J Med Sci 1951;221:176–82.

2. Jimenez Diaz C, Lopez Garcia E, Merchante A, Perianes J. Treatment of rheumatoid arthritis with nitrogen mustard. Preliminary report. JAMA 1951; 147:1418-9.
3. Dameshek W, Schwartz R. Treatment of certain "autoimmune" diseases with antimetabolites; a preliminary report. Trans Assoc Am Phys 1960; 73:113-27.
4. Myles AB. 6-Mercpatopurine (6 M.P.) in the treatment of rheumatoid arthritis and related conditions. Ann Rheum Dis 1965; 24:179-80.
5. Elion GB. Biochemistry and pharmacology of purine analogues. Fed Proc 1967; 26:898-904.
6. Elion GB, Hitchings GH. Azathioprine. In: Sartorelli AC, Johns DG (eds). Antineoplastic and immunosuppressive agents. Part II. Berlin: Springer-Verlag, 1975; 404-25.
7. Lorenzen I, Videbaek A. Treatment of collagen diseases with cytostatics. Lancet 1965; 2:558-25.
8. Corley CC, Lessner HE, Larsen WE. Azathioprine therapy of "autoimmune" diseases. Am J Med 1966; 41:404-12.
9. Philips VK, Bergen W, Rothermich NO. Azathioprine therapy in twenty-five patients with rheumatoid arthritis (RA). Arth Rheum 1967; 10:305.
10. Mason M, Currey HLF, Barnes CG, Dunne JF, Hazleman BL, Strickland ID. Azathioprine in rheumatoid arthritis. Br Med J 1969; 1:420-2.
11. Harris J, Jessop JD, deSaintonge DMC. Further experience with azathioprine in rheumatoid arthritis. Br Med J 1971; 4:463-4.
12. Levy J, Paulus HE, Barnett EV, Sokoloff M, Bangert R, Pearson CM. A double-blind controlled evaluation of azathioprine treatment in rheumatoid arthritis and psoriatic arthritis. Arth Rheum 1972; 15:116-7.
13. Urowitz MB, Gordon DA, Smyth HA, Prozanski W, Ogryzlo MA. Azathioprine in rheumatoid arthritis. A double-blind, cross-over study. Arth Rheum 1973; 16:411-8.
14. Urowitz MB, Hunter T, Bookman AAM, Gordon DA, Smythe HA, Ogryzlo MA. Azathioprine in rheumatoid arthritis: a double-blind study comparing full dose to half dose. J Rheumatol 1974; 1:274-81.
15. Hunter T, Urowitz MB, Gordon DA, Smythe HA, Ogryzlo MA. Azathioprine in rheumatoid arthritis. A long-term follow-up study. Arth Rheum 1975; 18:15-20.
16. Pinals RS. Azathioprine in the treatment of chronic polyarthritis: Long-term results and adverse effects in 25 patients. J Rheumatol 1976; 3: 140-4.
17. DeSilva M, Hazleman BL. Long-term azathioprine in rheumatoid arthritis: a double-blind study. Ann Rheum Dis 1981; 40:560-3.
18. Thompson PW, Kirwan JR, Barnes CG. Practical results of treatment with disease-modifying antirheumatoid drugs. Br J Rheumatol 1985; 24: 167-75.

19. Austin HA III, Klippel JH, Balow JE, LeRiche NGH, Steinberg AD, Plotz PH, Decker JL. Therapy of lupus nephritis. Controlled trial of prednisone and cytotoxic drugs. N Engl J Med 1986; 314:614–9.
20. Steinberg AD, Decker JL. A double-blind controlled trial comparing cyclophosphamide, azathioprine and placebo in the treatment of lupus glomerulonephritis. Arth Rheum 1974; 17:923–37.
21. Decker JL, Klippel JH, Plotz PH, Steinberg AD. Cyclophosphamide or azathioprine in lupus glomerulonephritis. Controlled trial: results at 28 months. Ann Intern Med 1975; 83:606–15.
22. Decker JL, Steinberg AD, Reinertsen JL, Plotz PH, Balow JE, Klippel JH. Systemic lupus erythematosus: evolving concepts. Ann Intern Med 1979; 91:587–604.
23. Dinant HJ, Decker JL, Klippel JH, Balow JE, Plotz PH, Steinberg AD. Alternative modes of cyclophosphamide and azathioprine therapy in lupus nephritis. Ann Intern Med 1982; 96:728–36.
24. Carette S, Klippel JH, Decker JL, Austin HA, Plotz PH, Steinberg AD, Balow JE. Controlled studies of oral immunosuppressive drugs in lupus nephritis: A long-term follow-up. Ann Intern Med 1983; 99:1–8.
25. Sztejnbok M, Stewart A, Diamond H, Kaplan D. Azathioprine in the treatment of systemic lupus erythematosus. A controlled study. Arth Rheum 1971; 14:639–45.
26. Cade R, Spooner G, Schlein E, Pickering M, DeQuesada A, Holcomb A, Juncos L, Richard G, Shires D, Levin D, Hackett R, Free J, Hunt R, Fregly M. Comparison of azathioprine, prednisone, heparin alone or combined in treating lupus nephritis. Nephron 1973; 10:37–56.
27. Tsokos GC, Caughman SW, Klippel JH. Successful treatment of generalized discoid skin lesions with azathioprine. Its use in a patient with systemic lupus erythematosus. Arch Dermatol 1985; 121:1323–5.
28. Bunch TW, Worthington JW, Combs JJ, Ilstrup DM, Engel AG. Azathioprine with prednisone for polymyositis. A controlled, clinical trial. Ann Intern Med 1980; 92:365–9.
29. Benson MD, Aldo MA. Azathioprine therapy in polymyositis. Arch Intern Med 1973; 132:547–51.
30. McFarlin DE, Griggs RC. Treatment of inflammatory myopathies with azathioprine. Trans Am Neurol Assoc 1968; 93:244–6.
31. Bunch TW. Prednisone and azathioprine for polymyositis. Long-term followup. Arth Rheum 1981; 24:45–8.
32. Huskisson EC. Azathioprine. Clin Rheum Dis 1984; 10:325–32.
33. Bach J-F, Dardenne M. The metabolism of azathioprine in renal failure. Transplantation 1971; 12:253–9.
34. Clements PJ, Davis J. Cytotoxic drugs: their clinical application to the rheumatic diseases. Sem Arth Rheum 1986; 15:231–54.
35. Bertino JR. Chemical action and pharmacology of methotrexate, azathioprine and cyclophosphamide in man. Arth Rheum 1973; 16:79–83.

36. Bach J, Dardenne M. Serum immunosuppressive activity of azathioprine in normal subjects and patients with liver diseases. Proc Roy Soc Med 1972; 65:260-3.
37. Ware A J, Luby JP, Hollinger B, Eigenbrodt EH, Cuthbert JA, Atkins CR, Shorey J, Hull AR, Combes B. Etiology of liver disease in renal transplant patients. Ann Intern Med 1979; 91:364-71.
38. Maddocks JL. Clinical pharmacological observations on azathioprine in kidney transplant patients. Clin Sci Mol Med 1978; 55:20P.
39. Coffey JJ, White CA, Lesk AB, Rogers WI, Serpick AA. Effect of allopurinol on the pharmacokinetics of 6-mercaptopurine (NSC 755) in cancer patients. Cancer Res 1972; 32:1283-9.
40. Bailey RR. Leukopenia due to a trimethoprim-azathioprine interaction. N Zeal Med J 1984; 97:739.
41. LePage GA. Incorporation of 6-thioguanine into nucleic acids. Cancer Res 1960; 20:403-8.
42. Prince HE, Ettenger RB, Dorey FJ, Fine RN, Fahey JL. Azathioprine suppression of natural killer activity and antibody-dependent cellular cytotoxicity in renal transplant recipients. Transpl Proc 1984; 16:1475-7.
43. Al-Safi SA, Maddocks JL. Strength of the human mixed lymphocyte reaction (MLR) and its suppression by azathioprine or 6-mercaptopurine. Br J Clin Pharmacol 1985; 19:105-7.
44. Abdou NI, Zweiman B, Casella SR. Effects of azathioprine therapy on bone marrow-dependent and thymus-dependent cells in man. Clin Exp Immunol 1973; 13:55-64.
45. Maddocks JL, Al-Safi SA. Lack of inhibition of purine nucleoside phosphorylase and adenosine deaminase in patients treated with azathioprine. Br J Clin Pharmacol 1985; 19:108-11.
46. Hahn BH, Bagby MK, Hamilton TR, Osterland CK. Comparison of therapeutic and immunosuppressive effects of azathioprine, prednisolone and combined therapy in NZB/NZW mice. Arth Rheum 1973; 16:163-70.
47. Gelfand MC, Steinberg AD, Nagle R, Knepshield JH. Therapeutic studies in NZB/W mice. I. Synergy of azathioprine, cyclophosphamide and methylprednisolone in combination. Arth Rheum 1972; 15:239-46.
48. Berry H,Liyanage SP, Durance RA, Barnes CG, Berger LA, Evans S. Azathioprine and penicillamine in treatment of rheumatoid arthritis: a controlled trial. Br Med J 1976; 1:1052-4.
49. Whisnant JK, Pelkey J. Rheumatoid arthritis: treatment with azathioprine (IMURAN). Clinical side effects and laboratory abnormalities. Ann Rheum Dis 1982; 41(Supplement 1):44-7.
50. Dwosh JL, Stein HB, Urowitz MB, Smythe HA, Hunter T, Ogryzlo MA. Azathioprine in early rheumatoid arthritis. Comparison with gold and chloroquine. Arth Rheum 1977; 20:685-92.

51. Currey HLF, Harris J, Mason RM, Woodland J, Beveridge T, Roberts CJ, Vere DW, Dixon AStJ, Davies J, Owen-Smith B. Comparison of azathioprine, cyclophosphamide, and gold in treatment of rheumatoid arthritis. Br Med J 1974; 3:763-6.
52. Berry H, Liyanage SP, Durance R, Barnes CG, Berger L. Trial comparing azathioprine and penicillamine in treatment of rheumatoid arthritis. Ann Rheum Dis 1976; 35:542-3.
53. Woodland J, Chaput de Saintonge DM, Evans SJW, Sharman VL, Currey HLF. Azathioprine in rheumatoid arthritis: double-blind study of full versus half doses versus placebo. Ann Rheum Dis 1981; 40:355-9.
54. Paulus HE, Williams HJ, Ward JR, Reading JC, Egger MJ, Coleman ML, Samuelson CO Jr, Willkens RF, Guttadauria M, Alarcon GS, Kaplan SB, MacLaughlin EJ, Weinstein A, Wilder RL, Solsky MA, Meenan RF. Azathioprine versus D-penicillamine in rheumatoid arthritis patients who have been treated unsuccessfully with gold. Arth Rheum 1984; 27:721-7.
55. Halberg P, Bentzon MW, Crohn O, Gad I, Halskov O, Heyn J, Ingemann M, Junker P, Lorenzen I, Moller I, Hansen TM, Olsen N, Pedersen G, Sorensen SF, Stage P. Double-blind trial of levamisone, penicillamine and azathioprine in rheumatoid arthritis. Clinical, biochemical, radiological and scintigraphic studies. Dan Med Bull 1984; 31:403-9.
56. Cade R, Stein G, Pickering M, Schlein E, Spooner F. Low dose, long-term treatment of rheumatoid arthritis with azathioprine. South Med J 1976; 69:388-92.
57. Balow JE, Austin HA III, Tsokos GC, Antonovych TT, Steinberg AD, Klippel JH. Lupus nephritis. Ann Intern Med 1987; 106:79-94.
58. Fauci AS, Katz P, Haynes BF, Wolff SM. Cyclophosphamide therapy of severe systemic necrotizing vasculitis. N Engl J Med 1979; 301:235-8.
59. Weiner SR, Paulus HE. Treatment of Wegener's granulomatosis (WG) with cyclophosphamide (CTX): Outcome analysis. Arth Rheum 1983; 26:S65.
60. Hall S, Barr W, Lie JT, Stanson AW, Kazmier FJ, Hunder GG. Takayasu arteritis. A study of 32 North American patients. Medicine 1985; 64: 89-99.
61. Lanham JG, Elkon KB, Pusey CD, Hughes GR. Systemic vasculitis with asthma and esoinophilia: A clinical approach to the Churg-Strauss syndrome. Medicine 1984; 63:65-81.
62. Leib ES, Restivo C, Paulus HE. Immunosuppressive and corticosteroid therapy of polyarteritis nodosa. Am J Med 1979; 67:941-7.
63. Panush RS, Yonker RA, Dlesk A, Longley S, Caldwell JR. Weber-Christian disease: Analysis of 15 cases and review of the literature. Medicine 1985; 64:181-91.
64. Old CW, Flannery EP, Grogan TM, Stone WH, San Antonio RP. Azathioprine-induced pure red blood cell aplasia. JAMA 1978; 240:552-554.

65. Guillaume P, Grandjean E, Male PJ. Azathioprine-associated acute pancreatitis in the course of chronic active hepatitis. Dig Dis Sci 1984; 29:78–80.
66. Taft PM, Jones AC, Collins GM, Halasz NA. Acute pancreatitis following renal transplantation. A lethal complication. Am J Dig Dis 1978; 23:541–4.
67. Kawanishi H, Randolph E, Bull FE. Azathioprine-induced acute pancreatitis. N Engl J Med 1973; 289:357.
68. Zarday Z, Veith FJ, Gliedman ML, Soberman R. Irreversible liver damage after azathioprine. JAMA 1972; 222:690–1.
69. DePinho RA, Goldberg CS, Lefkowitch JH. Azathioprine and the liver. Evidence favoring idiosyncratic, mixed cholestatic-hepato-cellular injury in humans. Gastroenterology 1984; 86:162–5.
70. DuVivier A, Munro DD, Verbov J. Treatment of psoriasis with azathioprine. Br Med J 1974; 1:49–51.
71. Munro DD. Azathioprine in psoriasis. Proc Roy Soc Med 1973; 66:747–8.
72. Sparberg M, Simon N, De Greco F. Intrahepatic cholestasis due to azathioprine. Gastroenterology 1969; 57:439–41.
73. Bedrossian CWM, Sussman J, Conklin RH, Kahan B. Azathioprine-associated interstitial pneumonitis. Am J Clin Pathol 1984; 82:148–54.
74. Carmichael DJS, Hamilton DV, Evans DB, Stovin PGI, Calne RY. Interstitial pneumonitis secondary to azathioprine in a renal transplant patient. Thorax 1983; 38:951–2.
75. Sharon E, Jones J, Diamond H, Kaplan D. Pregnancy and azathioprine in systemic lupus erythematosus. Am J Obstet Gynecol 1974; 118:25–8.
76. Saarikoski S, Seppala M. Immunosuppression during pregnancy: Transmission of azathioprine and its metabolites from the mother to the fetus. Am J Obstet Gynceol 1973; 115:1100–6.
77. DeWitte DB, Buick MK, Cyran SE, Maisels MJ. Neonatal pancytopenia and severe combined immunodeficiency associated with antenatal administration of azathioprine and prednisone. J Pediatr 1984; 105:625–8.
78. Cote CJ, Meuwissen HJ, Pickering RJ. Effects on the neonate of prednisone and azathioprine administered to the mother during pregnancy. J Pediatr 1974; 85:324–8.
79. Leb DW, Weisskopf B, Kanovitz BS. Chromosome aberrations in the child of a kidney transplant recipient. Arch Intern Med 1971; 128:441–4.
80. Penn I, Halgrimson CG, Starzl TE. DeNovo malignant tumors in organ transplant recipients. Transplant Proc 1971; 3:773–8.
81. Hoover R, Fraumeni JF Jr. Risk of cancer in renal-transplant recipients. Lancet 1973; 2:55–7.

82. Kinlen LJ, Shiel AGR, Peto J, Doll R. Collaborative United Kingdom-Australian study of cancer in patients treated with immunosuppressive drugs. Br. Med J 1979; 2:1461-6.
83. Seidenfeld AM, Smythe HA, Ogryzlo MA, Urowitz MB, Dotten DA. Acute leukemia in rheumatoid arthritis treated with cytotoxic agents. J Rheumatol 1984; 11:586-7.
84. Tilson HH, Whisnant J. Pharmaco-epidemiology—drugs, arthritis, and neoplasms: Industry contribution to the data. Am J Med 1985; 78(Supplement 1A):69-76.
85. Prior P, Symmons DPM, Hawkins CF, Scott DL, Brown R. Cancer morbidity in rheumatoid arthritis. Ann Rheum Dis 1984; 43:128-31.
86. Symmons DPM, Ahern M, Bacon PA, Hawkins CF, Amlot PL, Jones EL, Prior P, Scott DL. Lymphoproliferative malignancy in rheumatoid arthritis: a study of 20 cases. Ann Rheum Dis 1984; 43:132-5.
87. Isomaki HA, Mutru O, Koota K. Death rate and causes of death in patients with rheumatoid arthritis. Scand J Rheumatol 1975; 4:205-8.
88. Prior P. Cancer and rheumatoid arthritis: Epidemiologic considerations. Am J Med 1985; 78(Supplement a!):15-21.
89. Symmons DPM. Neoplasms of the immune system in rheumatoid arthritis. Am J Med 1985; 78(Supplement 1A):22-8.
90. Kinlen LJ. Incidence of cancer in rheumatoid arthritis and other disorders after immunosuppressive treatment. Am J Med 1985; 78(Supplement 1A):44-9.
91. Lewis P, Hazleman BL, Hanka R, Roberts S. Cause of death in patients with rheumatoid arthritis with particular reference to azathioprine. Ann Rheum Dis 1989; 39:457-61.
92. Hazleman B. Incidence of neoplasms in patients with rheumatoid arthritis exposed to different treatment regimens. Am J Med 1985; 78(Supplement 1A):39-43.
93. Calabresi P, Parks RE Jr. Antiproliferative agents and drugs used for immunosuppression. In: Gilman AG, Goodman LS, Rall TW, Murad F. (eds). The pharmacological basis of therapeutics, 7th ed. New York: Macmillan, 1985:1247-1306.
94. Kovarsky J. Clinical pharmacology and toxicology of cyclophosphamide: Emphasis on use in rheumatic diseases. Sem Arth Rheum 1983; 12:359-72.
95. Pederson-Bjergaard J, Ersboll J, Hansen VL, Sorensen BL, Christoffersen K, Hon-Jenson K, Nissen NI, Knudsen JB, Hansen MM. Carcinoma of the Urinary Bladder after Treatment with Cyclophosphamide for Non-Hodgkins Lymphoma. N Engl J Med 1988; 1028-32.
96. Bagley CM Jr, Bostick FW, DeVita VT Jr. Clinical pharmacology of cyclophosphamide. Cancer Res 1973; 33:226-33.
97. McLean A, Newell D, Baker G. The metabolism of chlorambucil. Biochem Pharmacol 1976; 25:2331-5.

98. Alberts DS, Chang SY, Hsiao-Sheng GC, Larcom BJ, Jones SE. Pharmacokinetics and metabolism of chlorambucil in man: a preliminary report. Cancer Treatm Rev 1979; 6(Suppl):9-17.
99. McLean A, Woods RL, Catovsky D, Farmer P. Pharmacokinetics and metabolism of chlorambucil in patients with malignant disease. Cancer Treatm Rev 1979; 6(Suppl):33-42).
100. McLean A, Newell D, Baker G, Connors T. The metabolism of chlorambucil. Biochem Pharmacol 1980; 29:2039-47.
101. Clements PJ. Cytotoxic immunosuppressive drugs. In: Paulus HE, Furst DE, Dromgoole SH. (eds). Drugs for rheumatic disease. New York: Churchill Livingstone, 1987:135-57.
102. Boston Collaborative Drug Surveillance Program. Allopurinol and cytotoxic drugs. Interaction in relation to bone marrow depression. JAMA 1974; 227:1036-40.
103. Vesell EW, Passanati GT, Greene FE. Impairment of drug metabolism in man by allopurinol and nortriptyline. N Engl J Med 1979; 283: 1484-8.
104. Kovacs K, Steinberg AD. Cyclophosphamide. Drug interactions and bone marrow transplantation. Transplantation 1972; 13:316-21.
105. Gaudin D, Yielding KL. Response of a "resistant" plasmocytoma to alkylating agents and x-ray in combination with the "excision repair inhibitors" caffeine and chloroquine. Proc Soc Exp Biol Med 1969; 131:1413-6.
106. Alberts DS, vanDaalen Wetters T. The effect of phenobarbitol on cyclophosphamide anti-tumor activity. Cancer Res 1976; 36:2785-9.
107. Hart LG, Adamson RH. Effect of microsomal enzyme modifiers on toxicity and therapeutic activity of cyclophosphamide in mice. Arch Int Pharmacodyn 1969; 180:391-401.
108. Field RB, Gang M, Kline I, Venditti JM, Waravdekar VS. The effect of phenobarbitol or 2-diethyl-aminoethyl-2,2-diphenylvalerate on the activation of cyclophosphamide in vivo. J Pharmacol Exp Ther 1972; 180:475-83.
109. Sladek NE. Therapeutic efficacy of cyclophosphamide as a function of its metabolism. Cancer Res 1972; 32:535-42.
110. Hayakawa T, Kanai N, Yamada R, Kuroda R, Higashi H, Mogami H, Jinnai D. Effect of steroid hormone on activation of endoxan (cyclophosphamide). Biochem Pharmacol 1969; 18:129-35.
111. Cannon GW, Jackson CG, Samuelson CO Jr, Ward JR, Williams HJ, Clegg DO. Chlorambucil therapy in rheumatoid arthritis: Clinical experience in 28 patients and literature review. Sem Arth Rheum 1985; 15:106-18.
112. Williams HJ, Reading JC, Ward JR, O'Brien WM. Comparison of high and low dose cyclophosphamide therapy in rheumatoid arthritis. Arth Rheum 1980; 23:521-7.

113. Shand FL, Howard JG. Induction in vitro of reversible immunosuppression and inhibition of B cell receptor regeneration by defined metabolites of cyclophosphamides. Eur J Immunol 1979; 9:17-21.
114. Turk JL, Poulter LW. Selective depletion of lymphoid tissue by cyclophosphamide. Clin Exp Immunol 1972; 10:285-96.
115. Turk JL, Poulter LW. Effects of cyclophosphamide on lymphoid tissues labeled with 5-iodo-2-deoxyuridine-^{125}I and ^{51}Cr. Int Arch Allergy 1972; 43:629-9.
116. Stockman GD, Heim LR, South MA, Trentin JJ. Differential effects of cyclophosphamide on the B and T cell compartments of adult mice. J Immunol 1973; 110:277-82.
117. Winkelstein A. Effect of immunosuppressive drugs on T and B lymphocytes in guinea pigs. Blood 1977; 50:81-91.
118. Hurd ER, Guiliano VJ. The effect of cyclophosphamide on B and T lymphocytes in patients with connective tissue diseases. Arth Rheum 1975; 18:67-75.
119. Clements PJ, Yu DTY, Levy J, Paulus HE, Barnett EV. Effects of cyclophosphamide on B- and T-lymphocytes in rheumatoid arthritis. Arth Rheum 1974; 17:347-53.
120. Dale DC, Fauci AS, Wolff SM. The effect of cyclophosphamide on leukocyte kinetics and susceptibility to infection in patients with Wegener's granulomatosis. Arth Rheum 1973; 16:657-64.
121. Diamanstein T, Willinger E, Reiman J. T-suppressor cells sensitive to cyclophosphamide and to its in vitro active derivative 4-hydroperoxycyclophosphamide control the mitogenic response of murine splenic B cells to dextran suflate. A direct proof for different sensitivities of lymphocyte subsets to cyclophosphamide. J Exp Med 1979; 150: 1571-6.
122. Kaufmann SHE, Hahn H, Diamantstein T. Relative susceptibilities of T cell subsets involved in delayed-type hypersensitivity to sheep red blood cells to the in vitro action of 4-hydroperoxycyclophos-phamide. J Immunol 1989; 125:1104-8.
123. Ozer H, Cowens JW, Colvin M, Nussbaum-Blumenson A, Sheedy D. In vitro effects of 4-hydroperoxycyclophosphamide on human immunoregulatory T subset function. I. Selective effects on lymphocyte function in T-B cell collaboration. J Exp Med 1982; 155:276-90.
124. Feehally J, Beattie TJ, Brenchley PEC, Coupes BM, Houston IB, Mallick NP, Postlethwaite RJ. Modulation of cellular immune function by cyclophosphamide in children with minimal-change nephropathy. N Engl J Med 1984; 310:415-20.
125. Maguire HC. Specific acquired immune unresponsiveness to contact allergens with cyclophosphamide in the mouse. Int Arch Allergy 1976; 50:651-8.

126. Berenbaum MC, Brown IN. Prolongation of homograft survival in mice with single doses of cyclophosphamide. Nature 1963; 200:84.
127. Owens AH Jr, Santos GW. The effect of cytotoxic drugs on graft-versus-host disease in mice. Transplantation 1971; 11:378–82.
128. Steinberg AD, Daley GG, Talal N. Tolerance to polyinosinic-poly-cytidylic acid in NZB/NZW mice. Science 1970; 167:870–1.
129. Bontoux D, Kahan A, Brouilhet H, Amor B, DelBarre F, Jouanneau M, Gniazdowska E. Effect and mode of action of chlorambucil in rheumatoid disease. Value of the lymphoblast transformation test. Revue du Rhumatisme 1971; 38:759–64.
130. Maguire HC, Ettore VL. Enhancement of dinitrochlorobenzene (DNCB) contact sensitization by cyclophosphamide in the guinea pig. J Invest Dermatol 1967; 48:39–43.
131. Turk JL, Parker D, Poulter LW. Functional aspects of the selective depletion of lymphoid tissue by cyclophosphamide. Immunology 1972; 23:493–501.
132. Lagrange PH, MacKaness GB, Miller TE. Potentiation of T-cell-mediated immunity by selective suppression of antibody formation with cyclophosphamide. J Exp Med 1974; 139:1529–39.
133. Kerckhaert JAM, Hofhuis FMA, Willers JMN. Inflience of cyclophosphamide on delayed hypersensitivity and acquired cellular resistance to Listeria monocytogenes in the mouse. Immunology 1977; 32:1027–32.
134. Rollinghoff M, Starzinski-Powitz A, Pfizenmaier K, Wagner H. Cyclophosphamide-sensitive T lymphocytes suppress the in vivo generation of antigen-specific cytotoxic T lymphocytes. J Exp Med 1977; 145:455–9.
135. Ferguson RM, Simmons RL. Differential cyclophosphamide sensitivity of suppressor and cytotoxic cell precursors. Transplantation 1978; 25:36–8.
136. Kahn M, de Seze S. Immunosuppression agents in rheumatology. Indications, results, and long-term adverse effects. Annales du Medecine 1974; 125:449–506.
137. Alepa FP, Zvaifler NJ, Sliwinski AJ. Immunologic effects of cyclophosphamide treatment in rheumatoid arthritis. Arth Rheum 1970; 13:754–60.
138. Stevenson HC, Fauci AS. Activation of human B lymphocytes. XII. Differential effects of in vitro cyclophosphamide on human lymphocyte subpopulations involved in B-cell activation. Immunology 1980; 39:391–7.
139. Santos GW, Owens AH. 19S and 7S antibody production in the cyclophosphamide or methotrexate-treated rat. Nature 1966; 209:622–4.
140. Aisenberg AC. Immunosuppression by alklyating agents: tolerance induction. Transpl Proc 1973; 5:1221–6.

141. Kawaguchi S. Studies on the induction of immunological paralysis to bovine -globulin in adult mice. II. The effect of cyclophosphamide. Immunology 1970; 19:291–9.
142. Many A, Schwartz RS. On the mechanism of immunological tolerance in cyclophosphamide-treated mice. Clin Exp Immunol 1970; 6:87–99.
143. Turk JL, Parker D. Further studies on B-lymphocyte suppression in delayed hypersensitivity, indicating a possible mechanism for Jones-Mote hypersensitivity. Immunology 1973; 24:751–8.
144. Duclos H, Galanaud P, Devinsky O, Maillot MC, Dormont J. Enhancing effect of low dose cyclophosphamide treatment on the in vitro antibody response. Eur J Immunol 1977; 7:679–84.
145. Curtis JE, Sharp JT, Lidsky MD, Hersh EM. Immune response of patients with rheumatoid arthritis during cyclophosphamide treatment. Arth Rheum 1973; 16:34–42.
146. Hersh EM, Wong VG, Freireich EJ. Inhibition of the local inflammatory response in man by antimetabolites. Blood 1966; 27:38–48.
147. Fosdick WM, Parsons JL, Hill DF. Long-term cyclophosphamide therapy in rheumatoid arthritis. Arth Rheum 1968; 11:151–60.
148. Smyth CJ, Bartholomew BA, Mills DM, Steigerwald JC, Strong SJ, Recart S. Cyclophosphamide therapy for rheumatoid arthritis. Arch Intern Med 1975; 135:789–93.
149. Townes AS, Sowa JM, Shulman LE. Controlled trial of cyclophosphamide in rheumatoid arthritis. Arth Rheum 1976; 19:563–73.
150. Cooperating Clinics Committee of the American Rheumatism Association. A controlled trial of cyclophosphamide in rheumatoid arthritis. N Engl J Med 1970; 283:883–9.
151. Vignon G, Bied JC. Comparative study of the various immunosuppressive agents in rheumatoid arthritis. Revue du Rhumatisme 1971; 38: 785–95.
152. de Seze S, Bedoiseau M, Debeyre N, Kahn MF. Resultats de la therapeutique a visee immunodepressive chez 40 malades atteints de polyarthrite rhumatoide grave. Sem Hop Paris 1967; 43:3084–91.
153. Bedrossian CWM, Miller WC, Luna MA. Methotrexate-induced diffuse interstitial pulmonary fibrosis. South Med J 1979; 72:313–8.
154. Renier JC, Deshayes P, Besson J, Barazer C, Delahaye D, Bregeon C. Treatment of rheumatoid polyarthritis by means of chlorambucil (in relation to 48 cases). La Presse Medicale 1967; 75:2527–30.
155. Iannuzzi L, Dawson N, Zein N, Kushner I. Does drug therapy slow radiographic deterioration in rheumatoid arthritis? N Engl J Med 1983; 309:1023–8.
156. Snaith ML, Holt JM, Oliver DO, Dunnill MS, Halley W, Stephenson AC. Treatment of patients with systemic lupus erythematosus including nephritis with chlorambucil. Br Med J 1973; 2:197–201.

157. Lehman T, McCurdy D, Bernstein B, Turner M, Katz A, Hanson V. Intravenous bolus cyclophosphamide (IV-CP) therapy of lupus nephritis in children. Arth Rheum 1986; 29 (Supplement):S92.
158. Fries JF, Sharp GC, McDevitt HO, Holman HR. Cyclophosphamide therapy in systemic lupus erythematosus and polymyositis. Arth Rheum 1973; 16:154-62.
159. Fauci AS, Haynes BF, Katz P, Wolff SM. Wegener's granulomatosis: prospective clinical and therapeutic experience with 85 patients for 21 years. Ann Intern Med 1983; 98:76-85.
160. Scott DGI, Bacon PA. Intravenous cyclophosphamide plus methylprednisolone in treatment of systemic rheumatoid vasculitis. Am J Med 1984; 76:377-84.
161. Shelhamer JH, Volkman DJ, Parrillo JE, Lawley TJ, Johnston MR, Fauci AS. Takayasu's arteritis and its therapy. Ann Intern Med 1985; 103:121-6.
162. Skoglund RR, Schanberger JE, Kaplan JM. Cyclophosphamide therapy for severe juvenile rheumatoid arthritis. Am J Dis Child 1971; 121: 531-3.
163. Buriot D, Prieur AM, leBranchu Y, Messerschmitt J, Griscelli C. Leucemie aigue chez trois enfants atteints d'arthrite chronique juvenille traites par le chlorambucil. Arch Fr Pediatr 1979; 36:592-8.
164. El-Ghobarey A, Balint G, DeCeulaer K, Dick WC, Buchanan WW, Hadidi T, Hassan TA. Dermatomyositis: observations on the use of immunosuppressive therapy and review of the literature. Postgrad Med J 1978; 54:516-27.
165. Geltner D, Kohn RW, Gorevic P, Franklin EC. The effect of combination therapy (steroids, immunosuppressives, and plasmapheresis) on 5 mixed cryoglobulinemia patients with renal, neurologic, and vascular involvement. Arth Rheum 1981; 24:1121-7.
166. O'Duffy JD, Robertson DM, Goldstein NP. Chlorambucil in the treatment of uveitis and meningoencephalitis of Behcet's disease. Am J Med 1984; 76:75-84.
167. Mishima S, Masuda K, Izawa Y, Mochizuki M, Namba K. Behcet's disease in Japan: ophthalmological aspects. Trans Am Ophthalmol Soc 1979; 77:225-79.
168. Tabbara KF. Chlorambucil in Behcet's disease: a re-appraisal. Ophthalmology 1983; 90:906-8.
169. Erickson SB, Kurtz SB, Donadio JV Jr, Holley KE, Wilson CB, Pineda AA. Use of combined plasmapheresis and immunosuppression in the treatment of Goodpasture's syndrome. Mayo Clin Proc 1979; 54:714-20.
170. Grupe WE, Heymann W. Cytotoxic drugs in steroid-resistant renal disease. Alkylating and antimetabolic agents in the treatment of

nephrotic syndrome, lupus nephritis, chronic glomerulonephritis, and purpura nephritis in children. Am J Dis Child 1966; 112:448–58.

171. Tolchin SF, Winkelstein A, Rodnan GP, Pan SF, Nankin HR. Chromosome abnormalities from cyclophosphamide therapy in rheumatoid arthritis and progressive systemic sclerosis (scleroderma). Arth Rheum 1974; 17:375–82.

172. Dau PC, Kahaleh MB, Sagebiel RW. Plasmapheresis and immunosuppressive drug therapy in scleroderma. Arth Rheum 1981; 24:1128–36.

173. Renier JC, Deshayes P, Houdent G, Bernat M, Bastard J, Bregeon C. Le traitement de la polyarthrite rhumatoide par le chlorambucil. Etude de 113 observations. Arch Med de l'ouest 1971; 1:47–58.

174. Cayla J, Rondier J. The treatment of 67 cases of rheumatoid arthritis with chlorambucil. Revue du Rhumatisme 1971; 38:765–70.

175. Arlet J, Mole J, Debrock J. Our experience of the treatment of chronic rheumatoid arthritis with immunosuppressive drugs: with reference to 41 cases. Revue du Rhumatisme 1971; 38:771–4.

176. Sauvezie B, Rampon S, Bussiere JL, Doly J, Flori B. Value of the lymphoblastic transformation test (LTT) with incorporation of titrated thymidine in the supervision of immuno-suppressive treatments in rheumatology. Rev Rhum Mal Osteoartic 1972; 39:609–16.

177. Renier JC, Bregeon C, Bonnette C. Results of immunodepressant treatment in 78 patients suffering from rheumatoid polyarthritis and having undergone treatment for more than four years. Revue du Rhumatisme 1975; 42:399–407.

178. Krel AA, Trifonov YI, Bolotin EV, Kanavskaya MZ. Cytopenic syndrome in patients with rheumatoid arthritis treated with leukeran and azathioprine. Sov Med 1979; (9):68–72.

179. Amor B, Herson D, Cherot A, DelBarre F. Follow-up study of patients with rheumatoid arthritis over a period of more than 10 years (1966–1978): analysis of disease progression and treatment in 100 cases. Annales Medecine Interne 1981; 132:168–73.

180. Renier JC, Bregeon C, Bonnette C, Boasson M, Bernat M, Basle M, Besson J, Wellinger C, Bourgeois B, Teisseire N. The evolution of patients with rheumatoid arthritis receiving immunosuppressors between 1965 and 1973. Revue du Rhumatisme 1978; 45:453–61.

181. Deshayes P, Renier JC, Bregeon C, Houdent G. Side-effects and complications of immunosuppressive therapy in rheumatoid arthritis. Revue due Rhumatisme 1971; 38:797–806.

182. Aymard JP, Lederlin P, Witz F, Rumilly F, Eisemann JC, Buisine J, Gregoire MJ, Guerci O, Streiff F. Acute leukemia following prolonged chlorambucil treatment of non-neoplastic disease: a study of two cases and literature review. Acta Clin Belg 1983; 38:228–35.

183. Kahn MF, Bedoiseau M, Six B, LeGoff P, deSeze S. Chlorambucil in rheumatoid arthritis. Revue du Rhumatisme 1971; 38:741–8.
184. Thorpe P, Hassall JE, York JR. Rheumatoid arthritis treated with chlorambucil. A five-year follow-up. Med J Aust 1976; 2:197–9.
185. Rudd P, Fries JF, Epstein WV. Irreversible bone marrow failure with chlorambucil. J Rheumatol 1975; 2:421–9.
186. Mullins GM, Colvin M. Intensive cyclophosphamide (NSC-26271) therapy for solid tumors. Cancer Chemother Rep 1975; 59:411–9.
187. Schein PS, Winokur SH. Immunsuppressive and cytotoxic chemotherapy: long-term complications. Ann Intern Med 1975; 82:84–95.
188. Marsh FP, Vince FP, Pollock DJ, Blandy JP. Cyclophosphamide necrosis of bladder causing calcification, contracture and reflux: treated by colocystoplasty. Br J Urol 1971; 43:324–32.
189. Johnson WW, Meadows DC. Urinary-bladder fibrosis and telangiectasia associated with long-term cyclophosphamide therapy. N Engl J Med 1971; 284:290–4.
190. Wall RL, Clausen KP. Carcinoma of the urinary bladder in patients receiving cyclophosphamide. N Engl J Med 1975; 293:271–3.
191. Pearson RM, Soloway MS. Does cyclophosphamide induce bladder cancer? Urology 1978; 11:437–47.
192. Fairchild WV, Spence CR, Solomon HD, Gangai MP. The incidence of bladder cancer after cyclophosphamide therapy. J Urol 1979; 122: 163–4.
193. Scheef W, Klein HO, Brock N, Burkert H, Gunther U, Hoefer-Janker H, Mitrenga D, Schnitker J, Voigtmann R. Controlled clinical studies with an antidote against the urotoxicity of oxazaphosphorines: preliminary results. Cancer Treatm Rep 1979; 63:501–5.
194. Fairley RF, Barrie JU, Johnson W. Sterility and testicular atrophy related to cyclophosphamide therapy. Lancet 1972; 1:568–9.
195. Kumar R, Biggart JD, McEvoy J, McGeown MG. Cyclophosphamide and reproductive function. Lancet 1972; 1:1212–4.
196. Miller DG. Alkylating agents and human spermatogenesis. JAMA 1971; 217:1662–5.
197. Jacobson RJ, Sagel J, Distiller LA, Morley JE. Leydig cell dysfunction in male patients with Hodgkins disease receiving chemotherapy. Clin Res 1978; 26:437A.
198. Chapman RM, Sutcliffe SB, Rees LH, Edwards CRW, Malpas JS. Cyclical combination chemotherapy and gonadal function. Retrospective study in males. Lancet 1979; 1:285–9.
199. Hinkes E, Plotkin D. Reversible drug-induced sterility in a patient with acute leukemia. JAMA 1973; 223:1490–1.
200. Blake DA, Heller RH, Hsu SH, Schacter BZ. Return of fertility in a patient with cyclophosphamide-induced azoospermia. Johns Hopkins Med J 1976; 139:20–2.

201. Greenburg LH, Tanaka KR. Congenital anomalies probably induced by cyclophosphamide. JAMA 1964; 188:423–6.
202. Toledo TM, Harper RC, Moser RH. Fetal effects during cyclophosphamide and irradiation therapy. Ann Intern Med 1971; 74:87–91.
203. Sokal JE, Lessmann EM. Effects of cancer chemotherapeutic agents on the human fetus. JAMA 1960; 151:1765–71.
204. Shotton D, Monie IW. Possible teratogenic effect of chlorambucil on a human fetus. JAMA 1963; 186:74–5.
205. Blatt J, Mulvihill JJ, Ziegler JL, Young RC, Poplack DG. Pregnancy outcome following cancer chemotherapy. Am J Med 1980; 69:828–32.
206. Cooper JA, Matthay RA. Drug-induced pulmonary disease. Disease-a-Month, 1987; 33:61–120.
207. Bacon AM, Rosenberg SA. Cyclophosphamide hepatoxicity in a patient with systemic lupus erythematosus. Ann Intern Med 1982; 97:62–3.
208. Thorpe P, Hassall J, York J. Cytotoxic therapy in rheumatoid disease. Med J Aust 1971; 2:796–8.
209. Lakin JD, Cahill RA. Generalized urticaria to cyclophosphamide: type I hypersensitivity to an immunosuppressive agent. J Allergy Clin Immunol 1976; 58:160–71.
210. Menkes CJ, Levy JP, Weill B, Delrieu F, Mathiot C, Delbarre F. Acute megacaryloblastic leukemia after immunodepressive treatment of rheumatoid arthritis. Nouv Presse Med 1975; 4:2869–71.
211. Kahn MF, Arlet J, Bloch-Michel H, Cariot M, Chaouat Y, Renier JC. Acute leukaemias after treatment using cytotoxic agents for rheumatologic purposes. 19 cases among 2006 patients. Nouv Presse Med 1979; 8:1393–7.
212. Zittoun R, Debre P, Gardais J, Thuau FP, Renier JC, Simon F. Small intestine lymphosarcoma after treatment of rheumatoid arthritis by chlorambucil. Nouv Presse Med 1972; 1:2477–9.
213. Prieur AM, Balafrej M, Griscelli C, Mozziconacci P. Results and long-term risks of immuno-suppressive treatment in chronic juvenile arthritis. A 40 case study. Revue du Rhumatisme 1979; 46:85–90.
214. Lebrancha Y, Drucker J, Nivet H, Rolland JC, Grenier B, Lejars O, Lamagnere JP, Buriot D. Acute monoblastic leukaemia in child receiving chlorambucil for juvenile rheumatoid arthritis. Lancet 1980; 1:649.
215. Dumont J, Thiery JP, Mazabraud A, Natali JC, Trapet P, Vilcoq JR. Acute meyloid leukemia following non-Hodgkin's lymphoma. Danger of prolonged use of chlorambucil as maintainance therapy. Nouv Rev Fr Hematol 1980; 22:391–404.
216. Berk PD, Goldberg JD, Silverstein MN, Weinfeld A, Donovan PB, Ellis JT, Landaw SA, Laszlo J, Najean Y, Pisciotta AV, Wasserman LR. Increased incidence of acute leukemia in polycythemia vera associated with chlorambucil therapy. N Engl J Med 1981; 304:441–7.

217. Aymard JP, Frustin J, Witz F, Colomb JN, Lederlin P, Herbeuval R. Acute leukemia after prolonged chlorambucil treatment for non-malignant disease: report of a new case and literature survey. Acta Haematol 1980; 63:283-5.
218. Fiere D, Felman P, Van HV, Coiffier B. Leucemies aigues myeloides apres administration de chlorambucil. Deux observations. Nouv Presse Med 1977; 7:756.
219. Chaplin H. Lymphoma in primary chronic cold hemagglutinin disease treated with chlorambucil. Arch Intern Med 1982; 142:2119-23.
220. Baltus JAM, Boersma JW, Hartman AP, Vandenbroucke JP. The occurrence of malignancies in patients with rehumatoid arthritis treated with cyclophosphamide: a controlled retrospective follow-up. Ann Rheum Dis 1983; 42:368-73.
221. Palmer RG, Dore CJ, Denman AM. Chlorambucil-induced chromosome damage to human lymphocytes is dose dependent and cumulative. Lancet 1984; 1:246-9.
222. Baker GL, Kahl LE, Medsger TA. Stolzer BL, Eisenbeis CH Jr, Agarwal AK. Malignancy in cyclophosphamide-treated rheumatoid arthritis patients: a long-term followup study (abstract). Arth Rheum 1985; 28: S37.
223. DeFronzo RA, Braine H, Colvin OM, Davis PJ. Water intoxication in man after cyclophosphamide therapy. Time course and relation to drug activation. Ann Intern Med 1973; 78:861-9.
224. Herman EH, Mhatre RM, Waravdekar VS, Lee IP. Comparison of the cardiovascular actions of NSC-109, 724 (ifosfamine) and cyclophosphamide. Toxicol Appl Pharmacol 1972; 23:178-90.
225. Karchmer RK, Hansen VL. Possible anaphylactic reaction to intravenous cyclophosphamide. Report of a case. JAMA 1977; 237:475.
226. Arena PJ. Oropharyngeal sensation associated with rapid intravenous administration of cyclophosphamide (NSC-26271). Cancer Chemother Rep 1972; 56:779-80.
227. Ehrlich GE. Heroic treatment for nonmalignant disease. JAMA 1982; 248:1743-4.
228. Sievers K, Hurri L. Combined therapy of rheumatoid arthritis with gold and chloroquine. I. Evaluation of the therapeutic effect. Acta Rheum Scand 1963; 9:48-55.
229. McCarty DJ, Carrera GF. Intractable rheumatoid arthritis. Treatment with combined cyclophosphamide, azathioprine, and hydroxychloroquine. JAMA 1982; 248:1718-23.
230. Csuka ME, Carrera GF, McCarty DJ. Treatment of intractable rheumatoid arthritis with combined cyclophosphamide, azathioprine, and hydroxychloroquine. A follow-up study. JAMA 1986; 255:2315-9.

231. Bunch TW, O'Duffy JD, Tompkins RB, O'Fallon WM. Controlled trial of hydroxychloroquine and d-penicillamine singly and in combination in the treatment of rheumatoid arthritis. Arth Rheum 1984; 27:267–76.
232. Bitter T. Combined disease-modifying chemotherapy for intractable rheumatoid arthritis. Clin Rheum Dis 1984; 10:417–28.
233. Taggart AJ, Hill J, Astbury C, Dixon JS, Bird HA, Wright V. Sulphasalazine alone or in combination with d-penicillamine in rheumatoid arthritis. Br J Rheumatol 1987; 26:32–6.
234. Butler D, Tiliakos N. Low-dose cytotoxic drug combination therapy in intractable rheumatoid arthritis (abstract). Arth Rheum 1985; 28:S15.
235. Biro JA, Segal AM, Mackenzie AH, Mazanec DJ, Wilke WS. The combination of methotrexate (MTX) and azathioprine (AZA) for resistant rheumatoid arthritis. Arth Rheum 1987; 30(Suppl):S18.

3

Cyclosporine in Rheumatoid Arthritis

Andrea Kowal and John H. Carstens, Jr.
Sandoz Research Institute, East Hanover, New Jersey

Thomas J. Schnitzer
Rush-Presbyterian-St. Luke's Medical Center, Chicago, Illinois

I. CHEMISTRY

Cyclosporine is a potent immunosuppressive agent extracted from the mycelia of the fungal species *Tolypocladium inflatum gams* recovered in soil samples from the Hardanger Vidda (Norway). Initial isolation and purification of this metabolite occurred in the early 1970s; its structure has since been established via chemical degradation together with X-ray crystallographic analysis of an iododerivative (1,2). Cyclosporine (Fig. 1) is a neutral, hydrophobic cyclic peptide with a MW of 1202.6 D. It is composed of 11 amino acid residues, all having the S configuration of the natural L-amino acids except for the D-alanine in position 8, which has the R configuration. The seven amino acids in positions 1, 3, 4, 6, 9, 10, and 11 are N-methylated; 10 of the amino acids are aliphatic: α-aminobutyric acid in position 2, sarcosine in position 3, *N*-methylleucine in positions 4, 6, 9, and 10, valine in position 5, alanine in position 7, D-alanine in position 8, and *N*-methylvaline in position 11. The unique structural feature of this molecule is the presence of an unsaturated C9 amino acid in position 1. This amino acid, found for the first time in cyclosporine, had never been previously isolated or known in free form. The successful synthesis of the complete molecule occurred in 1980 (3).

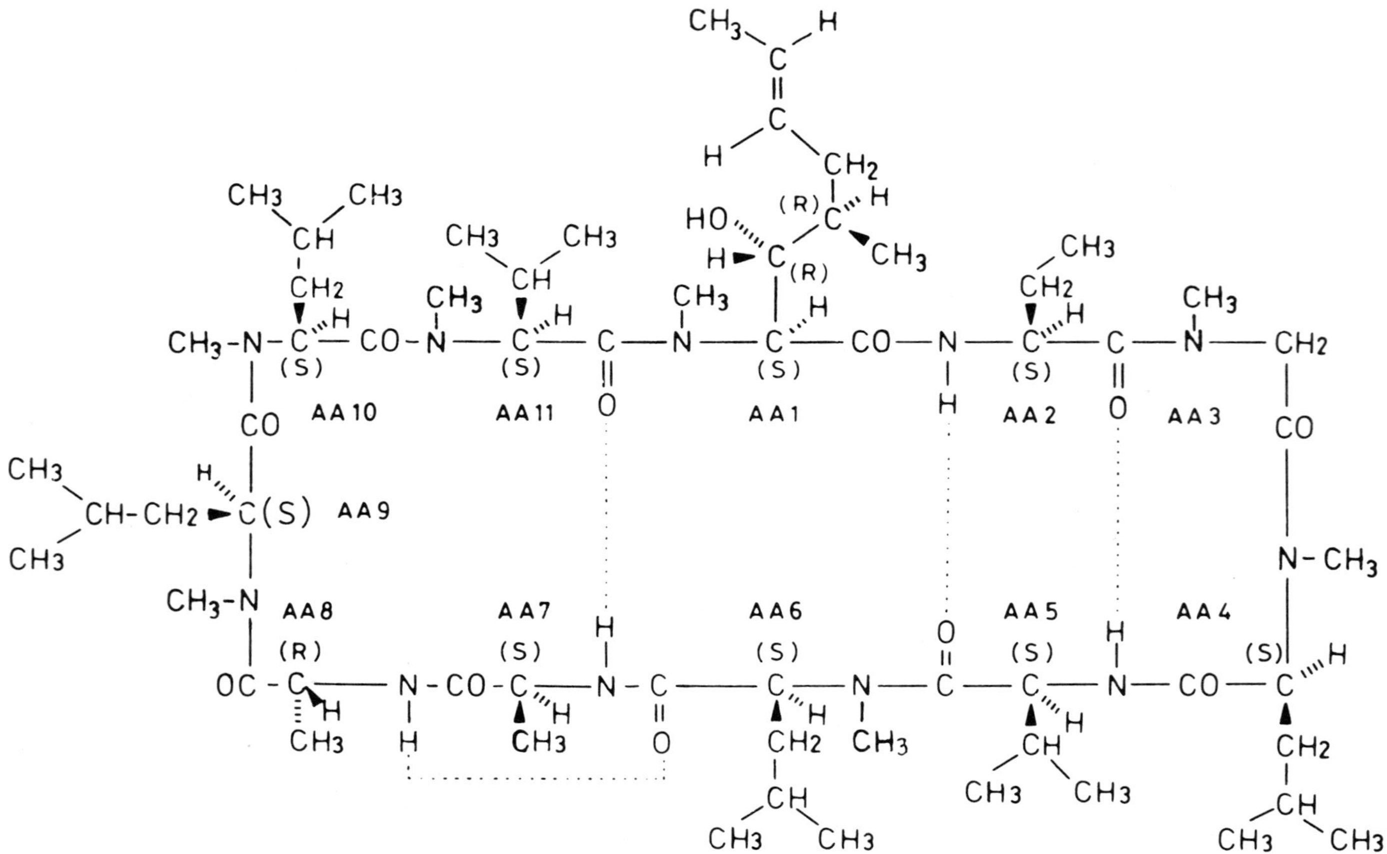

Figure 1 Structure of cyclosporine.

II. PRECLINICAL PHARMACOLOGY

A. Introduction

The Sandoz (Basel) search for new antifungal agents led to the isolation of the fungus *Tolypocladium inflatum gams*. A mixture of metabolites was separated from the original crude extracts. This mixture was chemically characterized and found to contain novel neutral polypeptides. These were then subjected to biological screening assays which demonstrated that this fungal extract possessed a narrow spectrum of in vitro antifungal activity and marginal in vivo fungistatic activity. In January 1972 Borel discovered the marked immunosuppressive properties of cyclosporine. Using a murine model, he examined both inhibition of hemagglutinin formation against sheep erythrocytes and survival time following inoculation of the murine leukemic cell line L1210. Interestingly, in these first experiments the immunosuppressive activity was impressive while no effect was seen on the survival of leukemic mice, indicating that the immunosuppressive properties were not linked to general cytostatic activity. These first results were irreproducible; the reason, assessed years later, was due to the compound's water insolubility. Cyclosporine was dissolved in an ethanol, Tween 80, and saline mixture in the preliminary tests; later assays utilized a suspension in 0.5% tragacanth. By the end of 1973, however, the immunosuppressive effect of cyclosporine A on both humoral and cell-mediated immunity and its strong activity in Freund's adjuvant arthritis were firmly established.

A profile of its pharmacological properties are as follows: selective activity on lymphocytes (principally T-helper cells), dose-dependent reversible suppression of humoral and cell-mediated immunity, suppression of chronic but not acute inflammatory reactions, inhibition of lymphocyte proliferation induction phase without mitotic disturbance, nonlymphotoxic, hematopoietically incompetence, and effectiveness in many species for a variety of organ transplantations (4). Cyclosporine A also inhibits lymphokine production and release including interleukin-2 (IL-2) or T-cell growth factor (5). These unique pharmacological characteristics of cyclosporine A encouraged the initiation of studies of the drug's effect in autoimmune diseases.

B. Animal Studies

1. Studies of Immunomodulation

Since the initial observations, numerous experiments utilizing animal models have demonstrated cyclosporine A to be effective in both the prevention and treatment of autoimmune disease. In young autoimmune (NZB x NZW) F1 mice this immunosuppressive agent was found to prevent the development of autoantibodies, and in older mice it reduced the level of autoantibodies, thus demonstrating that autoantibodies in this model can be pharmacologically controlled (6). Other investigations in the MRL-1pr/1pr mice which spontaneously develop massive T-cell lymphadenopathy with a marked expansion of an unusual L3T4-, Lyt-2, 6B2+ T-cell population, autoantibodies, and immune-mediated pathology further demonstrated the potential of cyclosporine for the treatment of autoimmune disease (7). Administration of cyclosporine prevented lymphadenopathy and expansion of their unique T-cell population in the peripheral lymph nodes and in the thymus. The increased expression of the c-myb and T-cell receptor β-chain genes associated with these unique cells was also corrected. Treated mice demonstrated a marked decrease in arthritis and glomerulonephritis and significantly prolonged survival. These beneficial effects of cyclosporine treatment occurred without a reduction in anti-DNA antibodies, circulating immune complexes, rheumatoid factor titers, or immunoglobulin concentrations.

Studies of the effectiveness of cyclosporine A in animal models of rheumatoid arthritis have suggested that this drug may be efficacious in the treatment of this disease process as well. In the type II collagen arthritis rat model, cyclosporine A reduced both joint swelling and collagen antibody titers when administered prior to antigen challenge (8-10); however, an enhanced inflammatory response was observed when administered after antigen introduction (8). In the Freund's adjuvant-induced model, cyclosporine A was effective in decreasing joint swelling when administered either before or after the adjuvant injection (9,11). In demonstrating that the immunological unresponsiveness observed in rats receiving concomitant treatment of cyclosporine and either type II collagen or complete Freund's adjuvant for a duration of 14 days is antigen-specific, cyclosporine-protected rats were rechallenged with either type II collagen or complete Freund's adjuvant after cessation of cyclosporine treatment (12). Type II collagen-immunized, cyclosporine-protected rats did not develop arthritis upon reimmunization with the same antigen; however, they did develop arthritis upon subsequent injection of Freund's adjuvant. Similarly, Freund's adjuvant-immunized, cyclosporine-protected rats showed a suppressed arthritic response upon reinjection with the same antigen, but developed arthritis upon subsequent injection of type II collagen.

Cyclosporine is also effective at inhibiting later stages of proliferation and erosive synovitis. In the group A streptococcal cell wall model of human rheumatoid arthritis induced by injection of female LEW/N rats, cyclosporine A was found to prevent disease despite the persistence of cell wall antigen in the joints (13,14). Cyclosporine A treatment must be begun, however, prior to sensitization. In contrast, cyclosporine A has been observed to be ineffective in the non-immune-mediated inflammatory models such as the carageenan-induced paw edema (15).

2. Toxicity

In comparison to later studies in man, earlier studies in rats of the nephrotoxicity of cyclosporine failed to demonstrate significant nephrotoxicity at therapeutic levels of the drug. Nephrotoxicity represented a major observation only at doses six times or greater than those required to produce optimal immunosuppression (16). Daily or every second day administration of 100 mg/kg of cyclosporine to Sprague-Dawley rats for a 3-week duration produced a progressive increase of serum urea, serum creatinine, and urinary *N*-acetyl- D-glucosaminidase activity. At the 100 mg/kg/day dose, morphological changes in the kidney were observed which included vacuolation and necrosis of proximal tubular epithelial cells with relatively minimal glomerular involvement (17). Cyclosporine-induced histological alterations of the kidney have mainly been found in the proximal tubule, particularly in the S2 and S3 segments. These changes are dose-dependent, develop a few days after taking cyclosporine A, and are almost completely reversible. On the ultrastructural level (18,19), dilation of the endoplasmic reticulum and an increased number of lysosomes and myeloid bodies have been observed.

The exact mechanism of cyclosporine A-induced nephrotoxicity has not yet been well elucidated. Evidence indicates that this immunosuppressant has an adverse effect on renal blood flow either by producing anatomical changes in the renal vasculature or by promoting physiological responses which lead to an increase in renal vasculature resistance. In Kyoto spontaneously hypertensive rats cyclosporine administration resulted in dose-dependent exudative and proliferative vascular damage (20,21). The vascular exudative lesions were more commonly observed at doses below 50 mg/kg/day, while the proliferative changes, along with a decrease in glomerular filtration rate, were more commonly observed at higher doses. The magnitude of hypertension did not significantly correlate with the severity of the vascular changes. In other investigations of pathogenetic factors involved in cyclosporine-induced renal dysfunction, renal tubular function and afferent arteriolar morphology were studied in male Fisher rats during severe experimental cyclosporine-induced reduction in globerular filtration rate (22). Administration of 50 mg/kg of cyclosporine for a period of 3–14 days resulted in a progressive decline in glomerular filtration rate with no difference in fractional sodium excretion, fractional lithium excretion, enzymuria, or in vitro renal cortical slice uptake of tetraethylammonium. Evidence of tubular necrosis was observed at 7 and 14 days via light microscopy; electron microscopy revealed a dramatic decline in the luminal diameter of the afferent arterioles in the cyclosporine-treated group versus control animals. The mechanisms causing these effects are thus far unknown.

Reversible biochemical abnormalities of liver function have been observed in animals receiving cyclosporine (17,23). Hepatotoxicity was exhibited in Sprague-Dawley rats administered cyclosporine at high doses of 100 mg/kg/day for a duration of 3 weeks and was manifested as significant increases in serum liver enzymes and bilirubin and a decrease in serum albumin (24). The morphological correlate consisted of centroacinar fatty change in hepatocytes with acidophilic degeneration and centroacinar necrosis after prolonged treatment. The presence of 1.0 μg/ml of cyclosporine in a cell-free system inhibited the microsomal incorporation of [^{14}C] leucine into total protein by 36% (25). Intraperitoneal treatment of rats with 5-50 mg/kg/day for 1-7 days showed a dose- and treatment duration-dependent inhibition of protein synthesis by liver microsomes (25). Because this immunosuppressant has been shown to cause dose-dependent weight loss due to anorexia in the early treatment period, the possibility of malnutrition contributing to hepatotoxicity in cyclosporine-treated rats has also been explored (26).

In rats, an atrophic gingivitis with loosening and divergent growth of incisor teeth was observed after a 10-week duration of 30 mg/kg/day of cyclosporine administration. In dogs a nonspecific hypertrophic gingivitis and periodontitis with abundant mononuclear cell infiltration was present after prolonged administration of 50 mg/kg/day (24). Another frequent finding in beagle dogs was generalized papillomatosis unlike the well-known oral papillomatosis commonly observed in this species (27). Histological examination of skin taken during this study revealed hyperkeratotic acanthopapillomatosis with cytoplasmic inclusions and numerous plasma cell infiltrates. No viral particles could be demonstrated in these lesions and spontaneous regression occurred with continued cyclosporine treatment. No cases of malignant transformation were observed.

The incidence of bacterial infections did not increase with cyclosporine treatment in animal studies (24). Utilizing functional studies of the reticuloendothelial system, cyclosporine-treated mice showed normal carbon clearance and organ distribution of sheep erythrocytes (28), supporting the view that cyclosporine does not impair nonspecific defense mechanisms. Neither a decrease of nucleated bone marrow cell count nor an inhibition of in vitro stem cell proliferation was seen in mice administered with 200 mg/kg/day of cyclosporine for 6 days (29).

Early rabbit and rat teratology experiments with cyclosporine demonstrated the occurrence of embryo and fetotoxicity at doses which were toxic to the mother; however, no teratological effect was detected (24). Upon prolonged administration of high doses, inhibition of meiosis was reported (30). Administration of cyclosporine at doses which did not produce general toxicity demonstrated no adverse effects on the fertility of randomly selected F1 rats. There was no increased incidence of malfunction and no significant effect on rat embryo implantation, embryonic survival, litter size, or body weights (27). No malignancies occurred in dogs, sheep, pigs, rabbits, and rodents that received prolonged treatment of cyclosporine (31). Assessment of cyclosporine's mutagenic potential by the Ames and micronucleus tests proved negative (24).

Neurological complications associated with the use of cyclosporine have been well recognized, but the cause of this toxicity remains unclear. Rats treated with high doses of cyclosporine exhibited dystonic and catatonic posturing, repetitive head nodding, and/or tonic-clonic seizures, and some died in status epilepticus; behavioral testing revealed delayed exploring, escape, and climbing behavior (32). In dogs, a recent study demonstrated that the acute administration of cyclosporine resulted in severe changes in cardiovascular hemodynamics along with decreased cerebral perfusion pressure, suggesting that in this situation cyclosporine's central nervous system side effects may be due to a decreased cerebral perfusion pressure (33).

Stimulation of hair growth, another complication observed in man, has also been seen in nude mice receiving 80 mg/kg/day after 5-6 days of treatment. Hair growth decreased after 3-4 days of drug discontinuation and resumed with subsequent treatment (34).

III. CLINICAL PHARMACOLOGY

A. Pharmacokinetics and Metabolism

Absorption of oral cyclosporine A from the GI tract has been found to be erratic and incomplete, thus explaining the wide variability between individuals in blood concentrations with fixed dose regimens based on body weight. Peak concentration (C_{max}) in blood and plasma is achieved at about 3.5 hr (35). C_{max} and area under the plasma or blood concentration/time curve are a function of the administered dose; this relationship is linear for plasma levels up to 1400 mg and nonlinear or parabolic for blood levels. As determined by specific assay, C_{max} is approximately 0.95 ng/ml/mg of dose for plasma and 2.7-1.4 for blood (35). Compared to intravenous infusion, the absolute bioavailability of the oral solution from a previous study is at best 20-50% at a steady state (35). In patients unable to take oral cyclosporine, intravenous preparation may be administered with doses reduced to approximately one-third of the oral doses.

Cyclosporine A is largely distributed outside the blood volume. Body fat, liver, pancreas, lungs, kidneys, adrenal glands, spleen, and lymph nodes have higher cyclosporine A concentrations than serum (36,37). The drug persists in body tissues for a considerable time after therapy is discontinued. Very low cyclosporine A concentrations found in the brain and cerebrospinal fluid suggest that cyclosporine A does not readily penetrate the blood-brain barrier (36,37). During pregnancy, cyclosporine A crosses the placenta and can be isolated from amniotic fluid. Cyclosporine has been detected in an infant's blood up to 48 hr after birth and also in the breast milk of mothers receiving the drug (38). Although the concentration of cyclosporine A is low in mother's milk, breastfeeding is not recommend for infants of mothers receiving cyclosporine A.

In blood, distribution is concentration dependent. The drug is highly bound to plasma proteins, erythrocytes, and lipoproteins. Approximately 33-47% is in the plasma, 4-9% in leukocytes, 5-12% in granulocytes, and 41-58% in erthrocytes. Uptake by leukocytes and erythrocytes becomes limited at higher concentrations; this explains the nonlinear dose proportionality of C_{max} and AUC in blood. In plasma, 90% is bound to proteins. Cyclosporine A is primarily dissolved in the lipid portion of serum lipoproteins and tightly bound to triglycerides. Ultracentrifugal fractionation of human serum subsequent to incubation with cyclosporine A demonstrated that in healthy, fasting individuals, 8% of the drug was found in the very-low-density lipoproteins (VLDL), 31% in the low-density lipoproteins (LDL), 46% in the high-density lipoproteins (HDL), and 15% in the nonlipoprotein fraction. In nonfasted healthy and nonfasted lipemic individuals 6 and 7% of cyclosporine A was found in the chylomicrons, 9 and 13% in VLDL, 28 and 30% in LDL, 39 and 37% in HDL, 12 and 13% in the nonlipoprotein protein fraction, respectively. In patients receiving cyclosporine A, the distribution varied: 12-19% in VLDL, 21-28% in LDL, 33-43% in HDL, and 13-20% in nonlipoprotein proteins. Isolated normal human lipoproteins exhibited a nonsaturable, low-affinity, high-capacity uptake for cyclosporine A (39).

Drug disposition is biphasic with cyclosporine A having a half-life of approximately 19 hr (range 10-27 hr). The elimination of cyclosporine A is primarily via the biliary system in humans with only 6% of the administered dose being excreted in the urine. Cyclosporine A is metabolized in the liver by the cytochrome P450 mixed function oxidase to at least 12 known metabolites, some of which also have immunosuppressive properties (40).

Compounds and drugs that induce hepatic enzyme metabolism (such as rifampicin, phenobarbital, and phenytoin) may lower cyclosporine concentrations (41-43). Drugs that inhibit hepatic metabolism (such as ketoconazole) raise the blood concentrations of cyclosporine; this may result in nephrotoxicity without dose adjustment (44). Hence, liver dysfunction may predispose the patient to cyclosporine-induced nephrotoxicity due to impaired cyclosporine metabolism.

There is no single pathway for the biotransformation of cyclosporine A (45). Only 0.1% of the dose is excreted in the urine as unchanged drug. Fifteen metabolites have been characterized in human urine; nine of these have been assigned structures. The major metabolic pathways consist of hydroxylation of the C carbon of the two leucine residues, C-carbon hydroxylation and cyclic ether formation in the side chain of the amino acid 3-hydroxyl-*N*,4-dimethyl-L-2-amino-6-octenoic acid, and N-dimethylation of one *N*-methylleucine residue. Hydrolysis of the cyclic peptide chain or conjugation of the above metabolites does not appear to be an important biotransformation pathway (45,46).

Cyclosporine therapy can be monitored clinically by the use of radioimmunoassays. The nonselective polyclonal radioimmunoassay (RIA) method measures the parent compound and cross-reacts with cyclosporine metabolites. Whole-blood values are approximately three times greater than plasma levels as a result of red cell cyclosporinc. High-performance liquid chromatography (HPLC) methods, though labor-intense, are specific for parent cyclosporine. A monoclonal antibody (Mab) RIA kit has recently been developed to provide an alternative to HPLC for specific measurements of cyclosporine concentrations and to allow investigation of the contribution of metabolites, as measured by the nonselective assay: one antibody selectively recognizes cyclosporine among the bioconversion products of the drug, thereby providing the specific measurement of the drug concentration in blood and other biological fluids; the other antibody recognizes structural elements of both cyclosporine and metabolites, thereby measuring the parent compound plus its bioconversion products such as metabolites 1 and 17 (47). Studies have shown that the specific Mab yields cyclosporine concentrations identical to those of HPLC in normal volunteers and in patients following oral doses of cyclosporine; the nonselective Mab provides concentration values parallel to those obtained with the polyclonal RIA (48).

There are numerous potential technical problems with cyclosporine A blood level monitoring (49). Blood collected at room temperature may show lower cyclosporine A concentrations unless adequate time is allowed for redistribution of the drug from red cells. Usually 2-3 hr is recommended prior to separation of plasma. There is a relatively narrow range of blood cyclosporine A concentrations that define adequate immunosuppression while avoiding the high concentrations associated with an increased incidence of side effects.

B. Effects on the Immune System

The exact manner in which cyclosporine modifies the immune response has not yet been identified; however, it is known that this interaction involves multiple factors. The most well-characterized effect of cyclosporine is on the T-lymphocyte helper/inducer subpopulations. Experimental evidence suggests that the effectiveness of cyclosporine is due to specific and reversible inhibition of immunocompetent lymphocytes, preferentially T lymphocytes, in the G0 or G1 phase of the cycle; this is most frequently demonstrated during mitogenic triggering of immunocompetent cells by an antigen stimulus (50, 51). Cyclosporine A may also affect the initial recognition of the antigen-MHC II (major histocompatability locus II) complex on the antigen-presenting cell (APC) by the T-helper cell and the sequential events that lead to T-cell activation. The binding of the T-helper cell to APC expressing the antigen-MHC II complex results in the release of interleukin-1 (IL-1) from the APC, which stimulates the release of IL-2 from the T-helper cells and leads to the expression of IL-2 receptor on select subpopulations of T cells (52,53). The IL-2 released from the T-helper cells subsequently stimulates the proliferation of cells expressing IL-2 receptors. Interleukin-2 also promotes the production of γ-interferon. Utilization of an anti-interleukin 2 receptor assay directly indicates that cyclosporine does not prevent the expression of IL-2 receptors of activated T cells (54). This is strongly supported by the demonstration that exogenous IL-2 reverses the inhibitory activity of cyclosporine (54,55).

In other experiments, cyclosporine A has been demonstrated to interfere not only with the production and release of IL-1 from antigen-activated macrophages but, more significantly, to inhibit IL-2 release from T-helper cells (52,53,56). Although it does not impair macrophage responsiveness to lymphokine (51) by this mechanism, it can block amplification of cellular immune responses and the generation of T-cell effector (helper and cytotoxic) (57) cells and functions which are dependent on the production of IL-2. Cyclosporine A can therefore impair the excretion of γ-interferon (58), an effect partially linked to drug-induced inhibition of natural killer activity (59), without affecting the synthesis of α- or β-interferons (58). Although cyclosporine interferes with the differentiation of cytotoxic T-cell precursors into mature cytotoxic T lymphocytes (53,60,61), it does not affect the recognition of IL-2 by cytotoxic T lymphocytes or reduce the cytotoxic activity of cytotoxic T cell already generated (62,63). Existing data also suggest that cyclosporine A may interfere with the lysosomal processing of antigens by the APC (64-66).

Interestingly, lymphocytes from alloantigen-sensitized mice treated with cyclosporine did not reactivate on exposure to the same alloantigen in mixed lymphocyte culture; however, their exposure to a third-party antigen remained intact (67). Cyclosporine's inhibition of the T cells' proliferative response has also been observed with certain lectin mitogens in vitro and is believed to be due to binding to the receptor sites for conconavalin A, phytohemagglutinin, and HLA-DR (50,68,69).

Natural suppressor cell activity has been attributed to a subset of cells present in hematopoietic tissues which can suppress a variety of lymphocyte responses without MHC restriction. Increasing evidence indicates that one of cyclosporine's critical mechanisms of action in experimental animals involves the relative sparing of T-suppressor cells (62). These cells are nonphagocytic and nontumoricidal, possess granulocyte/macrophage surface markers, and have monoblast-promonocyte morphology. In culture, these cells can differentiate into phagocytic macrophages. Rats on long-term cyclosporine therapy have increased numbers of natural suppressor cells as well as a doubling of natural suppressor cell activity (70). In vitro, cyclosporine induces an increase in macrophage number and proliferation rate. Because monocyte subpopulations exist at the bone marrow precursor level and can be selectively induced by inflammatory mediators, it has been suggested that cyclosporine A can induce the monocyte precursor to differentiate into a subpopulation of macrophages which may alter lymphocyte T4/T8 ratios during an immunological challenge (70). This may be representative as a novel mechanism by which cyclosporine exerts its immunomodulatory effects.

In comparison to other currently available immunosuppressive drugs, cyclosporine has been shown to have selective and specific cytotoxic effects. When its effects on murine spleen cells and mastocytoma cells (P-815) were examined, cyclosporine A was shown to affect lymphoid cell proliferation 300 times more potently than that of tumor cells (71). Repeated treatment with even toxic doses of cyclosporine A marginally decreased the number of bone marrow cells and did not impair the number or the proliferative capacity of the hematopoietic myeloid stem cells (29). These results demonstrated the selective activity of cyclosporine A on lymphoid cells and supported the concept that this agent is a prototype of a new generation of immunosuppressants.

C. Studies of Cellular Mechanism of Action

The effects of cyclosporine A at the cellular and subcellular level have been extensively investigated over the past several years. Cyclosporine A binds readily to lymphocyte membranes with a K_D of approximately 10^{-7} M (72). Cyclosporine has also been shown to bind to macrophages, granulocytes, erythrocytes, hepatocytes, and other cells (72,73). In examining the binding specificity of cyclosporine to lymphocyte membranes, several ligands were tested: mitogens (OKT3), HLA-DR, IL-1, IL-2, insulin, and prolactin. Although cyclosporine A and OKT3 recognition sites are closely associated with the T-cell receptor, there is not interference between the two since binding of OKT3 is not reduced by cyclosporine A and labeled cyclosporine A is not displaced by OKT3 (74). In contrast, cyclosporine A inhibits OKT3-induced proliferation of human peripheral T cells (75). Evidence indicates that the presence of cyclosporine does not affect the HLA-DR antigen receptor recognition (69). Some studies indicate that cyclosporine inhibits IL-1 binding to the T cell (76,77). Since IL-2 and insulin receptors are not expressed on quiescent lymphocytes (78,79), they are highly unlikely to be receptors for cyclosporine A. However, cyclosporine A has been demonstrated to have a very high affinity for the prolactin binding site and to displace the prolactin molecule from its binding site and vice versa (80,81). Furthermore, administration to rats of agents which lower prolactin levels has permitted cyclosporine A dosage to be decreased without a concomitant decrease in its efficacy (80). Interestingly, prolactin itself is believed to function as a lymphokine because it appears to modulate the immunoreactivity of lymphocytes by rendering them susceptible to antigenic stimuli (80).

When cells are incubated in the presence of cyclosporine, intracellular concentrations of the drug follow biphasic kinetics. Cyclosporine passively diffuses across the cell membrane and then becomes tightly bound to intracellular proteins. One of these, cyclophilin, has been characterized as a thymocyte cytosolic receptor for cyclosporine with a MW of 16,000 D (82). Furthermore, the immunosuppressive activity of cyclosporine and its analogs, measured by inhibition of IL-2 production and T-cell proliferation, correlates directly with cyclophilin binding. Except for *O*-acyl derivatives, binding of cyclosporine and its analogs to cyclophilin has been shown to be a necessary condition for the expression of immunosuppressive activity (83). By studying the binding of cyclophilin to more than 80 cyclosporine A derivatives, it was shown that cyclophilin binds to cyclosporine A residues 1, 2, 10, and 11; these are known contributors of the immunosuppressive activity of cyclosporine A (84). In addition to cyclophilin, cyclosporine has been demonstrated to bind to calmodulin and inhibit regulation of cGMP-dependent biological pathways which are responsible for signal regulation of nucleic acid and protein biosynthesis. Cyclosporine A may also bind to protein kinase C, which could result in modulating effects on calmodulin-cGMP pathways and inositol triphosphate pathways (85). Calcium ion influx is not influenced by the presence of cyclosporine (86). The early uptake of nucleoside which occurs simultaneously with calcium influx in mitogen-stimulated lymphocytes is also unaffected by this drug (87). However, mitogen-induced increase of mitochondrial and lysosomal activity is strongly reduced by cyclosporine A (64).

At the nuclear level, cyclosporine selectively inhibits the synthesis of mRNA encoding for IL-2 and potentially inhibits several other lymphokines (88). Transcription of these specific lymphokine mRNAs normally appears within a few hours after stimulation of resting T lymphocytes (89) and reaches a high concentration during the transition from the G0/G1 to the S phase of T-cell growth. Observations of inhibition of this activity further support the crucial influences of cyclosporine during this phase. In other experiments examining nuclear activity, cytoplasm derived from phytohemagglutinin A (PHA)-activated cells was shown to trigger DNA synthesis in nuclei derived from cells treated with cyclosporine A and PHA significantly less than in nuclei derived from the cells treated with PHA alone, suggesting that cyclosporine impairs the ability of the nucleus to respond to cytoplasmic activation signals (90). Cyclosporine A has also been implicated as having direct inhibitory effects on the nucleus by demonstrating a decrease in nuclear incorporation of [^{3}H] thymidine upon exposure to cyclosporine A at various time intervals after activation (90).

IV. EFFICACY

A. Introduction

Rheumatoid arthritis is a chronic, multisystem inflammatory disease process that exhibits articular and extra-articular manifestations which include pulmonary involvement, pericarditis, vasculitis, subcutaneous nodules, and keratoconjuctivitis sicca. The etiology of this disease remains unknown. Because of the increased prevalence of HLA-Dw4 and HLA-DRw4 in patients with rheumatoid arthritis, it is possible that rheumatoid disease is the expression of an immunological response to an as yet unidentified antigen in a genetically susceptible host. As of now, research has failed to produce any direct evidence for an infectious origin of rheumatoid arthritis.

Theoretically, cyclosporine can induce clinical remission in autoimmune disease by inhibiting lymphocyte activation and preventing the occurrence of an acute inflammatory response. The rationale for the use of cyclosporine A in rheumatoid arthritis is based on the following observations regarding both humoral and cellular immune mechanisms in relation to rheumatoid joint pathology:

1. T lymphocytes are found to infiltrate hyperplastic rheumatoid synovial cells along with lesser numbers of polymorphonulcear cells, macrophages, B lymphocytes, and plasma cells (91). Approximately 90% of the infiltrating T lymphocytes have T4 surface antigen. This is a significantly higher percentage than that observed in peripheral T lymphocytes. Most T4 cells have helper function.
2. Depressed T-cell suppressor function has been noted in patients with rheumatoid arthritis (92).
3. Decreased delayed hypersensitivity response to skin tests antigens and diminished mitogen responsiveness have been observed in rheumatoid arthritis patients (92).
4. Immunoglobulin IgG and IgM are found in synovium and synovial fluid of rheumatoid ptients (92).
5. Complement levels are decreased in rheumatoid arthritis patients, indicating continued activation of the immune system (93).
6. Many T cells are found to be in close association with synoviocytes which are noted to be macrophage-like cells (94).
7. In part the inflammatory response in rheumatoid arthritis is characterized by macrophage-monocyte and lymphocyte interactions which result in the production of lymphokines and monokines including interleukin-1, interleukin-2, macrophage inhibitor factors, macrophage-monocyte activating factors, and chemotactic factors (94-96).

Initial clinical studies with cyclosporine A in patients with rheumatoid arthritis were undertaken by several different investigations and tended to involve small groups of patients with cyclosporine being administered in an open label fashion. In 1979 Hermann and Muller studied six patients considered therapeutic failures to chloroquine, gold, and penicillamine, and reported significantly favorable improvement after 6 months of cyclosporine treatment (97). Side effects such as nephrotoxicity, gastrointestinal disturbances, and hirsutism were common but reversible. In another early series of pilot studies, Amor and Dougados reported that six patients suffering from stage I to stage III chronic rheumatoid arthritis displayed clinical improvement within 15 days of cyclosporine treatment at 9 mg/kg/day; patients continued to demonstrate improvement in morning stiffness, grip strength, and the Ritchie index after 2 months of treatment (98). Although a follow-up study by the same investigators utilizing a lower dose of cyclosporine A (5 mg/kg/day) in 12 rheumatoid arthritis patients demonstrated only a slight clinical improvement after 30 days of treatment, a good overall efficacy was demonstrated after 4 months (98). Improvement was observed in the same parameters as seen with the higher dose. The onset of drug efficacy appeared to be dose-related.

In further early uncontrolled studies, 15 patients with severe rheumatoid arthritis, refractory to conventional treatment, were administered a lose dose of cyclosporine (max. 5 mg/kg/day) in combination with a low dose of prednisone for a duration of 6 months (99). After an average of 7.5 weeks, 12 of these patients displayed clinical improvement. Clinical evaluation after 6 months of therapy showed 12 of these patients to be virtually free of symptoms, two of these patients showed no satisfactory response, and one patient dropped out of the study because of hypertension. Clinical improvement correlated only slightly with humoral and cellular laboratory parameters. Preliminary results of an open study in which 20 patients with progressive classical or definite rheumatoid arthritis were administered cyclosporine, at an initial dose of 5 mg/kg/day which was gradually increased to 10 mg/kg/day over a 2-month period, demonstrated improvement in morning stiffness, articular index, function and pain scores (100). These patients did not receive steroid therapy during the study and discontinued all second-line drugs 3 months before the study began; nonsteroidal anti-inflammatory drugs (NSAIDs) were permitted throughout the study. The significant clinical benefit of cyclosporine was maintained for 2 years (101).

A study by Bowles et al. at the Mayo clinic in which 10 patients with seropositive rheumatoid arthritis were treated for 6 months with 6 mg/kg/day in divided doses (bid) demonstrated this drug's efficacy at low dose. Nine of the ten patients responded to cyclosporine with significant reduction in morning stiffness and the total number of tender and swollen joints (102).

In an open, randomized comparison of cyclosporine and azathioprine in the treatment of rheumatoid arthritis, patients who took cyclosporine (10 mg/kg/day) for a duration of 26 weeks demonstrated significant improvement in the 50-ft walking time, circumferences of proximal interphalangeal joints, Ritchie articular index, global assessment by investigator, and strength, when compared with baseline findings (103). The azathioprine group (2.5-3 mg/kg/day) demonstrated improvement only in strength.

Table 1 refers to an open label pilot study by Weinblatt et al., in which 10 patients with active rheumatoid arthritis were administered oral cyclosporine for a 24-week period (104). The initial cyclosporine dosage was 6 mg/kg/day;

Table 1 CyA: Open Study (10 Patients, 36 Weeks, Cyclosporine Dose: Initial 6 mg/kg/day, Maximum 8 mg/kg/day)

Results	0 weeks	24 weeks
Painful joints	32	17[a]
Swollen joints	24	19[a]
Joint pain index	55	22[a]
Joint swelling index	33	25[b]
Global		
patient	4.3	2.8[b]
physician	3.4	2.9[b]
Morning stiffness	150	87
Toxicity: 10		
increased creatinine	10	
high blood pressure	7	
gastrointestinal	7	
tremor	4	
paresthesias	3	
flushing	2	
Withdrawals	2 (GI, LFTs)	
Washout period:		
flare of arthritis		
resolution of ADR		
elevated creatinine 7		

[a] $p < 0.05$.
[b] $p < 0.01$.
Source: Ref. 104.

this was increased at week 8 to 8 mg/kg/day in seven patients because of lack of efficacy. At week 12, the mean cyclosporine dosage was 7.3 mg/kg/day (range 5-8), and at week 24, the mean dosage was 6.1 mg/kg/day (range 4-8). The 24-week cyclosporine administration period was followed by a 12-week washout period. A significant improvement was observed at week 12 and continued through week 24 in the number of painful joints, number of swollen joints, joint pain index, joint swelling index, duration of morning stiffness, and patient and physician global assessments. No significant change was observed in the 50-ft walk time or grip strength. Rheumatoid factor, erythrocyte sedimentation rate (ESR), blood mononuclear subsets, and mitogen/antigen proliferation responses did not change significantly at weeks

12 and 24. Four weeks after discontinuing cyclosporine A treatment, a marked flare of arthritis activity (defined as a 30% or more increase in joint pain and swelling indices as compared with the last visit during the cyclosporine regimen) was observed and was sustained during the remainder of the 12-week washout period. This study was extended when seven of these patients elected to restart cyclosporine therapy upon the end of the 12-week washout period because of arthritic flares (105). The reentry dose of cyclosporine was 3 mg/kg/day due to the toxicity experienced in the initial study. After 12 weeks of this low-dose cyclosporine, significant improvement occurred only in the physician's global assessment and patient's global assessment with slight improvement observed in the number of painful joints and joint pain index. Nephrotoxicity was also observed at this dose.

Table 2, a comparison of several open label cyclosporine studies in rheumatoid arthritis patients, portrays the effectiveness of cyclosporine in the treatment of this autoimmune disease. Promising results from these open studies demonstrated the need for future studies to include placebo-controlled patient groups to clearly demonstrate cyclosporine's efficacy in the treatment of rheumatoid arthritis. Van Rijthoven and colleagues undertook a study in which 36 patients with active and erosive, definite or classical rheumatoid arthritis were administered cyclosporine or a placebo for a dura-

Table 2 Cyclosporine (CyA): Open Studies in Rheumatoid Arthritis

Investigator[a]	No.	Weeks duration	Initial dose	Results	Withdrawals
Dougados	6	12	8.5	Efficacy	5
Dougados	12	52	5.0	Efficacy	2
Madhok	20	18	5.0	Efficacy	0
Forre	24	26	10.0	Efficacy	2
Weinblatt	10	36	6.0	Efficacy	2
Weinblatt	7	12	3.0	Less efficacy	0
Bowles	10	36	6.0	Efficacy	0

[a]Dougados M, Amor B. Cyclosporin A in rheumatoid arthritis: preliminary clinical results of an open trial. Arth Rheum 1987; 30:83–7.

Forre O, Bjerkhoel F, et al. An open, controlled, randomized comparison of cyclosporine and azathioprine in the treatment of rheumatoid arthritis: a preliminary report. Arth Rheum 1987; 30:88–92.

Bowles CA, Gabriel S, et al. Cyclosporine (CsA) treatment for rheumatoid arthritis (RA). Arth Rheum 1987; 30:Supplement 58:S58.

tion of 6 months (106). Their data showed significant improvement in the cyclosporine group as measured by the number of swollen joints, Ritchie articular index, pain at rest, and active movement, versus the placebo group. In this study, the initial dosage of cyclosporine was 10 mg/kg/day for 2 months; if satisfactory therapeutic response was obtained, the dose was reduced to 7.5 mg/kg/day (months 3 and 4) and to 5 mg/kg/day (months 5 and 6). The dosage was effectively adjusted to clinical response and side effects. Final analysis of these results demonstrated that cyclosporine improved the clinically manifested symptoms, i.e., the number of swollen joints, Ritchie articular index, pain at active movement and at rest; however, no significant improvement in morning stiffness or laboratory parameters was found, and the placebo group showed a significant rise in ESR (107). No evidence of retardation or of deterioration via radiography was found in the cyclosporine group or the placebo group.

In a 4-month, double-blind, placebo-controlled study of 52 patients with active rheumatoid arthritis, Dougados et al. reported significant improvement in the cyclosporine group compared to the placebo group in the clinical assessment criteria (108). Clinical improvement of patients with rheumatoid arthritis on cyclosporine therapy was shown to correlate with a decrease in C-reactive protein, α_1-glycoprotein levels, and platelet counts, but not with ESR or rheumatoid factor titers.

In a similarly conceived study, Yocum et al. at the NIH enrolled 31 treatment-refractory, seropositive, rheumatoid arthritis patients in a 6-month, double-blind, randomized study comparing the efficacy of high-dose cyclosporine (10 mg/kg/day) with low-dose cyclosporine (1 mg/kg/day) (109). The patients' clinical and immunological status revealed that 10 of the 15 patients in the high-dose group and four of the 16 patients in the low-dose group displayed a significant decrease in articular score. Immunological evaluation of these 14 clinical responders showed that 12 of these patients had no in vitro proliferative responses to a variety of soluble recall antigens or responded minimally to a single antigen. A decrease in T-lymphocyte helper/suppressor ratio and an increase in natural killer cell population (as compared to clinical nonresponders) correlated with this immunosuppression. All of the high-dose patients who displayed anergy or responded to only one antigen demonstrated clinical improvement with cyclosporine. In contrast, patients with intact immune functions experienced less therapeutic benefit of either high- or low-dose cyclosporine. The immunomodulatory role of cyclosporine in rheumatoid arthritis was reflected by the reversal of anergy seen in the responder patients when the anergic status was reversed during therapy.

In these studies, it has been observed that the onset of action of cyclosporine is rapid and dose-dependent. Once clinical remission is induced, the dose may be decreased to a lower level than that initially required for induction. If one begins at these lower levels of cyclosporine (i.e., 6 mg/kg/day), it may take up to 8-12 weeks to see a clinical response. Presently, a target window of 400-600 ng/whole-blood RIA is being utilized as the starting dose in autoimmune disease indications. Because of the erratic absorption of cyclosporine, unpredictable blood levels may be observed at any one particular dose. Patients in whom the drug is quickly metabolized may require a higher oral dose to reach the therapeutic window. However, fundamental laboratory immunological parameters indicative of autoimmune disease often do not show a change at the therapeutic window required for clinical improvements, suggesting that cyclosporine has effects on other parameters of the immune system.

B. Other Related Autoimmune Indications

1. Systemic Lupus Erythematosus

Because cyclosporine was shown to improve the life span of (NZB X NZW) F1 female mice with lupus (110,111) and decrease anti-DNA antibody production in male mice of this strain, its clinical and immunomodulatory effects in patients with systemic lupus erythematosus (SLE) have been examined. In one early trial, two of five patients with SLE who received 10 mg/kg/day of cyclosporine for a duration of 7 weeks demonstrated clinical improvement (112). Results of another open label study of cyclosporine's efficacy in 10 SLE patients demonstrated the possibility of tapering the steroid dose without increasing the disease activity in cases of severe, steroid-dependent SLE (113). Data obtained from a 12-month open trial of cyclosporine administration (average dose 5 mg/kg/day) to patients with severe steroid-resistant and steroid-dependent SLE demonstrated beneficial clinical effects, allowing for a significant reduction in steroid dosage (114). In most cases improvement was assessed on a clinical basis. In contrast, the immunological abnormalities were not corrected, i.e., anti-double-stranded DNA and antinuclear antibodies and complement titers remained unchanged, while IgG levels increased significantly (the latter may have been due to a decrease in steroid dose). Clinical improvement persisted in only two patients at 6 and 15 months after discontinuation of treatment; three patients relapsed by month 6 after discontinuation of cyclosporine and two patients worsened by months 15 and 24 after discontinuation of cyclosporine.

Results of these and other studies have demonstrated that cyclosporine has been successfully used to treat patients with active SLE. However, it should be noted that some patients with very severe and potentially fatal SLE do not respond favorably (115).

Positive short-term results observed in four patients with lupus skin involvement resistant to steroids, cytotoxic agents, and hydroxychloroquine who were administered cyclosporine in combination with steroids led to the investigation of this drug combination with 20 patients with severe cases of SLE that had not responded well to conventional therapy (116). Cytotoxic agents were replaced by cyclosporine at 5 mg/kg/day in all patients studied. The combined steroid/cyclosporine administration favorably influenced this disease in the majority of patients. Of the initial four patients with skin involvement, one patient did not respond after 8 weeks of therapy, skin eruptions in two patients diminished in intensity, and the fourth patient, who also had arthralgia, demonstrated a disappearance of skin lesions and the arthralgias. Immunological data available from 16 patients after cyclosporine treatment showed the following: in eight patients there was a marked decrease in antibody activity against double-stranded DNA; in 10 patients the level of C3d decreased; in 11 patients the antibody level to single-stranded DNA decreased; in four patients the antibody level to single-stranded DNA increased; and the titer varied in one patient.

2. Psoriatic Arthritis

Initial experience with cyclosporine in four patients with psoriatic arthritis, reported in 1979, found this drug to be effective in producing a rapid and dramatic improvement in the psoriatic lesions of the skin; however, these improvements regressed upon discontinuation of the drug and resolved upon the restart of treatment (117). Administration of oral cyclosporine produced a dramatic response in a 56-year-old man crippled by severe psoriatic arthropathy (118). This patient was unresponsive to previous forms of immunomodulatory therapy. Upon the initial administration of 5 mg/kg/day of cyclosporine, the patient was effectively chair-bound, in continuous pain, and 75% of his total body area was covered in active psoriasis with acral pustulation. After 10 days, significant clearing of the skin lesions was observed; at 6 weeks, the patient's arthritis and synovitis improved to the extent that the patient was able to walk freely.

Clinical studies of the effectiveness of cyclosporine in psoriatic arthritis are too limited in number for one to conclude that this drug is a useful therapeutic agent at this time. Further trials are needed for conclusive evidence as to the therapeutic value of cyclosporine in this disease indication.

3. Polymyositis

Cyclosporine has been found to produce a favorable response in several patients with polymyositis (PM). An early study reports on three patients experiencing improvement of this disorder after addition of cyclosporine to regular prednisone therapy (119). These patients were considered therapeutic failures on other immunosuppressive regimens. Improvements were noted in muscle strength, general feeling of well being, functional disability grade, ability to walk, and muscle pain. In another case report, a patient with PM having progressive clinical deterioration was initially administered 10 mg/kg/day of cyclosporine with prednisone because previous immunosuppressive therapy had to be discontinued (120). The dose was reduced to 5 mg/kg/day by week 4. This patient felt better within 2 weeks; muscle strength gradually increased and serum muscle enzyme levels returned to normal within 2 months. The effectiveness of using cyclosporine alone was reported in a patient with PM in whom steroids had to be discontinued because of side effects (121). A few weeks after initiation of cyclosporine monotherapy, the patient's clinical condition improved and serum creatinine kinase gradually decreased. Thus, administration of cyclosporine to patients with PM not only induced favorable improvement but also allowed for a reduction of prednisone dose. These few cases clearly demonstrate the need for further clinical investigation to examine the effectiveness of cyclosporine in suppressing this disease.

4. Uveitis and Behçet's Disease

As a consequence of the observed effectiveness of cyclosporine in the S-antigen-induced experimental autoimmune uveitis model (122), it was examined as therapy for patients with uveitis. Over 70 patients with clinically active bilateral intermediate or posterior uveitis of a noninfectious etiology were enrolled in an open trial of cyclosporine (123,124). The initial cyclosporine dose was 10 mg/kg/day. Several patients demonstrated an increase in visual acuity within the first month of therapy, followed by an improvement in the vitreous haze and cellular activity. Continued effectiveness of cyclosporine therapy on these parameters was observed in 35 patients who reached the 18-month follow-up.

In another study which included seven patients with Behçet's disease, cyclosporine was shown to be effective in the control of acute attacks of posterior uveitis. Rapid decrease in the inflammatory activity in the vitreous body and the retina correlated with a significant increase in visual acuity 1-2 weeks after initiation of therapy (125). Cyclosporine did not appear to influence the disease activity in the anterior chamber. However, relapse was observed upon 1-2 weeks of drug cessation: increased inflammatory activity was present in the posterior and anterior segments and was accompanied by an increase in the number, frequency, and severity of mucocutaneous lesions.

Thirty patients with active bilateral sight-threatening intermediate and/or posterior uveitis refractive to treatment with corticosteroids and/or cytotoxic drugs were treated in a 3-year study with cyclosporine at an initial dose of 10 mg/kg/day and demonstrated a rapid initial decrease in the intensity of the intraocular inflammatory reaction accompanied by improvement in visual acuity in all patients (126). The initial cyclosporine dose was tapered to 7.5 mg/kg/day upon cessation of intraocular inflammatory processes; further reduction was aimed at a maintenance dose of 2 mg/kg/day. The tapering of cyclosporine dosage to less than 5 mg/kg/day was achieved in 14 patients without evidence of flare-up for up to 21 months. The cyclosporine dose was gradually decreased and totally discontinued in six patients. Although two of these patients demonstrated intraocular inflammation within 3 weeks of drug discontinuation, four remained free of symptoms with excellent vision during a 6- to 16-month follow-up without any treatment.

These promising results from open-trial cyclosporine studies have led to the initiation of randomized double-masked studies comparing the effectiveness of cyclosporine A to that of existing conventional therapy in uveitis patients. A 4-month, double-masked study of the use of cyclosporine was carried out in 96 patients with Behçet's disease; 47 patients received an initial dose of 10 mg/kg/day of cyclosporine and 49 patients received an established effective dose of 1.0 mg/day of colchicine (127). The cyclosporine group demonstrated a significantly greater reduction in the frequency and severity of ocular attacks along with a greater improvement in visual acuity versus the colchicine group. Eighty-nine percent of the cyclosporine patients showed significant disease amelioration versus 31% of the patients treated with colchicine. Deterioration was found in 18% of the colchicine group while no deterioration occurred in the cyclosporine group.

In another study comparing the efficacy of cyclosporine with conventional therapy (corticosteroids/Leukeran) in the treatment of Behçet's disease with active ocular inflammatory reactions, Ben Ezra et al. demonstrated cyclosporine to be more effective in decreasing the active ocular inflammatory processes and arresting the deterioration of visual acuity (128). Thirty-seven patients, randomized to a conventional or a cyclosporine regimen, were treated for 32 months. No obvious differences occurred in the extraocular symptoms between the two groups. Analysis of data from an extension of this study to 36 months showed the following: ocular inflammation was better controlled by cyclosporine therapy; improvement of visual acuity and/or preservation of vision at study entry were more often observed in the cyclosporine group; and the systemic manifestations (especially skin and articular lesions) of the disease were less prominent in the corticosteroid group (129).

V. SIDE EFFECTS OF CYCLOSPORINE ADMINISTRATION IN HUMANS

The majority of data concerning side effects observed during cyclosporine administration have been obtained from studies of transplant recipients receiving this immunomodulatory agent. Studies examining the efficacy of cyclosporine in the treatment of rheumatoid arthritis and other autoimmune disorders have demonstrated that the overall adverse reaction incidence was considerably less than that found in organ transplant patients. Side effects such as nephrotoxicity, gastrointestinal disturbances, and hirsutism are generally mild and may be reversible at low doses of cyclosporine (130). Cyclosporine-induced side effects appear to be more frequent and more severe at higher doses.

The principle adverse reaction, dose-dependent nephrotoxicity, has frequently been observed and correlated with an elevated serum creatinine and blood urea nitrogen. Dose-related decreases in glomerular filtration rate are common during cyclosporine immunosuppression. An adequate understanding of the mechanism of cyclosporine nephrotoxicity has been hindered by the lack of a suitable animal model. Initial short-term studies in various animal species failed to show major functional or structural abnormalities in the kidney. Studies utilizing large doses of cyclosporine in the rat have shown enzymuria, mild renal dysfunction, and proximal tubular cytoplasmic vacuolization (131). Increased numbers of lysosomes, cytosegresomes, and myeloid bodies observed along the length of the proximal tubule on electron microscopy suggest a direct toxic mechanism; however, the functional characterisics of the proximal tubule appear to be largely preserved. The increased fractional reabsorption in the proximal tubule is cyclosporine dose-dependent (132).

The morphological alterations of acute cyclosporine nephrotoxicity appear to be tubular lesions characterized by inclusion bodies, isometric vacuolization, and microcalcification (133). The striped interstitial fibrosis and tubular atrophy seen in man with high doses of cyclosporine has not yet been reproduced in any experimental model; this alteration is probably related to cyclosporine-associated arteriolopathy, predominantly found in human kidneys (134). Cyclosporine has been demonstrated in renal parenchymal cells by indirect immunofluorescence in fine-needle aspiration biopsies of renal allografts from patients with evidence of nephrotoxicity; these immunofluorescent deposits disappeared and transplant function improved upon dose reduction (135).

Cyclosporine nephrotoxicity has been reported in many studies of patients with rheumatoid arthritis. In a double-blind, randomized, 6-month study in which patients with rheumatoid arthritis were initially administered placebo or cyclosporine at 10/mg/kg/day for 2 months, the dose gradually being reduced to 5 mg/kg/day by month 5 upon satisfactory response, serum creatinine levels rose significantly (more than 30% from the initial level) during and after cyclosporine therapy whereas no changes occurred in the placebo group (136). The cyclosporine group also demonstrated a significant decrease in creatinine clearance which persisted after the end of the treatment. The gradual increase in serum creatinine observed during cyclosporine therapy did not correlate with the mean cyclosporine blood level or with the initial creatinine level; however, relative to the pretreatment value, the postcyclosporine therapy increase in creatinine significantly correlated with the increase during cyclosporine administration. From the results of this study, it was concluded that cyclosporine therapy, for not more than 6 months and at a maximum dosage of 10 mg/kg/day for 2 months, leads to an irreversible loss of more than 10% of renal function in rheumatoid patients.

In a safety and efficacy study using lower doses of cyclosporine, patients with rheumatoid arthritis were treated with 6 mg/kg/day of cyclosporine plus nonsteroidal anti-inflammatory agents for 6 months with dose adjustments made if the serum creatinine rose more than 50% above baseline values (137). Nine of 10 patients demonstrated significant clinical improvement, but nephrotoxicity remained a dose-limiting factor. A significant rise in serum creatinine and a decline in inulin and PAH clearances occurred at 6 months. One month after cyclosporine withdrawal, renal function improved but creatinine did not return to baseline. Renal insufficiency was evident upon cyclosporine continuation. Renal clearance studies improved with time (by week 100) and there appeared to be no deterioration in renal function with the same maintenance dose of cyclosporine, suggesting a stabilization with long-term cyclosporine use. Although data from this study suggest that low-dose cyclosporine is effective therapy for rheumatoid arthritis, it must be acknowledged that low-grade renal insufficiency occurs and may even be a dose-limiting factor.

Hypertension is another common side effect of cyclosporine therapy. Mild or moderate hypertension is more frequently encountered than severe hypertension and the incidence decreases over time. Previous hypertension has been reported to become exacerbated by cyclosporine therapy (136). New-onset hypertension was reported in 25% of a group of autoimmune patients treated with cyclosporine (138). Although lacking definitive evidence, the mechanism is presumed to be renal because plasma renin activity is increased during the acute states of experimental cyclosporine treatment (139). Systemic hypertension was the most frequently observed side effect in a trial of the efficacy of cyclosporine in 12 patients with rheumatoid arthritis, being seen in seven of these patients, five of whom had new-onset hypertension (114). Hypertension was also observed in patients with normal creatinine values. The elderly and patients treated with nonsteroidal anti-inflammatory drugs seem to exhibit a higher risk of developing hypertension (140). Antihypertensive therapy may be required. Although control of blood pressure can be accomplished with any antihypertensive agent, potassium-sparing diuretics should not be used because cyclosporine may cause hyperkalemia. Significant hyperkalemia, out of proportion to reductions in the glomerular filtration rate and associated with hyperchloremic metabolic acidosis and hyperuricemia, has been observed in individual patients. It has been suggested that hypoaldosteronism and tubular damage produce defects in potassium and hydrogen ion secretion (141) in the cortical collecting duct (142). Care should also be taken with the administration of calcium antagonists in the treatment of cyclosporine-associated hypertension since interference with cyclosporine metabolism may require a dosage adjustment.

A number of other side effects are seen infrequently with administration of cyclosporine to patients with autoimmune disease. Significant hepatotoxicity manifested as elevated hepatic enzymes and bilirubin has been observed during the early months of therapy when high doses of cyclosporine were employed. These chemistry elevations usually decreased with a reduction in dose. Gastrointestinal intolerance such as loss of appetite, nausea, and vomiting was also frequently observed. Occasionally, patients developed a syndrome of thrombocytopenia and microangiopathic hemolytic anemia, which was normochromic and normocytic; resolution occurred after dose reduction, drug discontinuation, and administration of streptokinase and heparin or plasmapheresis. As in patients receiving other immunosuppressants, patients receiving cyclosporine are at an increased risk compared to the normal population for the development of lymphomas and of other malignancies, particularly those of the skin. This increased risk appears related to the intensity and duration of immunosuppression rather than to the use of specific agents. To date, in nontransplant indications, no lymphomas or lymphoproliferative disorders have developed. Tremor, hirsutism, and gum hyperplasia have also been observed with cyclosporine administration. Hirsutism, prominent over the face and trunk, occurs more often in dark-complexioned individuals

Table 3 Adverse Reactions of Cyclosporine Treatment

	Randomized kidney patients		All autoimmune patients		
Body system/ adverse reaction	Autoimmune (N = 227) %	Azathioprine (N = 228) %	Kidney (N = 705) %	Heart (N = 112) %	Liver (N = 75) %
Genitourinary					
renal dysfunction	32	6	25	38	37
Cardiovascular					
hypertension	26	18	13	53	27
cramps	4	<1	2	<1	0
Skin					
hirsuitism	21	<1	21	28	45
acne	6	8	2	2	1
Central nervous system					
tremor	12	0	21	31	55
convulsions	3	1	1	4	5
headache	2	<1	2	15	4

Gastrointestinal					
gum hyperplasia	4	0	9	5	16
diarrhea	3	<1	3	4	8
nausea/vomiting	2	<1	4	10	4
hepatotoxicity	<1	<1	4	7	4
abdominal discomfort	<1	0	<1	7	0
Autonomic nervous system					
paresthesia	3	0	1	2	1
flushing	<1	0	4	0	4
Hematopoietic					
leukopenia	2	19	<1	6	0
lymphoma	<1	0	1	6	1
Respiratory					
sinusitis	<1	0	4	3	7
Miscellaneous					
gynecomastia	<1	0	<1	4	3

Note: The following reactions occurred in 2% or less of patients: allergic reactions, anemia, anorexia, confusion, conjunctivitis, edema, fever, brittle fingernails, gastritis, hearing loss, hiccups, hyperglycemia, muscle pain, peptic ulcer, thrombocytopenia, tinnitus. The following reactions occurred rarely: anxiety, chest pain, constipation, depression, hair breaking, hematuria, joint pain, lethargy, mouth sores, myocardial infarction, night sweats, pancreatitis, pruritis, swallowing difficulty, tingling, upper GI bleeding, visual disturbance, weakness, weight loss.

(143). Although troublesome, this can be treated via topical dipilatory agents. Dose-related gingival hyperplasia is more commonly seen in children and can be of such severity as to require gingivectomy. The incidence of gingival hyperplasia can be decreased if patients with poor dentition have their teeth corrected and plaque removed. Table 3 displays the adverse reactions occurring in 3% or greater of 892 patients involved in clinical trials of kidney, heart, and liver transplants.

Thus, although cyclosporine A has been demonstrated to possess significant therapeutic value in patients with rheumatoid arthritis and associated autoimmune disease, one must be aware of the potential side effects of this therapy. The incidence of adverse reactions may be decreased through the careful monitoring of cyclosporine blood levels, renal function parameters, liver enzymes, and blood pressure. The necessity of individual dose modification in accordance with the patient's exhibited safety parameters must be recognized. As a general recommendation at this time, the dose of cyclosporine should not exceed 5 mg/kg/day in the treatment of autoimmune disease. The gradual reduction of cyclosporine dose upon demonstration of efficacy will reduce the frequency of cyclosporine-manifested side effects.

REFERENCES

1. Ruegger A, Kuhn M, Lichti H, Loosli HR, Huguenin R, Quiquerez C, von Wartburg A. Cyclosporine A, in immunosuppressiv wirksamer Peptidmetabolit aus Trichoderma polysporum (Link ex Pers.) Rifai Helv Chim Act 1976; 59:1075–92.
2. Petcher TJ, Weber HP, Ruegger A. Crystal and molecular structure of an iododerivative of cyclic undecapeptide cyclosporine A. Helv Chim Act 1976; 59:1480–8.
3. Wenger R (1982) Chemistry of cyclosporine A. Proceedings of an international conference on cyclosporine A. Cambridge, September 1981.
4. Borel JF. The history of cyclosporine A and its significance. In: White DJG, ed. Cyclosporine A: proceedings of an international conference on cyclosporine A. Amsterdam: Elsevier, 1982:5–17.
5. NDA Submission, Volume 2.1, page 17, 196–201.
6. Gunn HC. Successful treatment of autoimmunity in NZB x NZW) F1 mice with cyclosporine and (Nva^2)-cyclosporine. I. Reduction of autoantibodies. Exp Immunol 1986; 64(2):225–33.
7. Mountz JD, Smith HR, Wilder RL, Reeves JP, Steinberg AD. CSA therapy in MRL-lpr/lpr mice: amelioration of immunopathology despite antibody production. J Immunol 1987; 38(1):157–63.
8. Kaibara N, Hotokebuchi T, Takagashi K, Katsuki I. Paradoxical effects of Cyclosporine A on collagen arthritis in rats. J Exp Med 1983; 158:2007–15.

9. Kaibara N, Hotokebuchi T, Takagashi K, Katsuki I, Morinaga M, Arita C, Jingushi S. Pathogenetic difference between collagen arthritis and adjuvant arthritis. J Exp Med 1984; 159:1388-96.
10. Henderson B. The anti-arthritic and immunosuppressive effects of cyclosporine on arthritis induced in the rat by type II collagen. Clin Exp Immunol 1984;57:51-6.
11. Borel JF, Feurer C, Gubler HV, Stahelin H. Biological effects of cyclosporine A: a new anti-lymphocytic agent. Agents and Actions 1976; 6(4):468-75.
12. Kaibara N, Hotokebuchi T, Takagishi K, Katsuki I, Morinaga M, Arita C, Jingushi S. Pathogenic difference between collagen arthritis and adjuvant arthritis. J Exp Med 1984; 159:1388-96.
13. Allen JB, Malone DG, Wahl SM, Calandra GB, Wilder RL. Role of the thymus in streptococcal cell wall-induced arthritis and hepatic granuloma formation. Comparative studies of pathology and cell wall distribution in athymic and euthymic rats. J Clin Invest 1985; 76:1042-56.
14. Yocum DE, Allen JB, Wahl SM, Calandra GB, Wilder RL. Inhibition by cyclosporine A of streptococcal cell wall-induced arthritis in rats. Arth Rheum 1986; 29:262-73.
15. White DJG. Cyclosporine A: clinical pharmacology and therapeutic potential. Drugs 1982;24:322-34.
16. Homan WP, Fabre JW, Williams KA, Millard PR, Morris PJ. Studies of immunosuppressive properties of cyclosporine A in rats receiving renal allografts. Transplantation 1980;29:361-6.
17. Thomson AW, Whiting PH, Cameron ID, Lessels SE, Simpson JG. A toxicological study in rats receiving immunotherapeutic doses of cyclosporine A. Transplantation 1981; 31:121-4.
18. Blair JT, Thomson AW, Whiting PH, Davidson RJL, Simpson JG. Toxicity of the immune suppressant cyclosporine A in the rat. J Pathol 1982; 138(2):163-78.
19. Ryffel B, Donatsch P, Hauser R. In: White DJG, ed. Cyclosporine A. New York: Elsevier, 1982.
20. Siegl H, Ryffel B, Petric R, et al. Transpl Proc 1983; 15:2719 (suppl 1).
21. Siegl H, Ryffel B, Donatsch P. Human Toxicol 1984; 3:418.
22. English J Evan A, Houghton DC, Bennett WM. Cyclosporine-induced acute renal dysfunction in the rat. Evidence of arteriolar vasoconstriction with preservation of tubular function. Transplantation 1987; 44(1).
23. Calne RY, White DJG, Pentlow BD, Rolles K, Syrakos T, Ohtawa T, Smith DP, McMaster P, Evans DB, Herbertson BM, Thiru S. Cyclosporin A: preliminary observations in dogs with pancreatic duodenal allografts and patients with cadaveric renal transplants. Transpl Proc. 1979; 11:860-4.

24. Ryffel B. Experimental toxicological studies with cyclosporine A. In: White DJG, ed. Cyclosporine A. New York: Elsevier, 1982.
25. Backman L, Appelkvist E-L, Ringden O, Dallner G. Effects of cyclosporine on hepatic protein synthesis. Second International Congress on Cyclosporine A. Washington, D.C., Nov. 4–7, 1987.
26. Farthing MJG, Clark ML. Nature of the toxicity of cyclosporine A in the rat. Biochem Pharmacol 1981; 30:3311–6.
27. Ryffel B, Donatsch P, Madorn M, Matter BE, Ruttiman G, Schon H, Stoll R, Wilson J. Toxicological evaluation of cyclosporine A. Arch Toxicol 1983; 53(2):107–41.
28. Lesley. Experimental toxicological studies with Cyclosporine A. In: White DJG, ed. Cyclosporine A. New York: Elsevier, 1982:71.
29. Borel JF, Feurer C, Magnee C, Stahelin H. Effects of the new anti-lymphocytic peptide cyclosporine A in animals. Immunology 1977; 32: 1017–25.
30. Zschauer A, Hodel Ch. Drug induced changes in rat seminiferous tubular epithelium. Arch Toxicol 1980; Suppl. 4:466–70.
31. Thiru S, Calne RY, Nagington J. Lymphomas in renal allograft patients treated with cyclosporine A as one of the immunosuppressive agents. Transpl Proc 1981; 13:359–64.
32. Racusen L, Famiglio L, Fivush B, Olton D, Fisher R, Solez K. Neurological abnormalities and mortality in rats treated with cyclosporine. Second International Congress on Cyclosporine A, Washington, D.C., 4–7 Nov 1987.
33. Toung T, Santos G, Fraizer C, McPherson R, Baumgardner W, Reitz B, Traystman R. Central nervous system effect on cyclosporine infusion in dogs. Second International Congress on Cyclosporine A. Washington, D. C., Nov. 4–7, 1987.
34. Pendry A, Alexander P. Stimulation of hair growth on nude mice by cyclosporine A. In: White DJG, ed. Cyclosporine A. New York: Elsevier, 1982.
35. NDA Submission, Vol. 3.74, chap. IV, pages 46–75.
36. Atkinson K, Boland J, Britton K, Biggs J. Blood and tissue distribution of cyclosporine in humans and mice. Transpl Proc 1983; 15:2430–49.
37. Rieo M, Gibbons S, Kwok D, Van Buren CT, Flechner S, Kahan BD. Cyclosporine levels in human tissues of patients treated for one week to one year. Transpl Proc 1983; 15:2434–7.
38. Flechner SM, Katz AR, Rogers AJ, Van Buren C, Kahan BD. The presence of cyclosporine in body tissue and fluids during pregnancy. Am J Kidney Dis 1985; 5:60–3.
39. Sgoutas D, MacMachon W, Love A, Jerkunica I. Interaction of cyclosporine A with human lipoproteins. J Pharm Pharmacol 1986; 38(8): 583–8.

40. Maurer G, Loosli HR, Schrier E, Keller B. Disposition of cyclosporine in several animal species and man. Structural elucidation of its metabolites. Drug Disposal Metab. 1984; 12:120–6.
41. Keown PA, Laupacis A, Carruthers G, Stawecki M, Koegler J, McKenzie FN, Wall W, Stiller CR. Interaction between phenytoin and cyclosporine following organ transplantation. Transplantation 1984; 38(3): 304–6.
42. Modry DL, Stinson EB, Oyer PE, Jamieson SW, Baldwin JC, Shumway NE. Acute rejection and massive cyclosporine requirements in heart transplant recipients treated with rifampin. Transplanation 1985; 39(3): 313–4.
43. Freeman DJ, Laupacis A, Keown PA, Stiller CR, Carruthers SG. Evaluation of cyclosporine-phenytoin interaction with observations in cyclosporine metabolites. Br J Clin Pharmacol 1984; 18:887–93.
44. Ferguson RM, Sutherland DER, Simmons RL, Najarian JS. Ketoconazole, cyclosporine metabolism and renal transplantation. Lancet 1982; 2:882.
45. NDA Submission, Volume 3.77.
46. NDA Submission, Volume 3.75, page 31.
47. Quesniaux V, Tees R, Schreier MH, Mauer G, Van Regenmortel MHV. Potential of monoclonal antibodies to improve therapeutic monitoring of cyclosporine. Clin Chem 1987; 33(1):32–7.
48. Schran HF, Rosano TG, Hassell AE, Pell MA. Determination of cyclosporine concentrations with monoclonal antibodies. Clin Chem 1987; 33(12):2225–9.
49. Yatscoff RW, Rush DN, Jeffrey JR. Effect of sample preparation on concentrations of cyclosporine A measured in plasma. Clin Chem 1984; 30:1812–4.
50. White DJG, Plumb AM, Pawelec G, Brons G. Cyclosporine A: an immunosuppressive agent preferentially active against proliferating T cells. Transplantation 1979; 27:55.
51. Wiseinger D, Borel JF. Studies on the mechanism of action of Cyclosporine A. Immunobiology 1980; 156:454.
52. Hess AD, Tutschka PJ. Effect of cyclosporin A on human lymphocyte responses in vitro. J Immunol 1982; 128(1):335–67.
53. Bunjes D, Hardt C, Rollinghoff M, Wagner H. Cyclosporine A mediates immunosuppression of primary cytotoxic T-cell responses by impairing the release on interleukin-1 and interleukin-2. Eur J Immunol 1981; 11(8):657–61.
54. Miyawaki T, Yachie A, Ohzeki S, Nagoki T, Taniguchi N. Cyclosporine A does not prevent expression of Tac antigen, a probable TCGF receptor model, on mitogen stimulated human T cells. J Immunol 1983; 130: 2737–42.

55. Hess AD. Effect of interleukin 2 on the immunosuppressive action of cyclosporine. Transplantation 1985; 39:62–8.
56. Dos Reis GA, Shevach EM. Effect of cyclosporine A on T-cell function in vitro: the mechanism of suppression of T-cell proliferation depends on the nature of the T-cell stimulus as well as the differentiation state of the responding T-cell. J Immunol 1982; 129(6):2360–7.
57. Kerman R. Effects of cyclosporine immunosuppression in vivo in man. Second International Congress on Cyclosporine A. Washington, D.C., Nov. 4–7, 1987.
58. Kalman VK, Klimpel GR. Effects of cyclosporine on the production of various interferons. Transpl Proc 1983; 15:2383.
59. Introna M, Allavena P, Spreafico F, Mantovani A. Inhibition of human natural killer activity by cyclosporine A. Transplantation. 1981; 31:113.
60. Andrus L, Lafferty KJ. Inhibition of T-cell activation by cyclosporine A. Scand J Immunol 1982; 15:449.
61. Morris PJ, Mason DW, Hutchinson IV. The effect of cyclosporine A on lymphocytes in animal models of tissue transplantation. Transpl Proc 1983; 15:2287.
62. Morris PJ. Cyclosporine A. Transplantation 1981; 32:349.
63. Burckhardt JJ, Guggenheim B. Cyclosporin A: in vivo and in vitro suppression of rat-T lymphocyte function. Immunology 1979; 279:443.
64. Koponen M, Grieder A, Loor F. Interference of cyclosporine with lymphocyte activation: blockage of the mitogen-induced increases of lysosomal and mitochondrial activities. Immunology 1984; 53(1):55–62.
65. Uyemura K, Dixon JFP, Parker JW. Inhibitory effect of cyclosporine on adherent cells in the oxidation-induced lymphocyte mitogenesis. Transpl Proc 1983; 15:2376.
66. Manca F, Kunki A, Celeda F. Inhibition of the accessory functions of murine macrophages in vitro by cyclosporine. Transplantation 1985; 39:644–8.
67. Wang BS, Heacock EH, Chang-Xue Z, Tilney NL, Strom TB, Mannick JA. Evidence for the presence of suppressor T lymphocytes in animals treated with cyclosporine A. J Immunol 1982; 128:1382.
68. Leoni P, Garcia RC, Allison AC. Effects of cyclosporine A on human lymphocytes in culture. J Clin Lab Immunol 1978; 1:67.
69. Palacios R, Moller G. Cyclosporine A blocks receptors for HLA–DR antigens on T cells. Nature 1981; 290:792.
70. Noga S, Fischer A, Hess A. Cyclosporine enhances the natural suppressor monocyte precusor populations in the rat. Second International Congress on Cyclosporine A. Washington, D.C., Nov 4–7, 1987.
71. Borel JF, Wiesinger D. Effects of cyclosporine A on murine lymphoid cells. In: Lucus, ed. Regulatory mechanisms in lymphocyte activation. New York: Academic Press, 1977:716–8.

72. LeGrue SJ, Friedman AW, Kahan BD. Binding of cyclosporine in human lymphocytes and phospholipid vesicles. J Immunol 1983; 131(2): 712–8.
73. Ryffel B, Gotz V, Heuberger B. Cyclosporine receptors on human lymphocytes. J Immunol 1982; 129(5):1978–82.
74. Ryffel B. Cyclosporine: effects on human T lymphocyte activation and clinical application. Clin Immunol Newslett 1984; 5:164–8.
75. Suthanthiran M, Evelyn M, Rubin AL, Stenzel KH. A reappraisal of the effects of monoclonal antibodies directed at T cell differentation antigens. Transplantation. 1984; 38:720–6.
76. Bendtzen K, Dinarello CA. Mechanism of action of cyclosporine A. Effects of T-cell-binding of interluekin 1 and antagonizing effect of insulin. Scand J Immunol 1984; 20:43–51.
77. Palacios R. Mechanism of T cell activation: role and functional relationship of HLA-DR antigens and interleukins. Immunol Rev 1982; 63:73–110.
78. Helderman JH, Raskin P. The T-lymphocyte insulin receptor in diabetes and obesity. An intrinsic binding defect. Diabetes 1980; 29:551.
79. Uchiyama T, Broder S, Waldmann TA. A monoclonal antibody (anti-Tac) reactive with activated and functionally mature human T cells. I. Production of anti-Tac monoclonal antibody and distribution of Tac (+) cells. J Immunol 1981; 126:1393.
80. Heistand PC. Prolactin: an autocrine modulator of lymphocyte responsiveness. A possible mechanism of action of cyclosporin. Proc. Natl. Acad. Sci. USA. In press.
81. Linzer DIH, Nathans D. Nucleotide sequence of a growth-related mRNA encoding a member of the prolactin-growth hormone family. Proc. Natl. Acad. Sci. USA 1984; 81;4255-9.
82. Handschumacher RE, Harding MW, Rice J, Drugge RJ. Cyclophilin: a specific cytosolic binding protein for cyclosporine A. Science 1984; 22: 544–6.
83. Durette P, Boger J, Dumont F, Frankshun R, Koprak S, Lin C, Melino M, Pessolano A, Pisano J, Schmidt J, Sigal N, Staruch M, Witzel B. A study of the correlation between cyclophilin binding and in vitro immunosuppressive activity of cyclosporine and analogs. Second International Congress on Cyclosporine A, Washington, D.C., Nov. 4–7, 1987.
84. Quesniaux V, Schrier M, Wenger R, Hiestand P, Harding M, Van Regenmortel M. Cyclophilin binds to the region of cyclosporine involved in its immunosuppressive activity. Second International Congress on Cyclosporine A, Washington, D.C., Nov. 4–7, 1987.
85. Colombani PM, Robb A, Hess AD. Cyclosporine A binding to calmodulin: a possible site of action on T-lymphocytes. Science 1985; 228 (4697):337–9.

86. Metcalfe S. Cyclosporine does not prevent cytoplasmic calcium changes associated with lymphocyte activation. Transplantation. 1984; 38:161–4.
87. Kay JE, Benzie CR, Borghetti AF. Effect of cyclosporine A on lymphocyte activation by the calcium ionophore A23187. Immunology 1983; 50:441–6.
88. Kronke M, Leonard WJ, Depper J, Ayra SK, Wong-Stall F, Gallo RC, Waldman TA, Greene WC. Cyclosporine A inhibits T-cell growth factor gene expression at the level of mRNA transcription. Proc Natl Acad Sci USA 1984; 81(16):5214–8.
89. Wiskocil R, Weiss A, Imboden J, Kamin-Lewis R, Stobo J. Activation of human T cell line: a two-stimulus requirement in the pretranslational events involved in the coordinate expression of interleukin 2 and gamma-interferon genes. J Immunol 1985; 134:1599–1603.
90. Cihero F, Kahan BD. Effects of cyclosporine on the nuclear function. Second International Congress on Cyclosporine A. Washington, D.C., Nov. 4–7, 1987.
91. VanBoxel JA, Paget SA. Predominantly T-cell infiltrate in rheumatoid synovial membranes. N Engl J Med 1975; 293(11):517–20.
92. Yu D, Peter J. Cellular immunological aspects of rheumatoid arthritis. Semin Arth Rheum 1974; 4:25–52.
93. Ruddy S, Austen KF. The complete system in rheumatoid synovitis: an analysis of complement component activities in rheumatoid synovial fluids. Arth Rheum 1970; 13:713–23.
94. Jannossy G, Duke O, Poulter LW, Panayi G, Bofill M, Goldstein G. Rheumatoid arthritis: a disease of T-lymphocyte/macrophage immunoregulation. Lancet 1981; 839–42.
95. Paget S, Gibofsky A.Immunopathogenesis of rheumatoid arthritis. Am J Med 1979; 67:961–70.
96. Klares K, Forsum U, Schenynius A, Kabilitz D, Wizzill H. Evidence in support of self-perpetuation HLA-DR dependent delayed type cell reaction in rheumatoid arthritis Proc Natl Acad Sci USA 1982; 29:3623–36.
97. Herrmann B, Muller W. Die therapie der chronischen polyarthritis mit cyclosporine A, einem neven immunosuppressivum. Akt. Rheumatol. 1979; 4:173–86.
98. Amor B, Dougados M. Ciclosporin in rheumatoid arthritis: open trials with different dosages. In: Schindler R, ed. Cyclosporine in automimmune diseases. First International Symposium, Basel, March 18–29, 1985.
99. Herzog Ch, Gross D.Low dose ciclosporin and prednisone: a step in the direction of selective immunosuppression in rheumatoid arthritis refractory to treatment (6-month follow-up). In: Schindler R, ed.

Cyclosporine in autoimmune diseases. First International Symposium, Basel, March 18-20, 1985.

100. Madhok R, Capell HA. Ciclosporin in rheumatoid Arthritis: preliminary results. In: Schindler R, ed. Cyclosporine in Autoimmune Diseases. First International Symposium, Basel, March 18-20, 1985.

101. Madhok R, Capell H. Cyclosporine: a long-term evaluation in rheumatoid arthritis. Second International Congress on Cyclosporine A, Washington, D.C., Nov. 4-7, 1987.

102. Bowles CA, Gabriel S, Bunch TW, Handweiger BS. Cyclosporine treatment for rheumatoid arthritis. The 51st Annual Meeting of the American Rheumatism Association. June 9-13, 1987, Washington, D.C.

103. Forre O, Bjerkoel F, Salvesen CF, Berg KJ, Rugstad HE, Saelid G, Mellbye OJ, Kass E. An open, controlled, randomized comparison of cyclosporine and azathioprine in the treatment of rheumatoid arthritis: a preliminary report. Arth Rheum 1987; 30(1):88-92.

104. Weinblatt ME, Coblyn JS, Fraser PA, Anderson RJ, Spragg J, Trentham DE, Austen KF. Cyclosporine A treatment of refractory rheumatoid arthritis. Arth Rheum 1987; 30(1):11-7.

105. Weinblatt ME, Coblyn JS, Fraser PA, Spragg J, Austen KF. Cyclosporine A in refractory rheumatoid arthritis (RA): extended observations at 3 mg/kg/day. The 51st Annual Meeting of the American Rheumatism Association. June 9-13, 1987, Washington, D.C.

106. Van Rijthoven AWAM, Dijkmans BAC, Goei The HS, Montnor-Beckers ZLBM, Jacobs PCJ, Cats A. Ciclosporin treatment in rheumatoid arthritis: a preliminary report of a multicentre placebo-controlled double-blind study. In: Schindler R, ed. Cyclosporine in autoimmune diseases. First International Symposium, Basel, March 18-20, 1985.

107. Van Rijthoven AWAM, Dijkmans BAC, Goei The HS, Hermans J, Montnor-Beckers ZLMB, Jacobs PCJ, Cats A. Cyclosporin treatment for rheumatoid arthritis: a placebo controlled, double-blind, multicenter study. Ann Rheum Dis 1986;(45):726-31.

108. Dougados M, Awada H, Amor B. Cyclosporine in rheumatoid arthritis: a double-blind placebo controlled trial in 52 patients. Second International Congress on Cyclosporine A, Washington, D.C., Nov. 4-7, 1987.

109. Yocum DE, Dougherty S, Gerber NL, Austin HA, Minor JR, Lesko LJ, Yarboro CH, Berkebile CE, Klippel JH, Wilder RL, Wahl SM. Immunomodulatory effects of cyclosporine A in rheumatoid arthritis. The 51st Annual Meeting of the American Rheumatism Association. June 9-13, 1987, Washington, D.C.

110. Isreal-Biet D, Noel LH, Bach MA,Dardenne M, Bach JF. Marked reduction of DNA antibody production and glomerulopathy in thymulin

(FTS-ZN) or ciclosporin A treated (NZB x NZW) F1 mice. Clin Exp Immunol 1983; 54:359.

111. Jones MG, Harris G, Cowing G. Response of murine autoimmune disease to cyclosporine and thiols. Transpl Proc 15 (Suppl 1) 1983; 2904.
112. Isenberg DA, Snaith ML, Al-Khader AA, Cohen SL, Fisher C, Morrow WJW, Mowbray J. Cyclosporine relieves arthralgra, causes angioedema. N Engl J Med 1980; 303:754.
113. Deteix P, Lefrancois N, Laville M, Colon S, Zech P, Traeger J. Open therapeutic trial of cyclosporine in systemic lupus erythematosus: preliminary results in 4 patients. In: Schindler R, ed. Cyclosporine in autoimmune diseases. 1st International Symposium, Basel, March 18-20, 1985:361-5.
114. Feutren G, Querin S, Noel LH, Chatenoud L, Beaurain G, Tron F, Lesavre PH, Bach JF. The effects of ciclosporin in severe systemic lupus erythematosus. J Pediatr Dec. 1987; 1063-8.
115. Halloran PF, Cole EH, Bookman AA, Urowitz MB, Clarke WTW. Possible beneficial effect of ciclosporin in some cases of severe systemic lupus erythematosus. In: Schindler R, ed. Cyclosporine in autoimmune diseases. 1st International Symposium, Basel, March 18-20, 1985: 356-60.
116. Miescher PA, Miescher A. Combined ciclosporin-steroid treatment of systemic lupus erythematosus. In Schindler R, ed. Cyclosporine in Autoimmune Disease. 1st International Symposium, Basel, March 18-20, 1985: 337-45.
117. Muller W, Herman B. Cyclosporine for psoriasis. N Engl J Med 1979; 301:555.
118. Harper JI, Keat ACS, Staughton RCD. Cyclosporin for psoriasis. Lancet 1984; 981-2.
119. Bendtzen K, Tvede N, Anderson V, Mortensen SA. Ciclosporin (CyA) in the management of polymyositis/idiopathic cardiomyopathy. In: Schindler R, ed. Cyclosporine in Autoimmune Disease. 1st International Symposium, Basel, March 18-20, 1985:110-3.
120. Goei The HS, Jacobs P, Hooben H. Cyclosporine in the treatment of intractable polymyositis. Arth Rheum 1985; 28:1436-7.
121. Borleffs JCC. Cyclosporine as monotherapy for polymyositis. Second International Congress on Cyclosporine A. Washington, D.C., Nov. 4-7, 1987.
122. Nussenblatt RB, Rodrigues MR, Wacker WB, Cevavrio SJ, Salinas-Carmora MC, Gery I. J Clin Invest 1981; 67:1128.
123. Nussenblatt RB, Palestine AG, Rook AH, Scher I, Walker WB, Gery I. Treatment of intraocular inflammatory disease with Cyclosporine A. Lancet 1983; 1:238-56.
124. Nussenblatt RB, Palestine AG, Chan CC. Cyclosporine A therapy in the treatment of intraocular inflammatory disease resistant to

systemic corticosteroids and cytotoxic agents. Am J Ophthalmol 1983;96:275.
125. Muftuoglu AU, Pazarli H, Yurdakul S, Yazici H, Ulku B, Tuzun Y, Serdarglu S, Ozyazgan Y, Ahug E, Bachcecioglu H. Treatment of ocular involvement in Behcet's disease with ciclosporin (preliminary report). In: Schindler R, ed. Cyclosporine in autoimmune diseases. 1st International Symposium, Basel, March 18-20, 1985:147-51.
126. BenEzra D, Cohen E, Rakotomalada M, de Courten C, Harris W, Chajek T, Friedman G, Pizanti S. Introduction: effect of cyclosporine in endogenous uveitis. Second International Congress on Cyclosporine. Washington, D.C., Nov. 4-7, 1987.
127. Masuda K, Nakajima A. A double-masked study of cyclosporine treatment in Behcet's disease. In: Schindler, R, ed. Cyclosporine in autoimmune diseases. 1st International Symposium, Basel, March 18-20, 1985. pg:162-164.
128. Ben Ezra D, Chajek T, Cohen E, Pizanti S, Friedman G, de Courten C, Harris W. Conventional versus cyclosporine therapy in Behcet's disease. Second International of Congress on Cyclosporine. Washington, D.C., Nov. 4-7, 1987.
129. Ben Ezra D, Chajek T, Friedman G, Pizanti S, Cohen E. Cyclosporine A and conventional immunosuppressive therapy in Behcet's disease. Immunointervention in autoimmune diseases. Paris, June 15-17, 1988.
130. Graf U, Marbet U, Muller W, Thiel G. Cyclosporin A—wirkungen and nebenwirkungen bei der behandlung der chronischen polyarthritis und der psoriasiarthritis. Immunol Infekt 1981;9:20-8.
131. Whiting PH, Thomson AW, Blair JT, Simpson JG. Experimental cyclosporin A nephrotoxicity. Br J Exp Pathol 1982;63:88-94.
132. Dieperink H, Leyssac PP, Kemp E, Starklint H. Glomerulotubular function in cyclosporine A treated rats. Clin Nephrol 1986; 25 (Suppl L): S70.
133. Mihatsch MJ, Thiel G, Spichtin HP, Oberholzer M, Brunner FP, Harder I, Olivieri V, Bremer R, Ryffel B, Stöcklin E, Torhost J, Gudat F, Zollinger HV, Loertscher R. Morphological findings in transplants after treatment with cyclosporine. Transpl Proc. 1983; 15:2821.
134. Mihatsch MJ, Thiel G, Basler V, Ryffel B, Landmann J, Von Overbeck J, Zollinger HU. Morphological patterns in cyclosporine-treated renal transplant recipients. Transpl Proc 1985; 17:101.
135. Von Willebrand E, Hayry P. Cyclosporin-A deposits in renal allografts. Lancet 1983;2:189-92.
136. Dijkmans BAC, Van Rijthoven AWAM, Goei The HS, Montnor-Beckers ZLBM, Jacobs PCJ, Cats A. Effect of cyclosporine on serum creatinine in patients with rheumatoid arthritis. Eur J Clin Pharmacol 1987;31: 541-5.

137. Bowles, Caroline. Pers. commun. 1988.
138. Palestine AG, Nussenblatt RB, Chan CC. Side effects of cyclosporine in nontransplant patients. Am J Med 1984; 77:652–6.
139. Baxter CR, Duggin GG, Willis NS, Hall BM, Horvath JS, Tiller DJ. Cyclosporine A-induced increases in renin storage and release. Res Commun Chem Pathol Pharmacol 1982; 37:305–11.
140. Von Graffenreid B, Harrison WB. Ciclosporin in autoimmune disease—side effects (with emphasis on renal dysfunction) and recommendation for use. In: Schindler R, ed. Cyclosporine in autoimmune diseases. First International Symposium, Basel, March 18–20, 1985.
141. Adu D, Turney J, Michael J, McMaster P. Hyperkalaemia in cyclosporin-treated renal allograft recipients. Lancet 1983; 2:370–2.
142. Battle DC, Gutterman C, Tarka J, Prasada R. Effect of short term cyclosporine A administration on urinary acidification. Clin Nephrol 1986; 25 (suppl):S62.
143. European Multicentre Trial Group. Cyclosporine in cadaveric renal transplantation: one year follow-up of a multicenter trial. Lancet 1983; 2:986–9.

4

Retinoids as Immunomodulatory Agents for Rheumatic Diseases

Thasia G. Woodworth* **and John W. Coffey**
Hoffmann-La Roche Inc., Nutley, New Jersey

I. INTRODUCTION

Initial clinical indications of the potential beneficial effects of retinoids in rheumatic conditions occurred during early clinical trials of etretinate and tretinoin (all-trans-retinoic acid) in psoriasis, when it became evident that symptoms and signs of psoriatic arthropathy improved during therapy (1-7). Subsequently a number of collaborators have evaluated the efficacy and mechanism of action of several retinoid compounds in animal models of rheumatoid arthritis (8-16). Harris briefly reviewed these observations in early 1984, and suggested that retinoic acid inhibition of collagenase and prostaglandin E_2 (PGE_2) production and the demonstration of inhibitory activity of several retinoid compounds in rodent models of arthritis provided support for identification of a retinoid derivative with a reasonable therapeutic index for clinical trials in patients with rheumatoid arthritis (17). Work has continued in several laboratories including our own to identify retinoids which would have fewer direct dermatological effects and enhanced anti-inflammatory and immunoregulatory activity. In the meantime, these effects continue to be elucidated in clinical experience with etretinate and isotretinoin.

**Current affiliation*: Seragen, Inc., Hopkinton, Massachusetts

Recently, retinoids such as 4-hydroxyphenyl retinamide (4-HPR) (9--11) and (all-E)-3,7-dimethyl-9-[2-(trifluormethyl)-6-(nonloxy)phenyl]-2,4,6,8-noatetraenoic acid (Ro23-6457) (13) have been evaluated as immunomodulatory and anti-inflammatory agents in animal models, preliminary to consideration for clinical evaluation. Similar to other retinoids, these agents exacerbate rodent collagen arthritis (10,14), but show significant efficacy in adjuvant arthritis and streptococcal cell wall-induced (SCW) arthritis (11,12, 15,16). One of these agents, 4-HPR has recently been evaluated in normal volunteers and in patients with severe dermatoses, but the occurrence of dermatological and ophthalmic adverse effects apparently led to discontinuance of the development program (18,19). Thus, rheumatologists and other clinicians continue to await the identification in preclinical studies of retinoids with potential antirheumatic efficacy and an acceptable adverse effect profile.

In this chapter, the chemistry, pharmacokinetics and metabolism, and preclinical pharmacology of several retinoids are reviewed, along with the clinical experience which has demonstrated anti-inflammatory and immunoregulatory activity of retinoids already evaluated in human clinical trials.

II. DEFINITION OF A RETINOID

The definition of the term "retinoid" has evolved over the last several years. It was first popularized by Sporn (20) and Mayer and Bollag (21) in their early publications describing the potential anticancer and dermatological applications of these compounds. Originally the term referred to retinol (vitamin-A alcohol) and its natural or synthetic derivatives, including retinal, retinoic acid, and several esters which had been derived from the parent compound. Initially, the International Union of Pure and Applied Chemistry (IUPAC) and the International Union of Biochemistry (IUB) defined retinoids in a joint commission report as "substance(s) related to vitamin A (retinol), which is a diterpenoid derived from a monocyclic parent compound, containing 5 carbon-carbon double bonds and a functional group at the terminus of the acyclic portion" (22,23). This definition was based on the chemical structure of the sentinal effector substances, retinol and retinoic acid, and was also thought to recognize the ability of these agents to maintain growth in animals fed diets lacking in vitamin A (20). More than 1500 new retinoids have been synthesized, and this definition does not take into account many of these tricyclic or tetracyclic retinoidal benzoic acid derivatives which behave like retinoids in biological assays and, in fact, are more potent than retinol. Thus, Sporn and Roberts (22) proposed the following definition:

A retinoid is a substance that can elicit specific biological responses by binding to, and activating, a specific receptor or set of receptors. The classical ligands for these receptors are retinol and retinoic acid, but it is clear that synthetic ligands can have a better molecular fit to these receptors than either molecule. The program for the biological response of the target cell resides in the retinoid receptor, rather than in the retinoid itself (22).

Compounds with structures as diverse as those pictured in Fig. 1 have demonstrated biological activities characteristic of retinoids in a variety of biological assays. These assays range from those assessing the prevention of cancer in experimental animals (24,25), or the support of growth in vitamin A-deficient rodents (26), to others measuring regulation of a specific gene (27) and control of cell differentiation or cell proliferation in tissue culture (28) or potentiation of murine T-cell dependent mitogen responses (29). The chemistry of retinoids will continue to evolve, and thus the focus of research is now on developing compounds which elicit certain structure-activity relationships to be therapeutically useful for such diverse clinical targets as cancer therapy and chemoprevention, dermatological conditions, and rheumatic diseases.

III. PHARMACOKINETICS AND METABOLISM

The pharmacokinetics and absorption, distribution, metabolism, and excretion of several retinoids have been studied in both experimental and clinical settings. These compounds include tretinoin (all-*trans*-retinoic acid); isotretinoin (13-*cis*-retinoic acid); etretinate, with its major biologically active metabolite, acetretin; and 4-HPR. While these compounds have demonstrated distinct and important differences with regard to their therapeutic and toxicologic profiles, certain aspects of the pharmacokinetic and metabolic handling of these compounds can be generalized. Importantly, retinoids are sometimes metabolized to active substances, and thus the pharmacokinetics of the parent may be unrevealing with regard to therapeutic efficacy (30–33).

Tretinoin is used only topically, since its therapeutic index when administered orally is extremely narrow with regard to hypervitaminosis A-like adverse effects. Pharmacologically, oral isotretinoin, acetretin, and etretinate demonstrate several similarities with regard to dermatological efficacy but differ significantly when elimination half-life is considered—several days for isotretinoin and acetretin, versus 120 days for etretinate (31). These compounds are incompletely absorbed following oral administration, but bioavailability is significantly increased by administration in a lipid-containing vehicle

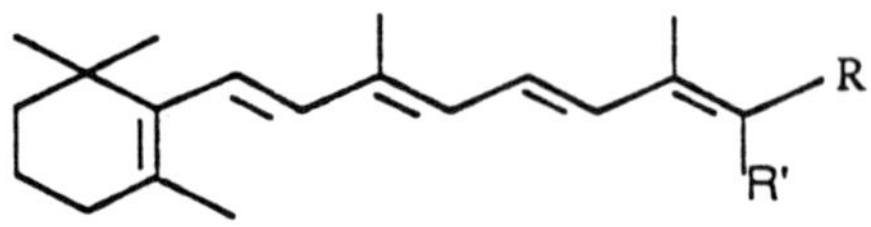

RETINOL (VIT A)	R = CH_2OH	
all-trans-retinoic acid	R = COOH	Manipulations of polar end
13-cis-retinoic acid (isotretinoin)	R' = COOH	
4-(hydroxyphenyl) retinamide (4-HPR)	R = CONH-C_6H_4OH	

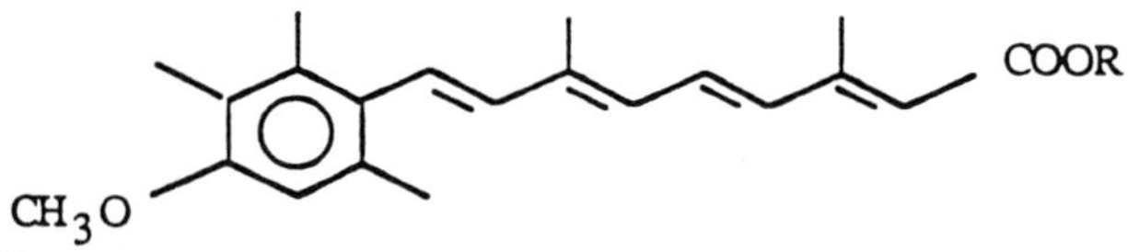

Etretinate (Ro10-9359)	R = C_2H_5	Replacement of cyclohexenyl moiety with substituted and non-substituted aromatic ring systems
Acetretin (Ro10-1670)	R = H	

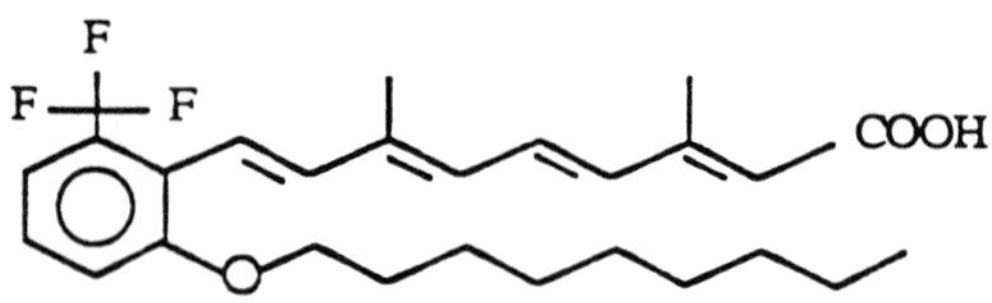

Ro23-6457

Replacement of cyclohexenyl moiety with substituted and non-substituted aromatic ring systems and addition of saturated side chain(s).

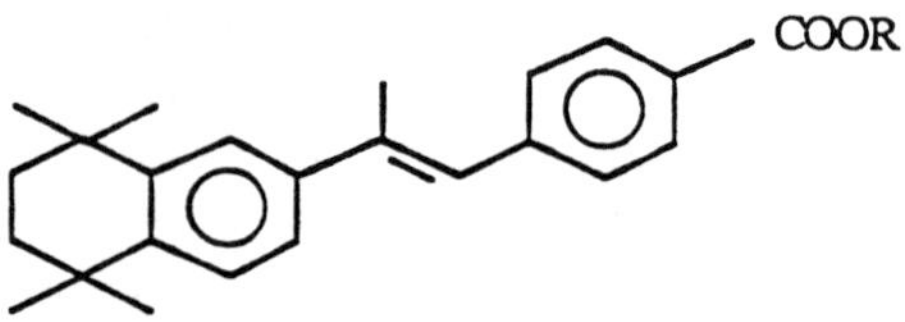

Arotinoids

Ro13-6298	R = C_2H_5	Cyclization of unsaturated side chain and addition of cyclohexane moiety to aromatic nucleus.
Ro13-7410	R = H	

Figure 1 Compounds that demonstrate retinoid activity.

or with meals, especially those containing fat. Isotretinoin also undergoes significant enterohepatic circulation, which adds to its bioavailability. Metabolic pathways include isomerization (which can also occur upon exposure to light), esterification, oxidation, hydroxylation, and glucuronidation. For isotretinoin, metabolism appears to take place mainly in the liver, whereas a significant amount of hydrolysis of etretinate to its free acid occurs in the gut, prior to absorption and liver metabolism (30).

The retinoids are quite lipophilic and significant uptake occurs via the lymphatics, in addition to the portal venous system. In the blood these agents are bound to plasma proteins. Acetretin and isotretinoin are carboxylic acid derivatives and are carried mainly by albumin, but a significant amount of etretinate, a lipophilic ester, is carried via lipoproteins (32). The majority of the clinically studied retinoids and their metabolites are excreted in the feces as a result of both incomplete absorption and biliary excretion. At the most, about 15-30% of metabolites are excreted in the urine, but in the case of 4-HPR none are detectable (30,33).

Pharmacokinetics of both parent retinoids and metabolites usually follow first-order kinetics (30-33), with the exception of etretinate, which seems to conform to three-compartment model (30–32). Steady-state concentrations of most retinoids can be predicted from single-dose data, providing indirect evidence that hepatic drug-metabolizing enzymes are not induced (30).

Very few studies have been performed to examine the pharmacokinetics of retinoids in the presence of coexisting renal or hepatic disease. In one recently published study (34) of etretinate in patients with chronic renal failure (CRF), levels of metabolites were similar to those of individuals with normal renal function, and the plasma half-life for all compounds was approximately the same in each group. However, CRF patients had lower serum albumin and elevated serum triglycerides, leading to higher peak levels of the free parent compound, suggesting that CRF patients are at higher risk for retinoid (hypervitaminosis A) adverse effects.

No detailed studies of tissue distribution of retinoids have been performed in humans. However, one study of etretinate in psoriatic patients (32) and several animal studies would suggest minimal accumulation in any tissue with the exception of adipose tissue (30–33), unlike retinol and its esters which are stored in the liver (20). In general, the plasma levels of retinoids are higher than those of tissue, and distribution is consistent with the pattern of circulation.

Descriptive pharmacokinetic parameters for representative compounds are summarized in Table 1.

Table 1 Pharmacokinetic Parameters for Representative Retinoids

	Tolerable C_{max} (ng/ml)	$T_{1/2}$ (min)	V_d (liters)	Ref.
Isotretinoin	200–500	6–36.5	N.R.	30–32
Etretinate	200–450	3–24[a]	150	30–32
4-HPR	N.R.[b]	16–20	N.R.	33

[a]Elimination $T_{1/2}$ = 120 days.
[b]N.R. = not reported.

IV. PRECLINICAL PHARMACOLOGY IN ANIMAL MODELS OF ARTHRITIS

13-*cis*-retinoic acid, etretinate, 4-HPR, and Ro23-6457 have been evaluated for their potential antiarthritic effects in rodent models of rheumatoid arthritis. Significant improvement in various arthritic parameters occurs in both adjuvant and streptococcal cell wall (SCW)-induced arthritis as well as in the arthritis of MRL/lpr (lupus) mice (8,9,11–13,15,16,35). In contrast, an interesting enhancement of collagen-induced arthritis in rats and mice has been seen, essentially unrelated to measurable suppression of prostaglandin E_2 (PGE_2) and collagenase production (16,14,35).

A. Adjuvant-Induced Arthritis

To induce adjuvant arthritis, one of the best characterized animal models of autoimmunity-associated arthritis, complete Freund's adjuvant, is injected into the footpad or the base of the tail. Over a period of about 3–4 weeks rats develop arthritis, characterized by swelling of the paws (especially of the hind limbs), which may also be associated with increased levels of acute phase proteins and tail inflammation. The arthritis peaks, then fades, leaving chronic ankylosis.(36,37).

Oral administration of 13-*cis*-retinoic acid to rats with either developing or established adjuvant arthritis significantly decreases inflammation and joint deformity. This effect is associated with a decrease in collagenase secreted in tissue culture by adherent cells isolated from the inflamed joints of these rats, but no affect on the amount of PGE_2 produced by the synovial cells. In addition, plasma fibrinogen, a representative acute phase reactant, is decreased five- to ten-fold in rats treated with 13-*cis*-retinoic acid, compared to vehicle-treated controls with arthritis. In comparison to indomethacin, 13-*cis*-retinoic acid is considerably less potent at maximally tolerated doses (37).

Similarly, Bradshaw demonstrated that oral administration of etretinate significantly decreased paw swelling in developing adjuvant arthritis and delayed its onset (35). However, compared to dexamethasone (0.5 mg/kg s.c.) and indomethacin (3 mg/kg p.o.), etretinate was only about half as effective. Collagenase and PGE_2 production were not assessed. Ro23-6457, a recently described retinoid derivative, shows similar effects in both the developing and established adjuvant arthritis models (16).

B. Streptococcal Cell Wall (SCW)-Induced Arthritis

4-HPR has been evaluated in SCW-induced arthritis. In this model, female LEW/N rats receive a single intraperitoneal injection of a saline suspension of streptococcal cell walls. This disease model is also biphasic, characterized by initial acute polyarticular inflammation that begins at 2–4 days postinjection and subsides within 7–10 days. Beginning at 10–14 days postinjection a chronic proliferative polyarticular synovitis becomes evident and persists for months, associated with the development of hepatic granulomas (11).

Haraoui et al. (11) have shown that treatment of SCW-induced arthritis with dietary 4-HPR from day 0 (i.e., the day SCW fragments are injected) has little effect on the acute polyarthritis, but that it produces a dose-dependent suppression of the chronic proliferative disease. Histologically, the inflammatory infiltrate in the synovium from the drug-treated animals is substantially reduced. In addition, there is a dose-dependent decrease in both collagenase and PGE_2 production by synovial cells removed from treated rats. Hepatic granuloma formation is unaffected in the 4-HPR-treated animals (11). In contrast, Ro-23-6457 was effective as an anti-inflammatory agent during both the acute and the chronic phase of SCW-induced arthritis (15). Cyclosporine A (CsA) treatment suppresses the chronic but not the acute arthritis in the SCW model (38). In addition, this agent inhibits hepatic granuloma formation (38).

C. Collagen-Induced Arthritis

Paradoxically, as demonstrated in studies by Trentham and Brinkerhoff, 13-*cis*-retinoic acid significantly enhances the inflammatory components in the collagen-induced arthritis model in rats, increases its severity, and may increase the incidence of the disease in collagen-challenged animals (10). In these studies native chick type II collagen in incomplete Freund's adjuvant is injected intradermally into outbred female Sprague-Dawley rats. Polyarticular arthritis develops within 14 days in up to 60% of the injected rats. This chronic proliferative synovitis is characterized by the occurrence of both anticollagen autoantibodies and probable cellular immune function defects, demonstrated by the development of delayed-type hypersensitivity to collagen (10,37).

Etretinate (35) and 4-HPR (9) also significantly enhance the frequency and severity of this arthritis in rats without altering the day of onset. In the case of 4-HPR, this enhancement of arthritis occurred despite a significant increase in anticollagen antibodies and a more than 80% decrease in PGE_2 production by cultured synovial adherent cells. The magnitude of delayed-type hypersensitivity to collagen was also unaffected by the retinoid. This effect is similar to that seen in some studies when collagen arthritis is treated with cyclophosphamide, gold, or *d*-penicillamine (35,42,43). Interestingly, in a murine model of collagen arthritis, the recently characterized immunosuppressive retinoid derivative Ro23-6457 significantly suppressed the acute polyarthritis when administered at or before the time of antigen challenge. However, this compound also exacerbates the disease when administered once arthritis develops (13). Treatment with cyclosporine A during the induction phase also suppresses the arthritis, whereas treatment later, during the preclinical phase of the proliferative arthritis, significantly enhances the condition (40,41).

Comparative effects of retinoids and other antirheumatic agents are summarized in Table 2.

V. RETINOID EFFECTS ON ANIMAL AND HUMAN IMMUNE FUNCTION

The effects of retinoids on animal and human immune function are variable depending on the response measured, the model studied, and whether the tests are performed in vitro or in vivo. Responses also vary depending on the concentration/dose of the retinoid, the delivery vehicle, and possibly the structure of the compound. In early studies, retinoids were commonly classified as immunostimulants, perhaps on the basis of the immunostimulatory role of retinol in immunization and the inhibition of tumor growth in mice. This classification was based on experiments of Medowar (49), as well as those of Saffiotti et al. (50), Cohen and Cohen (51), Bollag (52), Dennert and Lotan (53), and Sporn (54). Occasionally, immunization and tumor models in rodents and immune function assessment in patients being treated for acne, psoriasis, or disorders of keratinization have paradoxically identified

Table 2 Comparison of Effects of Retinoids and Current Therapeutic Agents in Animal Models of Rheumatoid Arthritis[a]

	NSAIDs	13-*cis* retinoic acid	Etretinate	Ro23-6457	4-HPR	Cortico-steroids	Cyclosporine	Cyclophos-phamide	*d*-Penicillamine (60–200 mg/kg/po)	Ref.
Adjuvant										
Developing[b]										
Acute	↓↓↓	↔	↔	↔	↓	↓↓	↓↓	↔	↔	8,12,16,37,43,45,46
Chronic	↓↓↓	↓	↓↓	↓↓	↓↓	↓↓↓	↓↓	↓↓	↔	
Established	↓	↓	↓	↓↓	↓↓	↓↓	↓↓	↓	↔	
Collagen										
Developing										
Chronic	↓↓	↑	↑	↓	↑	↓↓↓	↓	↓	↓,[c]	9,10,35,40–44
Established	↓↓	↑	↑↑	↑	↑↑	↓↓	↑	↑,↓,↔	↑,↓,↔	
Streptococcal cell-wall										
Developing										
Acute	N.A.	N.A.	N.A.	↓↓	↔,↓	N.A.	↔	N.A.	N.A.	9,15,38
Chronic	N.A.	N.A.	N.A.	↓↓↓	↓↓↓	N.A.	↓↓↓	N.A.	N.A.	
Established	N.A.	N.A.	N.A.	N.A.	↓↓↓	N.A.	↓↓↓	N.A.	N.A.	
MRL/1pr Spontaneous arthritis in autoimmune model of SLE	N.A.	N.A.	N.A.	↓↓	N.A.	↓↓	↓↓	↓↓	N.A.	13,47,48

[a]Adapted from Bradshaw et al. (35) and Coffey et al. (36)

[b]Developing disease indicates that drug therapy was initiated at the time that the eliciting agent was administered to induce the arthritis. Acute refers to the inflammation that develops during the first few days after administration of the eliciting agent, while chronic refers to the arthritis that develops over a period of weeks. Established disease indicates that the arthritis was allowed to develop over a period of weeks. Established disease indicates that the arthritis was allowed to develop untreated for a selected period of time prior to initiation of drug therapy.

[c]Conflicting results seen (see text).

Key for activity levels: ↑↑ > ↑/potentiation; ↓↓↓ > ↓↓ > ↓/suppression; ↔ no effect; N.A./not available.

immunosuppressive properties, often dependent on the response evaluated and the timing, dose, and duration of drug administration (13,55-59).

Immune effects of vitamin A and retinoids have recently been reviewed by Dennert (60), Shapiro and Edelson (61), and Nauss (62). The adjuvant properties of retinol have been demonstrated in several murine models (55,56,62) but have not been apparent in epidemiological studies in humans (63). Concurrent administration of retinol with tetanus toxoid or sheep red blood cell immunization increased antigen-specific antibody in mice, whereas no enhancement of antitetanus antibody production in humans could be shown in a comparative study. However, additional evidence for this effect has been noted in mice fed diets deficient in vitamin A, since these animals show markedly attenuated immune responses (62). Supplementation with either vitamin A or 13-*cis*-retinoic acid results in increased lymphoid tissue and enhanced accessory cell function (macrophage and dendritic cells) in alloproliferative and allocytotoxic assays (64), as well as oxazalone delayed-type hypersensitivity (65,66). Malkovsky and collaborators have shown further that the $Lytl^{+}2^{-}$ T-lymphocyte and IL-2 may play a major role in mediating retinoid-induced immunomodulation (66,67). These observations also appear to support earlier ones by Lotan and Dennert that treatment with several retinoids enhanced IL-2 production and cell-mediated cytotoxicity in mice. (53,60,68).

In contrast, in vitro studies of human peripheral blood lymphocytes and purified natural killer cells have shown little influence of retinoic acid (10^{-5} to 10^{-8} M) on cytotoxic potential. Rather, retinoic acid significantly reduces the sensitivity of some tumor targets to natural killing (69). Additional in vitro studies using retinoic acid at concentrations of 10^{-5} to 10^{-7} M have shown enhanced proliferation to mitogens by human thymocytes and tonsillar lymphocyte (70), but not by splenic or lymphoid lymphocytes (71). Human antibody responses in vitro are also augmented by similar concentrations of retinoic acid (72). Higher concentrations of retinoic acid (10^{-4} M), which also decrease cell viability, inhibit mitogenesis and E-rosette formation as well as natural killer activity of human peripheral blood lymphocytes (73).

In some murine immune response models, immunosuppressive properties of retinoids have become apparent, both with first-generation retinoids and, more importantly, with "third-generation" compounds. In studies by Barnett, treatment with 13-*cis*-retinoic acid, 3 mg per mouse weekly, completely suppressed the primary IgE response to ovalbumin, but upon reimmunization animals demonstrated increased titers of IgE antibody (55,56). Thus, a primary response was suppressed, but a secondary response was enhanced, in this case by a weekly dose of 13-*cis*-retinoic acid prior to and at the time of immunization. More recently, a retinoid-like agent of the nonatetraenoic acid family, Ro23-6457, has been shown to block the induction of murine cell-mediated immune responses, delayed-type hypersensitivity responses, and humoral immune responses. Rejection of murine skin transplants is also significantly suppressed by nontoxic doses. In addition, nephritis, anti-DNA antibody production, and arthritis in MRL/lpr mice, as well as diabetes in BB rats, is significantly attenuated (13). This compound has not been evaluated clinically.

In limited in vivo studies to examine the influence of retinoids on human immune function, both immune-enhancing and immunosuppressive properties have been observed. These findings are summarized in Table 3. Studies by Watson et al. (74) in healthy volunteers to determine possible immune effects of 13-*cis*-retinoic acid, prior to a cancer chemoprevention study, showed no significant effect on T-cell blastogenesis or surface markers. B-lymphocytes tended to decrease during drug administration and returned to normal after therapy ended. Plasma corticosteroids also decreased significantly with treatment. In contrast, in a study of patients with psoriatic arthropathy, Rosenthal observed an increase in total and activated T-lymphocytes with a decrease in B-lymphocytes after 6 months of etretinate therapy (1). It would appear that the retinoids in clinical use also have variable but quite limited effects on immune function, depending on dose, response studied, and whether or not healthy or ill individuals are evaluated. Effects seem to be immunoregulatory with modest changes in both T- and B-lymphocyte numbers and function.

In addition, anti-inflammatory effects have been seen in acne, psoriasis, and psoriatic arthropathy, as well as in other less common dermatological conditions with a rheumatic component (described in Sec. VII of this chapter). Effects associated with etretinate administration to patients with psoriasis include suppression of polymorphonuclear leukocyte antibody-dependent cell-mediated cytotoxicity (58), and normalization of increased chemotactic activity (2,75). Significant inhibition of superoxide production in vitro has been demonstrated along with a decrease in lysosomal enzyme release (76). Additional studies have shown that only OH^- generation appears to be inhibited (77). Nevertheless, these observations suggest a direct regulatory effect on the abnormal granulocyte function in psoriasis.

Significant challenges to interpretation of these often conflicting in vitro and in vivo experimental results include the need to determine the influence of the route of administration and the vehicle used to deliver the retinoid, as well as to assess the impact of changes in bioavailability and plasma concentration achieved with a particular dose. In addition, the timing of drug

Table 3 Retinoid Effects on Human Immune Function

Study (Ref.)	Design	Drug	Dose/duration	# Subjects	Lymphocyte subsets	Lymphocyte function	Comments
Healthy volunteers (74)	Open	13-*cis*-retinoic acid	0.13 mg/kg/d (9 mo)	10	↓B-lymphs at 5 months ($p < 0.05$) ↑$\frac{T4}{T8}$(2.1→4.3)	No change in Con A, PHA proliferation	2 F stopped 2 with bone pain, menstrual changes, irritability. ↓corticosteroid levels, persisted 45 days beyond end of study
Acne[a] (75)	Open[b]	13-*cis*-retinoic acid	0.5 mg/kg/qd (6 mo)	13	↑Fc receptors on B-lymphs ↑T4–8 wk ↑T4/T8	N.D.	↑IgG (wk 8) ↓IgG (wk 12) ↑IgA
Darier's disease[a] (76)	Open	13-*cis*-retinoic acid	10–20 mg/d (6 mo)	2	↓Total T-lymphs ↑T-suppressor	Lymphocyte hyperreactivity to Con A normalized	–
Nonmalignant skin disorders[a] (77)	Open	Etretinate	25–50 mg/d up to 11 mos. (mean = 8 mo)	11	N.D.	Tendency to ↑NK	No change in α-IFN or α-IFN NK activity
	Open[b]		25–75 mg/kg/d (up to 11 mo)		N.D.	↑NK at 2 mo, then return to baseline	–
Psoriasis[a] (1,56)	Open[b]	Etretinate	0.5–1 mg/kg/d (up to 11 mo)	27	↑T-lymphs ↓B-lymphs ↑active T lymphs	↑Con A proliferation NK and monocyte ADCC remain normal	↓PMN ADCC
(78)	Open[b]	Etretinate	50 mg/d (1 mo)	5	T3, T4, T8 lymphs remained normal	N.D.	–

[a]All patients improved clinically.
[b]Parameters assessed during run-in period (off drug), as well as on drug.
Abbreviations: ADCC-antibody-dependent cell-mediated cytotoxicity; Con-A, concanavalin A; IFN-interferons; NK-natural killer cell (activity); PHA-phytohemagglutinin; PMN, polymorphonuclear.

administration in relation to the immune challenge, as well as the duration of dosing, can significantly influence the effect seen. Due to the complexity of these interrelationships, the ultimate clinical use of retinoid agents will depend at least in part on the ability to measure specific in vivo immunopharmacodynamic parameters that can predict an appropriate clinical response.

VI. MECHANISM OF ACTION OF RETINOIDS

A. Cellular Binding Proteins and Receptors for Retinoids

Cystolic proteins that specifically bind retinol [cellular retinol binding protein (CRBP)] or retinoic acid [cellular retinoic acid binding protein (CRABP)] have been known for several years (79). The physiological function of CRBP has not been studied in detail; however, in the case of CRABP, the current hypothesis is that this protein probably plays a role in the transport, metabolism, and storage of retinoic acid, but that it is not the cellular receptor responsible for the biological actions of retinoic acid. Instead, the recently described α-, β-, and γ-retinoic acid receptors (RAR) are more likely to be the binding proteins that mediate the cellular effects of retinoic acid (80-83). These latter proteins belong to the family of steroid and thyroid nuclear receptors that characteristically have a domain that binds the small ligand and another domain that interacts with DNA in a specific fashion when the ligand binding site is occupied. It appears that this mechanism facilitates the regulation of expression of specific genes by the small ligand like (like retinoic acid). A recent study demonstrated that two synthetic retinoids with potent biological activity bind to an intracellular protein in HL-60 cells which has some properties which are similar to those of RARs (84), and the speculation is that synthetic retinoids may induce biological effects by binding to the nuclear RARs.

B. Effects of Retinoids on Cell Activity and Gene Transcription

Historically, retinoids have been viewed as antiproliferative agents which can induce cell differentiation, e.g., recall original observations of their role in cancer prevention (29) and in the differentiation of malignant cell lines (20, 21). Exploration of their role in the control of oncogene expression, though limited, suggests that retinoids may act at this level to regulate cell function by modulating the cellular pathways controlled by certain growth factors and their receptors. In studies by Jetten (85,86), retinoic acid has been shown in several cell systems to induce a nearly 10-fold increase in the number of available epidermal growth factor (EGF; transforming growth factor-α, TGF-α) receptors. The EGF receptor is partially encoded by the erb-B oncogene, and Earp et al. (87) have further shown that retinoic acid specifically enhances the synthesis of the mRNA for the EGF receptor.

Retinoids can have either a growth-stimulating or a growth-inhibitory effect, depending on the nature of EGF (TGF-α) receptor function for a particular cell line and the experimental conditions. When stimulation of the EGF receptor enhances proliferation, retinoic acid can stimulate cell proliferation, whereas when stimulation of the EGF receptor inhibits proliferation, retinoic acid has an inhibitory effect as well. These effects are highly concentration-dependent and occur typically at retinoic acid concentrations of 10^{-8} M or greater (88).

For rheumatoid synovial cells, retinoids antagonize the mitogenic effect of EGF and transforming growth factor β (TGF-β), as shown in studies by Brinkerhoff et al. (9,89). The complexity of such interactions is further demonstratred in studies by Roberts et al. (90) with c-myc-transformed Fischer rat 3T3 fibroblasts. Under normal conditions, these cells can be induced to grow and form colonies in soft agar by treatment with either EGF alone or by the combination of platelet-derived growth factor (PDGF) and TGF-β. Interestingly, retinoic acid is 100-fold more potent as a inhibitor of colony formation when a combination of PDGF and TGF-β is used to induce a colony growth, compared to its effect when EGF is used to stimulate colony growth.

There is also evidence that retinoid modulation of receptor expression/function and gene transcription may influence the generation and regulation of inflammatory or immune responses. For example, in the case of human monocytes and/or murine macrophages, receptor expression/function (e.g., the Fc receptor) on the cell membrane is modulated as a result of retinoid synergism with γ-interferon to induce tissue transglutaminase, an enzyme which induces crosslinking of membrane proteins (57,91). This effect is associated with suppression of monocytic cytostatic activation (57). Retinoic acid alone has been shown to induce rapid expression of the gene for transglutaminase in both normal and malignant monocytic cells (mouse peritoneal macrophages and human HL-60 cells) and to result in increased levels of transglutaminase in those cells (92-94).

Retinoic acid also suppresses the transcription of the gene for collagenase in human fibroblasts (95). Concurrently, the production of tissue inhibitor of metalloproteinase, a collagenase inhibitor, is upregulated (96). How these diverse effects might ultimately result in retinoid anti-inflammatory or immunosuppressive activities in vivo remains to be further explored.

Since retinoic acid can affect enzyme induction and also oncogene expression, the intracellular signals responsible for its action are of particular interest. Studies by Isakov and associates (97,98) have focused on the influence of some retinoids on protein kinase (PKC) activity, though the physiologic significance of these data is not clear at this time. For example, retinal, a retinoid whose only known function is in the visual cycle, inhibits T-lymphocyte PKC at 10^{-5} to 10^{-7} M by direct competition with phosphatidylserine (PS), while retinoic acid at high (non-physiologic) concentrations ($>10^{-5}$M) stimulates this same PKC by substituting for PS. It is difficult to attach biological significance to these observations since retinoic acid is known to antagonize the biological effects of phorbol esters (known activators of PKC) in a number of systems. Nevertheless, it remains possible that some retinoids may modulate T-lymphocyte-derived PKC activity, and perhaps T-cell function, via positive or negative cooperation with membrane phospholipids. The PKC effect appears to be dependent on both the concentration and structure of the particular retionid, e.g., retinol has no effect on PKC.

It is apparent from the foregoing discussion that retinoids can affect several cell functions which are critical to cellular activation and differentiation. The pivotal mechanism by which these effects are induced remains to be identified and may be related to the nature of the cell-specific recpetor. Nevertheless, the ultimate clinical expression of these effects is characterized by a concentration, schedule, and duration-dependent modulation of immune activity which can result in suppression of responses in some cases and enhancement of responses in others. Ultimately, the ability to use these agents clinically for immunoregulation in disease states will depend on a clearer understanding of their mechanism(s) of action.

C. Mechanisms Possibly Contributing to the Anti-Inflammatory Antirheumatic Activity of Retinoids

In vitro studies with intact inflammatory cells, i.e., ionophore-stimulated rat peritoneal macrophages (99), have shown that some anti-inflammatory retinoids (e.g., all-trans-retinoic acid and 13-*cis*-retinoic acid) at μM concentrations inhibit the conversion of arachidonic acid to proinflammatory eicosanoids via both the cyclooxygenase and the Δ^5 lipoxygenase pathways. These same retinoids also inhibit the production of PGE_2 by cultured rheumatoid synovial cells (100). 4-HPR, another anti-inflammatory retinoid, has been reported to inhibit PGE_2 production by confluent cultures of synovial cells from the joints of rats with SCW-and collagen-induced arthritis (10). Furthermore, monolayers of synovial cells from 4-HPR-treated arthritic rats (SCW-and collagen-induced) also produce less PGE_2 ex vivo than do monolayers from vehicle-treated control animals (10,11). In contrast, treatment with 13-*cis*-retinoic acid does not inhibit the ex vivo production of PGE_2 by synovial cells from rats with adjuvant-induced arthritis (8). Whether there is a relationship between the ex vivo/in vitro inhibitory effects of retinoids on arachidonic acid metabolism and the in vivo anti-inflammatory activity of retinoids remains to be determined. It is indeed possible that inhibitory effects on arachidonic acid metabolism may contribute to the anti-inflammatory activity of some retionoids but not to that of others.

Retinoids have also been shown to inhibit the production of collagenase by primary cultures of rheumatoid synovial cells and by later passages of rheumatoid synovial cells after stimulation with IL-1 (100). In addition, synovial cells isolated from the arthritic joints of rats with adjuvant-, collagen-, or SCW-induced arthritis that have been treated with retinoids produce less collagenase than do similar cells from vehicle-treated arthritic animals (8-11). Recent studies have demonstrated that freshly isolated synovial cells from rats with SCW-induced arthritis exhibit growth characteristics (such as anchorage-independent growth and lack of contact inhibition) usually associated with transformed cells. These abnormal growth patterns were reversed by retinoids (101).

Retinoids also inhibit the generation of chemotactic factors for neutrophils and possibly the diapedetic activity of these cells, and thus may inhibit their accumulation at sites of inflammation (102,103). The generation of reactive oxygen species is also suppressed (77,103).

Anti-inflammatory effects have also been seen in acne, psoriasis, and psoriatic arthropathy, as well as in other less common dermatologic conditions with a rheumatic component (described in section VII of this chapter). Effects associated with etretinate administration to patients with psoriasis include suppression of polymorphonuclear leukocyte antibody-dependent cell-mediated cytotoxicity (58) and normalization of increased chemotactic activity (2,102). These observations suggest a direct regulatory effect of etretinate on the abnormal granulocyte function in psoriasis.

Specific retinoid effects on immune function, assessed in various rodent arthritis models, also provide insights regarding the potential antirheumatic action of these agents. The observation that retinoids can exacerbate the development of adjuvant-and SCW-induced arthritis cannot be explained at this time. One could speculate, however, that a combination of retinoid immunoregulatory properties results in a shift towards apparent immune enhancement in the collagen-induced arthritis model. For example, IL-1 appears to play a more prominent role in the development of collagen arthritis, as reported by Phadke et al. (104) in their studies of the pathophysiology of various arthritis models. They observed that peritoneal macrophages from rats with collagen-induced arthritis spontaneously secrete about twice as much IL-1 as control rats and eight-fold more than those from rats with adjuvant arthritis. Since retinoic acid has been shown to enhance macrophage IL-1 production (105), this effect could contribute to exacerbation of collagen-induced arthritis.

In addition to the effect of retinoic acid on IL-1 production, lymphocytes and splenocytes from collagen arthritic rats spontaneously produce more IL-2 than do similar cells from adjuvant arthritic rats. Retinoid suppression of PGE_2 production may further enhance T-lymphocyte actions, since PGE_2 is not only proinflammatory but also immunoregulatory (106). Physiologic concentrations of PGE_2 (10^{-8} M), comparable to those found at inflammatory sites, have been shown to suppress most activated T-lymphocyte functions in vitro, including IL-2 production (107), the generation of cytotoxic T-lymphocytes (108), and antigenic stimulation (109). Furthermore, retinoic acid upregulates IL-2 receptor expression on activated human thymocytes, in association with enhanced blastogenic responses and significantly increased IL-2 dependent growth (110). However, peripheral blood lymphocytes are unaffected, suggesting that retinoic acid can affect only proliferating, activated blasts at restricted stages of development. These effects, in combination with the loss of PGE_2-negative feedback on IL-2 production may compound the enhancement of cellular immune responses by certain retinoids in collagen arthritis, and may provide an additional explanation for increased severity of this condition in retinoic acid-treated animals. It is important to note, however, that at least one retinoid-derivative, Ro 23-6457, can suppress developing collagen arthritis in mice (14).

Retinoid effects on cellular immune function have also been suggested by studies of passively transferred adjuvant arthritis in rats (111). This condition can be induced in naive rats by injection of sensitized spleen cells, provided the cells are further activated with concanavalin A. Treatment of rats receiving these sensitized cells with 13-*cis*-retinoic acid (starting 3 days prior to cell transfer and continuing for 19 days) suppresses the arthritis. When donor arthritic rats were treated instead, the passive arthritis is also suppressed, suggesting that retinoids may affect both induction and effector mechanisms (111).

VII. CLINICAL EXPERIENCE WITH RETINOID TREATMENT IN HUMAN DISEASES WITH AN INFLAMMATORY OR ARTHRITIS COMPONENT

Current reported human clinical experience with retinoid treatment of rheumatic conditions includes studies evaluating etretinate, Ro13-6298 (an arotinoid), and isotretinoin. Psoriatic arthropathy (1-7), Reiter's disease (112), rheumatoid arthritis (113), and various autoimmune or inflammatory skin diseases such as cutaneous lupus erythematosus (59), dystrophic epidermolysis bullosa (114), and cystic acne (115,116) have been studied. This clinical experience is summarized in Table 4 and includes observations regarding adverse drug effects, laboratory findings, and, in some cases, immune function studies.

A. Psoriatic Arthropathy

At least four clinical trials evaluating etretinate treatment for psoriatic arthropathy, and involving about 100 patients (1-5), have shown evidence of improvement in symptoms and signs as well as some parameters of inflammatory activity. These improvements are similar to those attained with nonsteroidal anti-inflammatory drug (NSAID) treatment.

In a 24-week, double-blind study comparing etretinate with ibuprofen, Hopkins and Bird evaluated 40 patients with psoriasis and psoriatic arthritis, 20 of whom received etretinate $\leq$0.5 mg/kg/day (3). Eleven of 20 patients completed 24 weeks of therapy with etretinate, but only one of 20 patients completed 24 weeks of therapy with ibuprofen alone. Statistically significant improvement was seen only for articular index at 16 weeks, and this beneficial effect was similar for both groups. Laboratory parameters also improved, but in the ibuprofen group only histidine increased, reflecting decreased disease activity, whereas in the etretinate-treated group there was a statistically significant decrease in erythrocyte sedimentation rate (ESR) and C-reactive protein (CRP), and a significant increase in hemoglobin and histidine, indicative of broader biochemical improvement in disease activity. Mucocutaneous dryness and slight elevations of cholesterol and triglycerides were the only adverse effects noted, but it is also important to note that etretinate, like vitamin A, is teratogenic. This study suggested the potential for antiarthritic activity of retinoids and encouraged continued evaluation of etretinate as well as other retinoid compounds and their derivatives in rheumatic conditions.

Open studies (1,2,4) have also suggested improvement in morning stiffness, as well as in numbers of swollen and painful joints, in psoriatic arthropathy treated with etretinate 0.5-1.0 mg/kg daily. Laboratory improvement also occurred with decreased ESR and CRP. In another study (1), further exploration of the specific immunological effects showed a relative decrease in T-lymphocytes, a relative increase in B-lymphocytes, and enhanced lymphocyte activation by concanavalin A.

A potent retinoid derivative, the arotinoid Ro13-6298, has also been evaluated in a pilot studies in more than 20 patients with severe psoriatic arthropathy unresponsive to nonsteroidal drugs (117-119). Because of potency demonstrated in animal models, this drug was administered at very low daily doses of 0.0005-0.01 mg/kg. Within 2-4 weeks clinical improvement occurred, characterized by a reduction in swelling and redness of the affected joints, an increase in joint mobility, a decrease in morning stiffness, and a substantial decrease in the daily dosage of analgesics. Radiological improvement was demonstrated by a decrease in the number of erosive and osteolytic bone lesions in two of 10 patients and a decrease in the number and intensity of bone scan foci in four of 10 patients. The ESR decreased in all patients. Two patients experienced a complete remission at 45 and 60 days, and in one patient remission was maintained for more than 6 months. Adverse effects were confined to modest mucocutaneous dryness without hair loss or skin fragility. No abnormalities of blood lipids, liver or renal function studies occurred.

B. Rheumatoid Arthritis

Only anecdotal and unpublished observations are available regarding clinical experience with retinoids and their derivatives in rheumatoid arthritis (113, 121,122). Efficacy in adjuvant and strep-cell wall animal models would suggest that 13-*cis*-retinoic acid or 4-HPR might be effective (8,9), and improvement in acne fulminans-associated arthritis (123) is also suggestive. However, the occasional occurrence during acne treatment of conditions characterized by immunological abnormalities, such as inflammatory bowel disease (124) and, rarely, arthritis and vasculitis (125,126), has discouraged further rheumatological evaluation of this agent.

In a recently published study of etretinate in rheumatoid arthritis (113), Hill et al. evaluated 15 patients with active rheumatoid arthritis, characterized by the presence of three of five criteria (tenderness of more than six joints, swelling of more than three joints, morning stiffness of more than 45 min, Ritchie articular index of >20, and ESR of >28 mm/hr). Six of 15 patients completed the study. Dropouts began to occur at week 4 with the majority dropping out by week 12, mainly because of mucocutaneous dryness and lack of efficacy. In the remaining patients, only joint circumfrence, sedimentation rate, hemoglobin, and sulfhydryl improved significantly. Total IgM also decreased.

A matrix of these parameters was constructed and compared to others developed previously for aspirin, aclofenac, *d*-penicillamine, and sodium aurothiomalate. The matrix for etretinate more closely resembled that for the nonsteroidal agents. These authors suggested that the dose of etretinate used,

Table 4 Clinical Experience with Retinoid Treatment of Rheumatic Conditions

Condition	Drug	Dose/duration	Design	# Patients	Clinical	Lab	ADEs	Ref.
Psoriatic arthropathy	Etretinate	0.5 mg/kg/d 24 wks	Double-blind vs. ibuprofen	20	11/20 completed imp. joints	↓ESR, CRP ↑Hgb.	Cheilitis, dry skin	3
	Etretinate	~30 mg 9d (20–45 mg) 13–24 wk	Open	13	11/13 completed ↓a.m. stiffness ↓Ritchie index	↑total T-cells ↑active T-cells ↑Con A blasts ↓B-cells ↓ESR	Mucocutaneous dryness	1
	Etretinate	1 mg/kg/d × 1 mo ~25 mg/d maint.	Open	20	"improved"	N.R.	"Acceptable"	2
	Etretinate	50 mg/d 24 wks	Open	40	26/40 completed ↓a.m. stiffness ↓no. of painful joints ↓no. of swollen joints	↓ESR	Mucocutaneous dryness	4
	Ro13-6298	0.5 to 1 μg/kg	Open (pilot)	12	↑joint mobility ↓swelling ↓a.m. stiffness	↓ESR	Pruritis-1/12 Cheilitis-3/12	117
	Ro13-6298	60 μg/day 12 wks	Open crossover to etretinate 50 mg/d	10	↑joint mobility ↓erythema ↑joint flexibility	↓ESR 2/10imp. X-ray	↑Transaminase-2/10 ↑triglyceride-1/10	118
Rheumatoid arthritis	Etretinate	1 mg/kg/d × 4 wks 0.5 mg/kg/d × 23 wks	Open-parallel group all on ibuprofen	15	6/15 completed ↓joint circumference trend towards ↓ joint index and ↑ grip strength (lack of efficacy 4/15)	↓IgM ↓ESR ↑Hgb	Mucocutaneous dryness pruritis 6/15 alopecia 2/15	113
Reiter's syndrome	Etretinate	0.75 mg/kg/d × 2 wks then 0.5–0.65 mg/kg × 10 wk	Double-blind placebo, with crossover to	60	53/60 completed skin lesions imp. "trend" to global point improvement	N.R.	Mucocutaneous dryness-70–100% headache-7%	112
Cutaneous lupus erythematosus	13-*cis*-retinoic acid	80 mg/d 16 wks	Open pilot	10	8/10 excellent ↓erythema ↓scaling ↓no. of lesions ↓scarring	↓skin inflammatory infiltrate ↓T-lymphocytes in skin	Mucocutaneous dryness sl. ↑triglyceride	59

1.0 mg/kg/day for 4 weeks, followed by 0.5 mg/kg/day for up to 20 weeks, might have been suboptimal, but in view of its limited tolerability further clinical trials were unwarranted. Other clinicians have observed suggestive indications of some efficacy at modestly tolerated doses of etretinate (121) and Ro13-6298 (122).

Phase I clinical trials of 4-HPR in normal volunteers (33) and in patients with severe psoriasis (19) or basal cell nevus syndrome (18), performed because of demonstrated efficacy in animal models of rheumatoid arthritis (9,11,12), were directed at eventual clinical development of this compound for treatment of rheumatoid arthritis. This program was apparently discontinued because of the development of skin and ophthalmic toxicity (128).

C. Reiter's Disease

The clinical symptoms of Reiter's disease, which include a psoriatic-like dermatitis, prompted the investigation by Lassus and associated in Finland of the potential efficacy of etretinate for the treatment of this condition (112). In a 12-week randomized study of etretinate versus placebo in 60 patients with documented Reiter's disease, patients were treated with etretinate, 0.75 mg/kg/day, during the first 2 weeks, with subsequent adjustments to 0.5-0.65 mg/kg/day. After 6 weeks of treatment with either placebo or active drug, all patients received etretinate. Since all patients improved during the study period, no statistically significant differences were seen, but the trend was in favor of etretinate (improvement in 50% placebo-treated, 76% placebo-etretinate, and 86% etretinate only).

D. Cutaneous Lupus Erythematosus

Cutaneous lupus erythematosus is often resistant to treatment with current therapies such as avoidance of sunlight exposure, and intralesional and topical corticosteroids. Recently, Newton and associates (59) described treatment of this disease with oral isotretinoin at a dose of 80 mg daily for 16 weeks. Eight of 10 patients treated experienced an excellent clinical response without significant side effects. Erythema and scaling decreased dramatically along with a decrease in the size and extent of the skin lesions, with total resolution of some skin lesions and minimal scarring. The only adverse experiences were mucocutaneous dryness and very slight elevations of serum triglycerides. Antinuclear antibody titers, if present before therapy, did not change. Dramatic improvement in the microscopic appearance of the skin lesions occurred, which was characterized by a reduction in the mononuclear inflammatory cell infiltrate, decreased hyperkeratosis, and a loss of characteristic dermoepidermal junction vacuolar interface changes.

Immunologically, no significant changes in mononuclear cell counts or in T4/T8 lymphocyte ratios were noted, but there was a striking decrease in the numbers of T-lymphocytes detectable at the dermoepidermal junction. These investigators considered isotretinoin to be effective short-term therapy for establishing rapid control in treatment-resistant lesions of cutaneous lupus erythematosus. Further studies are warranted.

E. Cystic Acne

13-*cis*-retinoic acid is dramatically effective in the treatment of several forms of severe acne. Efficacy was initially suggested by animal studies in which evidence of marked inhibition of sebaceous gland function was apparent, and, indeed, in patients treated with isotretinoin, sebum production is inhibited and sebaceous glands atrophy during treatment. Clinical studies (115,116) confirmed that this drug also exerts an anti-inflammatory effect, a property which may explain its efficacy in earlier stages of treatment.

Plewit and Wagner (115) studied the anti-inflammatory effects of isotretinoin specifically in 16 patients with various forms of severe cystic acne. They performed a patch test using 40% potassium iodide ointment under an occlusive dressing on the upper back, before and during treatment with isotretinoin. A statistically significant reduction in all inflammatory reaction parameters, including erythema, edema, and papule and pustule formation, was noted.

Subsequently, Holland et al. (116) evaluated the immune function of 13 acne patients being treated with 0.5 mg/kg/day of isotretinoin for 4 months. In all patients acne improved dramatically and, at 8 weeks there were statistically significant increases in T4 cells, immunoglobulins and, at 16 weeks in B-cells with surface immunoglobulin markers. There was no significant change in total T-cells or suppressor T-cells. However, these changes returned towards normal over the 4-month treatment period. Isolated occurrences of immunologically mediated conditions such as vasculitis (126,127) in patients receiving 13-*cis*-retinoic acid would suggest that a clinically significant change in immune function can be induced in a susceptible population of these patients.

F. Other Inflammatory Dermatoses

In recessive dystrophic epidermolysis bullosa, treatment with isotretinoin has been evaluated. Cooper and associates (114) evaluated three patients treated with low doses (approximately 0.4 mg/kg/day) and noted a significant reduction in the number of blistering lesions, while larger doses, up to 2 mg/kg/day, caused increased cutaneous fragility and a resultant poor response on that basis.

In other inflammatory or autoimmune skin diseases such as Behcet's syndrome, Duhring's disease, bullous pemphigoid with eosinophilia, and even necrotizing vasculitis with eosinophilia, treatment with etretinate 0.5-1 mg/kg/day resulted in improvement in skin lesions over a period of 1-3 weeks (129). In combination with prednisone, efficacy was even greater. Nevertheless, controlled clinical studies are needed to evaluate the potential therapeutic role that oral retinoids might play in these inflammatory dermatoses.

VIII. ADVERSE EFFECTS OF RETINOIDS

Retinoids have been defined as agents which bind to "retinoid receptors," for which retinol (vitamin A) or retinoic acid may be the prototypical ligands. Thus, a discussion of the hypervitaminosis A syndrome can provide important insights to facilitate an understanding of the adverse clinical effects of retinoids (130). Each new retinoid identified in preclinical investigations is screened to maximize the desired therapeutic effects and to minimize the toxic side effects. This therapeutic index is influenced by the changes in absorption, metabolism and tissue distribution which can occur secondary to changes in structure. The mode by which retinoids are transported in the plasma and are delivered to tissues can also contribute to the development of hypervitaminosis A toxicity.

For example, retinol is normally transported from the liver to peripheral tissues as a retinol • retinol binding protein (RBP) • transthyretin complex, and is apparently delivered to tissues in a controlled fashion via a specific interaction between the retinol-RBP complex and cell surface receptors. When retinol is present in unphysiologically large amounts, the transport capacity of the RBP system becomes saturated and the excess retinol/retinol ester becomes associated with other plasma proteins (mainly lipoproteins). As a result, retinol delivery to tissues is unregulated and can lead to retinol toxicity (130).

Unlike retinol, retinoic acid and a majority of the synthetic retinoids are transported in plasma bound to albumin and appear to enter cells from a small pool of free drug. This relatively unregulated mode of delivery may contribute to the observation that retinoic acid and some other synthetic retinoids produce hypervitaminosis A toxicity at lower doses than does retinol. While non-specific "membranolytic" effects of excess retinoid probably contribute to the symptoms of hypervitaminosis A toxicity, it is also likely that interactions with cytosolic retinol binding protein (CRBR), cellular retinoic acid binding protein (CRABP), and retinoic acid receptor (RAR) proteins, and subsequent activation of specific gene pathways are also involved. Furthermore, the observation that synthetic retinoids tend to bind to the cytosolic binding proteins for retinoic acid rather than those for retinol may also explain why many synthetic retinoids do not appear to interfere with normal vitamin A metabolism (131), except in subtle ways.

Acute toxicity can occur as a result of massive doses of retinol, natural retinol metabolites, and synthetic retinoids, but it is important to be aware that clinically significant toxicity occurs at single doses which are much greater than the cumulative dose required to produce chronic anorexia, headache, dizziness, fatigue, and irritability, followed within a few days by generalized skin desquamation. Physical findings include cheilitis, alopecia, hepatomegaly, splenomegaly, tenderness of the long bones, edema, and hemorrhagic manifestations. Neurologically, increased intracranial pressure is noted, at times associated with papilledema and changes in mentation. Calcium, alkaline phosphatase, and liver enzymes are elevated, and thrombocytopenia may occur.

In contrast, chronic retinoic toxicity can be manifest in virtually every organ system. Particularly important adverse effects include skin fragility and pruritis, alopecia, mucositis, papilledema, changes in vision (including poor night vision), hepatomegaly, at times leading to cirrhosis, muscle pain and cramps, paresthesias, arthralgias, and bone pain, with or without skeletal hyperostoses. Laboratory findings include elevation of liver enzymes, elevated alkaline phosphatase and serum calcium, and changes in lipoproteins, including elevated triglycerides. Changes in renal function may be manifested by the occurrence of edema and proteinuria with sterile pyuria (130,132).

The mechanism of these adverse effects is complex, related to the obvious multiplicity of metabolic effects of retinoids. Few studies have been performed to examine the mechanism of hypervitaminosis A toxicity. In one study by Hixson and Harrison (133), the effect of NSAID administration on retinoic acid toxicity in mice was evaluated to determine whether changes in prostaglandin metabolism influenced the occurrence of the skeletal adverse effects of retinoic acid. Mice receiving a toxic dose of retinoic acid (14 mg/kg i.p. daily for 21 days) were compared to mice receiving the same dose of retinoic acid with NSAID, (e.g., aspirin, ibuprofen, etc.) for 21 days. Seven of 20 mice receiving retinoic acid alone died, compared to three of 20 receiving retinoic acid with aspirin. Comparing the occurrence of fractures, the number of mice with three or more fractures was significantly greater in the retinoic acid alone group. In addition, there was less loss of body weight in the aspirin plus retinoic acid group. This study appears to support the possibility that the skeletal toxicity of retinoids is at least in part secondary to changes in prostaglandin synthesis.

Retinoids now in use clinically produce a range of these adverse effects at therapeutic doses (132,134). Thus, treatment with isotretinoin and etretinate, the only drugs approved and marketed, is reserved for severe forms of acne and pustular psoriasis, respectively, as well as disorders of keratinization. 4-Hydroxyphenyl retinamide, a retinoid derivative noted to have more specific anti-inflammatory and immunoregulatory effects, has apparently been removed from clinical trials because of the occurrence of night blindness and severe mucocutaneous toxicity during early clinical trials in both normal volunteers and patients with severe psoriasis and basal cell nevus syndrome (128). Thus, clinicians await the availability of retinoids with an improved therapeutic index.

IX. SUMMARY AND PERSPECTIVES

Isotretinoin and etretinate, drugs developed primarily for their efficacy in severe dermatological conditions, are the only retinoids currently marketed. Nevertheless, it is apparent from the preceding discussion that experiments performed with various retinoids have demonstrated outcomes highly suggestive of anti-inflammatory and immunomodulatory activity.

For this reason, intensive research programs are attempting to identify retinoids and derivative molecules with potent immunomodulatory and/or anti-inflammatory activity and decreased toxicity relative to the available retinoids. Based on studies from several laboratories, conflicting data have been obtained indicating both stimulatory and suppressive activities of various retinoid compounds, depending on the concentration, duration of incubation or exposure, and whether studies were in vivo or in vitro. In vivo effects are also influenced by route of administration and formulation. In addition, structure-activity relationships are likely. Because of these unique characteristics, the immunoregulatory activity of each new retinoid evaluated is potentially distinctive from other previously characterized molecules.

More than 1500 retinoid derivatives have been synthesized over the last several years and several of these are being screened in preclinical animal models designed to specifically identify anti-inflammatory and/or immunomodulatory activity, and to be able to separate these effects from the toxicity and teratogenicity. Several compounds are in late stages of preclinical evaluation (13,16), and the expectation is that at least one will become available clinically within the next few years.

REFERENCES

1. Rosenthal M, Ro 10-9359; an aromatic retinoid in the treatment of psoriatic arthritis. Drug Res 1982; 32 (II), Nr. 8:842–4.
2. Chieregato GC, Leoni A. Treatment of psoriatic arthropathy with etretinate: a two year follow-up. Acta Derm Venereol (Stockh) 1986; 66(4): 321–4.
3. Hopkins R, Bird HA, Jones H, Surrall KE, Astbury C, Miller A, Wright V. A double-blind controlled trial of etretinate (Tigason) and ibuprofen in psoriatic arthritis. Ann Rheum Dis 1985; 44:189–93.
4. Klinkoff AV, Gertner E, Chambers A, Gladman DD, et al. Pilot study of etretinate in psoriatic arthritis. J. Rheum 1989; 16:789–91.
5. Stollenwerk R, Fischer-Hoinkers H, Komenda K, Schilling F. Clinical observations in oral retinoid therapy for psoriatic arthropathy, (Ro 10-9359) In: Orafanos et al. (ed.). Retinoids. New York: Springer-Verlag, 1980: 205–209.
6. Rosenthal M. Retinoid in der behandlung vor psoriasis-arthritis. Schweiz Med Wschr 1979; 109:1912–4.
7. Bitter T, Bahous I, Rosenthal M. All-trans retinoic acid (R): a remission aim in the treatment of psoriatic arthritis (PA). Ann Rheum Dis 1981; 40:209.
8. Brinckerhoff CE, Coffey JW, Sullivan AC. Inflammation and collagenase production in rats with adjuvant arthritis reduced with 13-cis-retinoic acid. Science 1983; 221:756–8.
9. Brinckerhoff CE, Sheldon LA, Benoit MC, Burgess DR, Wilder RL. Effect of retinoids on rheumatoid arthritis, a proliferative and invasive non-malignant disease. In: Retinoids, differentiation and disease. Ciba Foundation Symposium 1985; 113:191–211.
10. Trentham DE, Brinckerhoff CE. Augmentation of collagen arthritis by synthetic analogues of retinoic acid. J. Immunol 1982; 129:2668–72.
11. Haraoui B, Wilder RL, Allen JB, Sporn MB, Helfgott RK, Brinkerhoff CE. Dose-dependent suppression by the synthetic retinoic, 4-hydroxyphenyl retinamide, of streptococcal cell wall-induced arthritis in rats. Int J Immunopharmac 1985; 7:903–16.
12. Fisher C, Persico F. Fenretinide [N-(4-hydroxyphenyl retinamide) 4-HPR] as an effective inhibitor of adjuvant arthritis in the Lewis female rat. Arth Rheum 1985; 28:S70.
13. Faherty D, Weissbach A, Rosenberger M, Benjamin W, Devens B. Activity of a novel immunomodulatory compound in murine models of skin transplantation and autoimmune disease. FASEB J 1988; 2:A910.
14. Sedgwick A. Personal communication.
15. Wahl S. Personal communication.
16. Hanglow AC, Rosenberger M, Lovey AJ, Nemzek R, Welton AF, Coffey JW. Antiinflammatory and immunoregulatory effects of novel

retinoid-like 2, 4, 6, 8 nonatetraenoic acids in adjuvant arthritis. Agents and Actions 1989; 27:347–50.

17. Harris E. Retinoid therapy for rheumatoid arthritis. Ann Intern Med 1984; 100:146–7.
18. Kaiser-Kupfer MI, Peck GL, Caruso RC, Jaffe MJ, DiGiovanna JJ, Gross EG. Abnormal retinal function associated with fenretinide, a synthetic retinoid. Arch Ophthalmol 1986; 104:69–70.
19. Kingston TP, Lowe NJ, Winston J, Heckenlively J. Visual and cutaneous toxicity which occurs during N-(4-hydroxyphenyl) retinamide therapy for psoriasis. Clin Exp Dermatol 1986; 11:624-7.
20. Sporn MB, Dunlop NM, Newton DL, Henderson WR. Relationships to structure and activity of retinoids. Nature 1976; 263:110–3.
21. Mayer H, Bollag W, Hanni R, Reugg R. Retinoids, a new class of compounds with prophylactic and therapeutic activities in oncology and dermatology. Experientia 1978; 34:1105–19.
22. Sporn MB, Roberts AB. Introduction: what is a retinoid? In: Retinoids. Differentiation and disease. Ciba Found Symp 1985; 113:1–5.
23. Sporn MB, Roberts AB, Roche NS, Kagechika H, Shudo K. Mechanism of action of retinoids. J Am Acad Dermatol 1986; 15:756–64.
24. Frickel F. Chemistry and physical properties of retinoids. In: Sporn MB., et al, eds. The Retinoids. Academic Press, Vol. 1. Orlando: 1984: 7–145.
25. Sporn MB, Roberts AB. Biological methods of analysis and assay of retinoids. In: Sporn MB, et al. eds. The Retinoids. Academic Press, Vol. 1. Orlando:1984: 235–79.
26. Stephens-Jarnagin A, Miller DA, Deluca HF. Growth supporting activity of a retinoidal benzoic acid derivative and 4,4-difluororetinoic acid. Arch Biochem Biophys 1985; 237:11–6.
27. Eckert RL, Green H. Cloning of cDNAs specifying vit. A-responsive human keratins. Proc Natl Acad Sci USA 1984; 81:4321–5.
28. Lotan R. Effects of vit. A and its analogs (retinoids) on normal and neoplastic cells. Biochim Biophys Acta 1980; 605:33–91.
29. Dillehay DL, Li W, Kalin J, Walia AS, Lamon E. In vitro effects of retinoids on murine thymus-dependent and thymus-independent mitogenesis. Cell Immunol 1987; 107:130–7.
30. Allen JG, Bloxham DP. The pharmacology and pharmacokinetics of retinoids. Pharmacol Ther. Submitted, 1988.
31. Lucek RW, Colburn WA. Clinical pharmacokinetics of the retinoids. Clin Pharmacokin. 1985; 10:38–62.
32. Paravicini U, Busslinger A. Etretinate and isotretinoin, two retinoids with different pharmacokinetic profiles. In: Cunliffe WJ, Miller AJ, eds. Retinoid Therapy. Lancaster: MTP Press, 1984: 11–23.
33. Disaraju RK, Scott V, Nayak RK, Minn FL. The pharmacokinetics of fenretinide in healthy volunteers. Clin Pharmacol Ther 1985; 37:190 (B33).

34. Vahlquist A. Etretinate pharmacokinetics in chronic renal failure. Dermatologica 1987; 175:224–8.
35. Bradshaw D, Cashin CH, Kennedy AJ. Further studies on the anti-inflammatory effects of retinoids. In: Saurat JH, ed. Retinoids: new trends in research and therapy. Basel: Karger, 1985: 204–18.
36. Coffey JW, Fiedler-Nagy C, Weisman SM, Woodworth TG, Welton AF. Retinoids as potential anti-rheumatic agents. In: Chemistry and biology of synthetic retinoids. Dawson N, Okamura Y, eds. Boca Raton: CRC Press, 1988.
37. Zwillich SH, Lipsky PE. Molecular mimicry in the pathogenesis of rheumatic diseases. In: Pathogenesis of chronic inflammatory arthritis, rheumatic disease clinics of NA. 1987; 13: 339–52.
38. Yocum DE, Allen JB, Wahl SM, Calandra GB, Wilder RL. Inhibition by cyclosporine A of streptococcal cell wall-induced arthritis and hepatic granulomas in rats. Arth Rheum 1986; 129:262–73.
39. Trentham DE, Townes AS, Kang AH. Autoimmunity to type II collagens: an experimental model of arthritis. J Exp Med 1977; 146:857–68.
40. Kaibara N, Hotokebuchi T, Takagishi K, Katsuki I. Paradoxical effects of cyclosporine A on collagen arthritis in rats. J Exp Med 1983; 158: 2007–15.
41. Kaibara N, Hotokebuchi T, et al. Pathogenic difference between collagen arthritis and adjuvant arthritis. J Exp Med 1984; 159:1388–96.
42. Phadke K, Carrol J, Nanda S. Effects of various anti-inflammatory drugs on type II collagen-induced arthritis in rats. Clin Exp Immunol 1982; 47:579–86.
43. Lewis AJ, Carlson RP, Chang, J.Experimental models of inflammation. In: Bonta IL, Bray MA, Parnham MJ. eds. The pharmacology of inflammation. Amsterdam: Elsevier, 1985: 371–97.
44. Yamaki K, Nakagawa H, Tsuruhiki S. Inhibitory effect of antiinflammatory drugs on type II collagen-induced arthritis in rats. Ann Rheum Dis 1987; 46:543–48.
45. Borel JF, Feurer C, Gubla HU, Stahelin H. Biological effects of cyclosporin A: a new anti-lymphocytic agent. Agents and Actions 1976; 6: 468–75.
46. Arrigoni-Martelli E, Bramm E. Investigations on the influence of cyclophosphamide, gold sodium thiomalate and D-penicillamine on mystatin edema and adjuvant arthritis. Agents and Actions 1975; 5:264–67.
47. Mountz JD, Smith HR, Wilder RL, Reeves JP, Steinberg AD. CsA therapy in MRL lpr/lpr mice: amelioration of immunopathology despite autoantibody production. J Immunol 1987; 138:157–63.
48. Smith HR, Chused TM, Steinberg AD. Cyclophosphamide-induced changes in the MRL-lpr/lpr mouse: effects on cellular composition, immune function and disease. Clin Immunol Immunopathol 1984; 30: 51–61.

49. Medowar PB, Hunt R. Anti-cancer action of retinoids. Immunology 1981; 42:349-53.
50. Saffiotti U, Montesano R, Sellakumar R, Borg SA. Experimental cancer of the lung. Inhibition by vitamin A of the induction of tracheobronchial squamous metaplasia and squamous cell tumors. Cancer 1967; 20: 857-64.
51. Cohen BE, Cohen IK. Vitamin A: adjuvant and steroid antagonist in the immune response. J Immunol 1973; 111:1376-80.
52. Bollag W. Prophylaxis of chemically-induced benign and malignant epithelial tumor by vitamin A acid. Eur J Cancer 1972; 8:689-93.
53. Dennert G, Lotan R. Effects of retinoic acid on the immune system: stimulation of T-killer cell induction. Eur J Immunol 1978; 8:23-9.
54. Sporn MB. Vitamin A and its analogues (retinoids) in cancer prevention. In: Winnick M, ed. Nutrition and cancer. New York: Wiley, 1977: 119-50.
55. Barnett JB. Immunopotentiation of the IgE antibody response by 13-cis retinoic acid. Int. Arch Allergy Appl Immunol 1982; 67:287-90.
56. Barnett JB. Immunomodulating effects of 13-*cis*-retinoic acid on the IgE response of BALB/C mice. Int Arch Allergy Appl. Immunol 1982; 69:368-73.
57. Mehta K, Claringbold P, Lopez-Berestein G. Suppression of macrophage cytostatic activation by serum retinoids: a possible role for transglutaminase. J Immunol 1987; 138:3902-06.
58. Ellis CN, Kang S, Grekin RC, LoBuglio AF, Vorhees JJ. Etretinate therapy for psoriasis: reduction of antibody-dependent cell-mediated cytotoxicity of polymorphonuclear leukocytes. Arch Dermatol 1985; 121:877-80.
59. Newton RC, Jorizzo JL, Solomon AR, Sanchez RL, Daniels JC, Bell JD, Cavallo T. Mechanism-oriented assessment of isotretinoin in chronic or subacute cutaneous lupus erythematosus. Arch Dermatol 1986; 122: 170-6.
60. Dennert G. Retinoids and the immune system: immunostimulation by vitamin A. In: The Retinoids. Vol. 2. Orlando: Academic Press, 1984; 373-90.
61. Shapiro PE, Edelson RL. Effects of retinoids on the immune system. In: Saurat JH, ed. Retinoids: new trends in research and therapy. Basel: Karger, 1985: 225-35.
62. Nauss KM. Influence of vitamin A status on the immune system. In: Bauernfeind JC, ed. Vitamin A deficiency and its control. 1986: 207-43.
63. Brown KH, Rajan MM, Clakraborty J, Aziz KMA. Failure of a large dose of vitamin A to enhance antibody response to tetanus toxoid in children. Am J Clin Nutr 1980; 33:212-17.

64. Katz KR, Drzymala M, Turton JA, Hicks RM, Hunt R, Palmer L, Malkovsky M. Regulation of accessory cell function by retinoids in murine immune responses. Br J Exp Pathol 1987; 68:343–50.
65. Katz DR, Mukherjee S, Maisey J, Miller K. Vitamin A acetate as a regulator of accessory cell functions in delayed-type hypersensitivity responses. Int Arch Allergy Appl. Immunol 1987; 82:53–6.
66. Colizzi V, Malkovsky M. Augmentation of interleukin-2 production and delayed hypersensitivity in mice infected with mycobacterium bovis and fed a diet-supplemented with vitamin A acetate. Infect Immunol. 1985; 48:581–83.
67. Malkovsky M, Edwards AJ, Hunt R, Palmer L, Medowar DB. T-cell-mediated enhancement of host-versus-graft reactivity in mice fed a diet enriched with vitamin A acetate. Nature 1983; 302:338–40.
68. Lotan R, Dennert G. Stimulatory effects of vitamin A analogues on induction of cell-mediated cytotoxicity in vivo. Cancer Res 1979; 39: 55–8.
69. Sidell N, Famatiga E, Shau H, Golub SH. Immunological aspects of retinoids in humans: III Effects of retinoic acid on the natural killing of tumor cells. J Bio Resp Mod 1985; 4:240–50.
70. Sidell N, Famatiga E, Golub SH. Augmentation of human thymocyte proliferative responses by retinoic acid. Exp Cell Biol. 1981; 49:239–45.
71. Sidell N, Rieber P, Golub SH. Immunological aspects of retinoids in humans. I. Analysis of retinoic acid enhancement of thymocyte responses to PHA. Cell Immunol 1984; 87:118–25.
72. Sidell N, Famatiga E, Golub SH. Immunological aspects of retinoids in humans: II. Retinoic acid enhances induction of hemolytic plaque-forming cells. Cell Immunol 1984; 88:374–81.
73. Moriguchi S, Jackson JC, Watson RR. Effects of retinoids on human lymphocyte functions in vitro. Human Toxicol 1985; 4:365–78.
74. Watson RR, Jackson JC, Alberts DS, Hicks MJ. Cellular immune functions of adults treated with a daily, long term, low-dose of 13-*cis*-retinoic acid. J Leuk Biol 1986; 39:567–77.
75. Holland DB, Gowland G, Cunliffe WJ. Inflammatory responses in acne patients treated with 13-*cis*-retinoic acid. Br J Dermatol 1984; 110:343–5.
76. Soppi A, Soppi E, Eskola J, Jansen CT. Cell-mediated immunity in Darier's disease: effect of systemic retinoid therapy. Br J Derm 1982; 106:140–52.
77. Yoshioka A, Miyachi Y, Imamura S, Niwa Y. Anti-oxidant effects of retinoids on inflammatory skin diseases. Arch Dermatol Res 1986; 278:177–83.

78. Lazzini C, Trevisan G, deLuyk S, Manglarotti M. Evaluation of lymphocyte subpopulations with monoclonal antibodies in five psoriatic patients treated with etretinate. La Ricerca Clin Lab 1984; 14:323–5.
79. Chytil F and Ong DE. Cellular retinoid binding proteins. In: Sporn MB, Roberts AB, and Goodman DS, eds. The Retinoids, Vol. 2, Orlando: Academic Press, 1984; 89–123.
80. Petkovich M, Brand N, Krust A, Chambon R. A human retinoic acid receptor which belongs to the family of nuclear receptors. Nature 1987; 330:444–50.
81. Giguere V, Ong ES, Sequi P, Evans RM. Identification of a receptor for the morphogen retinoic acid. Nature 1987; 330:624–9.
82. Brand N, Petkovich M, Krust A, Chamborn P, DeThe H, Marchio A, Tiollas P, Dejean A. Identification of a second human retinoic acid receptor. Nature 1988; 332:850–3.
83. Krust A, Kastner Ph, Petkovich M, Zelent A, Chambon P. A third retinoic acid receptor, hRAR-γ. Proc Natl Acad Sci (USA) 1989; 86:5310–4.
84. Hashimoto Y, Kagechika H, Kawachi E, Shudo K. Specific Uptake of retinoids into human promyelocytic cells HL-60 by retinoid-specific protein: possibly the true retinoid receptor. Jpn J Cancer Res (Gann) 1988; 79:473–83.
85. Jetten AM, Retinoids and their modulation of cell growth. In: Guroff G, ed. Growth and maturation factors. Vol. 3. New York: Wiley, 1985; 3:252–93.
86. Jetten AM. Effects of retinoic acid on the binding and mitogenic activity of epidermal growth factor. J Cell Physiol 1982; 110:234–40.
87. Earp HS, Lee LW, Raymond VW. EGF and retinoic acid stimulate EGF receptor biosynthesis. J Cell Biochem 1986; Suppl. 10C:12.
88. Roberts AB, Sporn MB. Transforming growth factors. Cancer Surveys 1985; 4:683–705.
89. Brinckerhoff CE. Morphologic and mitogenic responses of rabbit synovial fibroblasts to transforming growth factor-β requires transforming growth factor-α or epidermal growth factor. Arth Rheum 1983; 26: 1370–7.
90. Roberts AB, Roche NS, Sporn MB. Selective inhibition of the anchorage-independent growth of myc-transfected fibroblasts by retinoic acid. Nature 1985; 315:237–9.
91. Mehta K, Lopez-Berestein G, Moore WT, Davies PJA. Interferon-γ requires serum retinoids to promote the expression of tissue transglutaminase in cultured human blood monocytes. J Immunol 1985; 134:2053–6.
92. Moore WT, Murtaugh MP, Davies PJA. Retinoic acid-induced expression of tissue transglutaminase in mouse peritoneal macrophages. J Biol Chem 1984; 259:12794–802.

93. Chiocia, EA, Davies PJA, Stein JP. The molecular basis of retinoic action. J Biol Chem 1988; 263:11584–9.
94. Davies PJA, Murtaugh PM, Moore WT, johnson GS, Lucas D. Retinoic acid-induced expression of tissue transglutaminase in human promyelocytic leukemia (HL-60) cells. J Biol Chem 1985; 260:5166–74.
95. Brinckerhoff CE, Plucinska IM, Sheldon LA, O'Connor GT. Half-life of synovial cell collagenase mRNA is modulated by phorbol myristate acetate, but not all-trans-retinoic acid or dexamethasone. Biochemistry 1986; 25:6378–84.
96. Clark SD, Kobayashi DK, Welgus HG. Regulation of the expression of tissue inhibitor of metalloproteinase and collagenase by retinoids and glucocorticoids in human fibroblasts. J Clin Invest 1987; 80: 1280–8.
97. Isakov N. Regulation T-cell-derived of protein kinase C-activity by vitamin A derivatives. Cell Immunol 1988; 115:288–98.
98. Isakov N, Mally MI, Scholz W, Altman A. T-lymphocyte activation: The role of protein kinase C and the bifurcating inositol phosphate signal transduction pathway. Immunol Rev 1987; 95:89–111.
99. Fiedler-Nagy C, Wittreich BH, Georgiadis A, Hope WC, Welton AF, Coffey JW. Comparative study of natural and synthetic retinoids as inhibitors of arachidonic acid release and metabolism in rat peritoneal macrophages. Dermatologica 1987; 175 (suppl.1), 81–92.
100. Brinckerhoff CE, McMillan RM, Dayer JM, Harris ED. Inhibition by retinoic acid of collagenase production in rheumatoid synovial cells. N Engl J Med 1980; 303:432–6.
101. Yocum DE, Lafyatis R, Remmers EF, Schumacher HR, Wilder RL. Hyperplastic synoviocytes from with streptococcal-cell wall-induced arthritis exhibit a transformed phenotype that is thymic-dependent and retinoid inhibitable. Am J Path 1988, 132:38–48.
102. Ellis CN, Kang S, Grekin RC, Vorhees JJ, Silva J. Etretinate therapy reduces polymorphonuclear leukocyte chemotaxis-enhancing properties of psoriatic serum. J Am Acad Derm 1985; 13:437–43.
103. Camisa C, Eisenstat B, Ragaz A, Weissman G. The effects of retinoids on neutrophil functions in vitro. J Am Acad Derm 1982; 6:620–9.
104. Phadke K, Carlson DG, Gritter BD, Butler LD. Role of IL-1 and IL-2 in rat and mouse arthritis models. J Immunol 1986; 136:4085–91.
105. Trechsel V, Evequoz V, Flersch H. Stimulation of interleukin I and interleukin III production by retinoic acid in vitro. Biochem J 1985; 230:339–46.
106. Goodwin JS. Immunologic effects of non-steroidal anti-inflammatory drugs. Am J Med 1984; 77(48):7–15.
107. Rappaport RS, Dodge GR. Prostaglandin E_2 inhibits the production of human interleukin-2. J Exp Med 1982; 155:943–8.

108. Leung KH, Mihich E. Prostaglandin modulation of development of cell-mediated immunity in culture. Nature 1980; 288:597–06.
109. Muscoplat CC, Klausner DJ, Brunner CJ, Sloane ED, Johnson DW. Regulation of mitogen and antigen-stimulated lymphocyte blastogenesis by prostaglandin. Infect Immunol 1979; 26:311–5.
110. Sidell N, Ramsdell F. Retinoic acid upregulates interleukin-2 receptors on activated human thymocytes. Cell Immunol 1988; 115:299–309.
111. Weissman SM, Nemzek RD, Anderson CM, Coffey JW. One retinoid treatment alters the development of arthritis by the transfer of spleen cells from rats with adjuvant arthritis. Arth Rheum 1987; 30:566.
112. Lassus A, Eskelinin A, Saila K, Koenoenen M, Lauharanta J. Treatment of Reiter's disease with etretinate. In: Saurat JH, ed. Retinoids: new trends in research and therapy. Basel: Karger, 1985; 391–6.
113. Hill J, Bird HA, Sitton NG, Dixon JS, Miller A. A clinical and biochemical evaluation of etretinate in rheumatoid arthritis. J Rheum Internat 1988; 8(2):55–9.
114. Cooper TW, Tabas M, Bauer EA. Retinoic acid in recessive dystrophic epidermolysis bullosa. In: Saurat JH, ed. Retinoids: new trends in research and therapy. Basel: Karger, 1985; 219–224.
115. Plewig G, Wagner A. Anti-inflammatory effects of 13-*cis* retinoic acid. Arch Derm Res 1981; 270:89–94.
116. Holland DG, Gowland G, Cunliffe WJ. Inflammatory responses in acne patients treated with 13-*cis* retinoic acid (isotretinoin). Br J Dermatol 1984; 110:343–5.
117. Fritsch P, Rauschmeier W, Neuhofer J. Response of psoriatic arthropathy to arotinoid (RO13-6298): a pilot study. In: Cunliffe WJ, Miller AJ, eds. Retinoid Therapy. Lancaster: MTP Press, Ltd., 1984; 328–33.
118. Tsambos D, Orfanos CE. Antipsoriatic activity of a new synthetic retinoid, the arotinoid Ro13-6298. Arch Dermatol 1983; 119:746–51.
119. Fritsch P, Rauschmeier W, Zussner C. Arotinoid in psoriatic arthropathy. In: Saurat JH, ed. Retinoids: new trends in research and therapy. Basel: Karger, 1984: 384–90.
120. Lieciewicz J. Pers. commun.
121. Cziernetski, D. Pers. commun.
122. Klinkoff, A. Pers. commun.
123. Darley CR, Currey HLF, Baker H. Acne fulminans with arthritis in identical twins treated with isotretinoin. Royal Soc Med 1984; 77:328–30.
124. Accutane package insert, Hoffmann-La Roche, Inc.
125. Matsuoka L, Wortsman J, Pepper J. Acute arthritis during isotretinoin treatment for acne. Arch Intern Med 1984; 144:1870–1.
126. Epstein E, McNutt S, Beallo R, Thyberg W, Brody R, Hirsch A, LaBraico J. Severe vasculitis in two young men treated for acne with 13-*cis* retinoic acid. Arch Derm 1987; 123:1123–5.

127. Dwyer JM, Kenizer K, Thompson Taylor B, Chen D, Labraico J, Schiefferdecker R, Winkelmann RK. Vasculitis and Retinoids. The Lancet, 1989; Vol II, 494–6.
128. Venuti MC. Therapeutic approaches to rheumatoid arthritis and other autoimmune diseases. Annu Rep Med Chem 1986; 21:201–10.
129. Orfanos CE, Bauer R. Evidence of anti-inflammatory activities of oral synthetic retinoids: experimental findings in clinical experience. Br J Dermatol 1983; 109:55–60.
130. Silverman AK, Ellis CN, Vorhees JJ. Hypervitaminosis A syndrome: a paradigm of side effects. J Am Acad Dermatol 1987; 16:1027–39.
131. Goodman DS. Vitamin A and retinoids in health and disease. N Engl J Med 1984; 310:1023–31.
132. Kamm JJ, Ehmann CW, Ashenfelter KO. Preclinical and clinical toxicology of selected retinoids. In: Sporn MB, et al, eds. The Retinoids. Vol. 2. Orlando: Academic Press, 1984; 287–325.
133. Hixson EJ, Harrison SD. Effect of nonsteroidal anti-inflammatory drugs on the sublethal retinoic acid toxicity in Swiss mice. Biochem Pharm 1981; 30:1714–16.
134. Morison WL. Etretinate and psoriasis. Arch Dermatol 1987; 123:879–81.
135. Ney U, Ball IJ, Hill RP, Westmacott D, Bloxham DP. Anti-inflammatory effects of synthetic retinoids may be related to their immunomedulatory action, Dermatologica 1987; 175(suppl.1):93–9.

5

Apheresis

Steven Weiner
Olive View Medical Center and UCLA School of Medicine, Los Angeles, California

Harold E. Paulus
UCLA School of Medicine, Los Angeles, California

I. INTRODUCTION

Apheresis (from the Greek *aphairesis*, meaning "to take away") has been defined by John Klippel (1) as (a) removal of a component of the blood from the intravascular circulation; (b) a word termination denoting removal of the word stem to which it is affixed, as in plasmapheresis, leukapheresis, or cryapheresis.

The natural history of any new therapeutic approach may be divided into three phases. The first is the honeymoon period, when great enthusiasm for the use of the approach is shown. The second, a backlash-downswing, is a reaction to the disappointment that occurs when the initial, often unrealistic hopes and aspirations for the therapy have not been met. The third phase occurs when the therapy takes its appropriate place based on at least a modicum of controlled data. Apheresis had a meteoric rise in popularity at the time of its introduction as a treatment for rheumatic and immunologically mediated disorders during the mid-1970s (1-4). Over the next decade apheresis was used to treat over 150 diseases with results ranging from spectacular to abysmal (1-8). Unrealistic expectations, lack of controlled studies leading to misuse and overuse, and cost considerations resulted in the end of the first phase and the start of the second. We are now entering the third phase whereupon apheresis will assume a realistic place in the therapeutic armamentarium for the treatment of rheumatic diseases. This third phase of evolution was brought on by a number of developments.

First, apheresis has clear benefit against certain rheumatic diseases in certain situations. However, one can no longer assume the effectiveness of apheresis in all rheumatic diseases. Rather, one must determine the subsets in which it may work best and the factors that may be predictive of both positive and negative responses. Second, as rheumatological therapeutics follow oncologic therapeutics toward more complex regimens, it may become appropriate to combine treatment approaches into induction, consolidation, and maintenance regimens in which apheresis may play a selective role. Third, industry research and development in apheresis equipment and software has reduced its formerly prohibitive costs; further improved technology has added new dimensions to the potential accomplishments of apheresis. Last, as an age of specific immunotherapy begins, apheresis can help to implement such therapies. For example, it can be used to remove clonal cell populations, treating and altering them ex vivo and then reinfusing them.

Apheresis is therefore a therapeutic modality with an enlarging but more specific scope of application (9). Initial use of apheresis in immune-mediated glomerulonephritis (10) had suggested its application to rheumatic disorders. Technical improvements have made apheresis safe, rapid, and easy to perform, and its role as an immune modulator has been demonstrated (11). In the future, apheresis may play an integral role in rheumatic disease therapeutics (Table 1).

II. HISTORICAL DEVELOPMENT

The concept of apheresis was already inherent in the ancient Greek belief in evil humors and the value of purging or cleansing of a diseased system (13, 14). Again, the Greek word aphairesis means "to remove" or "to take away." Application of the Greek concept of removing evil humors led to the removal of noxious substances by purgation, often with drastic laxatives, induction of vomiting by certain herbs, or, even more dramatically, by bloodletting. Bloodletting was often done to such an extreme that it may have caused the deaths of the French king, Louis XIII, and our first president, George Washington (13,15,16). The reasons for bloodletting were much the same 300 years ago as the current indications for apheresis (16):

Table 1 Ready Reference Guide

	Thoracic duct	Plasmapheresis	Lympho-plasmapherisis	Special
Rheumatoid arthritis	2,21,65–70	5,71,81–85,90, 93,94,91,92[b]	72–77 78–80[b]	95–97
Systemic lupus erythematosus	137	109,111,112 114–136		138,139 141[a]
Vasculitis				
Small-vessel		143–149		
Medium-vessel		146,150,151, 15?	153	
Scleroderma				
Raynauds		179 (82,187)[b]		
Generalized	178	188–193, (194)[b]		
Cryoglobulinemia		179–181		
Myositis				
Poly- and dermatomyositis		220–224	223	
Juvenile dermatomyositis		217–219		
Juvenile rheumatoid arthritis		5,225		
Psoriatic arthritis		5		
Behçet's disease		226		
Scleromyxedema		227		
MCTD		222		

[a]Cryoapheresis, synchronization, immunoadsorption, etc.
[b]Controlled trials.

> It eliminates rheumatic ailments, warms the marrow, promotes digestion, cleans the mind, dries up the brain, cures various sicknesses and makes the urine clean and clear (17).

Robert Boyle in 1666 refined these concepts by suggesting that sick dogs might be cured by removing blood and exchanging it for the blood of a healthy dog (18). However, he could not decide if blood removal or replacement was the beneficial technique. Haden began the modern investigation of apheresis in 1902, when he bled rabbits and returned their washed red blood cells (RBCs) in artificial serum (12). Able and associates were the first to describe plasma removal with or without replacement with physiological solutions in humans. Able was also the first to use the term "plasmapheresis" but had little enthusiasm for the tremendous amount of effort and time involved (19). Modern plasmapheresis technique was first applied in 1960 by Schwab and Fahey in the treatment of Waldenstrom's macroglobulinemia and its complicating hyperviscosity syndrome (20). Plasma was manually removed and replaced with crystalloid solutions, thereby significantly lowering plasma viscosity.

The first machines to improve the efficiency of apheresis were developed to harvest white blood cells (WBCs).

The use of therapeutic apheresis in rheumatic disorders stems from work done using the technique of thoracic duct drainage (21). With thoracic duct drainage the thoracic duct was surgically cannulated, lymph drained (largely T lymphocytes), cells removed by centrifiguation, and then lymph reinfused (2,21). Huge numbers of lymphocytes were removed—5 X 1010 lymphocytes daily—10 times as many as were removed in more modern lymphocytapheresis studies. Excellent responses in rheumatoid arthritis (RA) and systemic lupus erythematosus (SLE) were noted with this technique (22,23). Thoracic duct drainage involved a surgical procedure and therefore had an attendant surgical risk, could not be repeated, and required prolonged hospitalization. Therapeutic plasma exchange and lymphocytapheresis, outgrowths of thoracic duct drainage, do not require an initial surgical procedure (though they may require a vascular access procedure) and allow more flexibility in the decision of what to remove and, consequently, what to replace (9,16,23-25). Clinical benefits may be seen with removal of 5 X 109 lymphocytes—far fewer than were removed by thoracic duct drainage (71,79).

III. TECHNICAL ASPECTS AND MECHANISMS OF ACTION

The technology of apheresis is an outgrowth of the technology of blood banking. In 1878 a Swedish inventor, De Laval, designed and patented the first open, continuous-flow centrifuge to separate cream and revolutionized the dairy industry (26). During World War II the dramatically increased need for plasma was met by Edwin J. Cohn by adapting De Laval's centrifuge to separate plasma from whole blood (26). Subsequently, Cohn became interested in the concept that blood would last longer if stored as its component parts. In 1949, he developed a machine to rapidly separate blood at low gravitational force as it passed through a closed system—Cohn's fractionator. By 1959, growing interest in separation and transfusion of WBCs stimulated new developments in cell separation. However, the modern technology of cell separation may stem from a collaboration between International Business Machines (IBM) and the National Cancer Institute (NCI) (26). A senior engineer at IBM (Judson) had a son with acute leukemia. He would bring his son weekly to NCI for cytodepletion. This process was arduous for both patient and technician. Judson at IBM and Freireich at NCI collaborated to develop three machines to simplify cytodepletion: a machine that automatically fractionated banked blood into plasma and packed RBCs, a density-gradient centrifuge to separate the fractions of blood, and a machine to separate cells (leukocytes) from blood obtained from healthy donors. In essence, they developed the forerunner of today's continuous-flow, automated cell separator (28). The current generation of IBM equipment can, during continuous flow, remove blood, centrifuge it, selectively separate components by means of concentric channels and collection ports, and then reinfuse any combination of component parts and replacement fluids. An alternative process, plasmapheresis, uses membrane filtration techniques adapted from dialysis, whereby plasma is removed from whole blood during extracorporeal perfusion.

Apheresis technology can accomplish four basic changes in immune-mediated and/or rheumatic diseases (1,3,5,6,8,9,25). First, one may remove an abnormal cell population which may then be either treated and reinfused, or discarded. Second, a new cell population that has been altered by treatment or depleted of an undesirable cell type may be added. Third, a specific plasma constituent may be removed, such as the autoantibodies due to Rh alloimmunization in pregnancy, the immune complexes of SLE, monoclonal proteins associated with hyperviscosity syndromes, cryoglobulins, toxins as in mushroom poisoning, or protein-bound drug in an overdosed patient. Last, a plasma constituent may be added, such as IgG in ITP or TTP. The difficulty in applying apheresis to rheumatic diseases is the incomplete understanding of the etiopathogenic factors and the complex interplay of cellular and protein components of the body's immune system. In addition, to paraphrase Paul Schmidt: while technology can easily do a 4-liter plasma exchange daily (50% of plasma proteins in the body), the problem is not the removal of 50% of "bad" things but often the removal of 50% of "good" things (16). The latter may include plasma proteins that maintain oncotic pressure, coagulation factors that maintain hemostasis (27), and inhibitory proteins (resulting in rebound production of antibodies, etc.) (28).

In a practical sense, apheresis may alter immunological parameters while concurrently improving the clinical condition. In Goodpasture's syndrome, autoantibody production appears limited and autoantibodies (antiglomerular basement membrane) will disappear in less than 8 weeks with aggressive plasmapheresis and cytotoxic drug therapy (29). With less aggressive therapy, disappearance of the antibodies will take longer. However, tissue damage in this usually fatal illness clearly is minimized. Unfortunately, not all autoimmune diseases have self-limited production of pathogenic proteins. Although apheresis will reduce levels of plasma proteins, immune complexes, and immunoglobulin in the short term (30), especially in disorders such as systemic lupus erythematosus, a rapid increase in concentrations of immune complexes and serum proteins may occur immediately after apheresis, suggesting an "antibody rebound" phenomenon (31). Thus apheresis may help to deplete circulating immune complexes or to alter the equilibrium between soluble antigen and antibody that is responsible for complex formation, but it is less effective in reducing circulating antibody levels in patients who continue to produce new antibody (32). Certain concentrations of a specific antibody in plasma may provide negative feedback for the synthesis of antibody of the same specificity; apheresis-induced antibody rebound, at least in part, may be due to proliferation of antibody-specific B cells (33,34). In theory, such proliferation of pathogenic clones may be abrogated by combining apheresis with the use of cytotoxic drugs (31).

Immune complexes are removed from the circulation by the mononuclear phagocytic system (MPS), formerly termed the reticuloendothelial system, using specific receptors for the Fc part of the immunoglobulin molecule (35). Should these receptors become saturated with soluble immune complexes, the complexes may deposit in other tissues and cause damage (36). By removing excess circulating immune complexes, apheresis may "unblock" the Fc receptors, allowing the MPS to function normally again. This theoretical mechanism may be operant in the treatment of rheumatic disease with apheresis (31).

To reiterate, the complex interplay of immunoactive proteins, immune complexes, and cellular components of the immune system makes a simple understanding of the action of apheresis treatment in any given rheumatic disease quite difficult. Klippel and others describe the net quantitative result of apheresis for removal and subsequent reconstitution of a plasma or cellular factor as a U-shaped concentration-time curve with a descent, a trough, and an ascent phase. Control of the curve is determined by factors such as volume of exchange, frequency and duration of exchanges, and nature of replacement fluids (1,37). A single extended (several hours) plasma exchange removing a standard circulating plasma volume calculated as 40 ml/kg of body weight will result in a 65% decrease in concentration of circulating plasma constituents if there is no net shift between the extravascular and intravascular space and not major synthesis or catabolism (38). Induction of benefits is usually accomplished by plasmapheresis every other day for three treatments. This schedule is often extended (a consolidation and then a maintenance period) to prevent rebound or reequilibration of bound or extravascular antibody, immune complexes, and other substances. An every-other-day schedule with crystalloid and albumin replacement will successfully deplete IgG, IgM, cholesterol, fibrinogen, and complement (38). A number of plasma factors detectable in rheumatic disease also may be removed, such as rheumatoid factors; interferon; vasoactive peptides; antibodies to nuclear, cytoplasmic, or membrane antigens; cryoproteins; complement; cytokines; lymphokines; as well as cytotoxic or proliferative factors. With cytapheresis, lymphocytes may be removed (1,5,6,8,9,11,14,16,20,24, 25,27,31,37,38).

Several problems confound interpretation of study results from apheresis treatment of rheumatic disease. First, the erythrocyte sedimentation rate may be lowered dramatically by removing fibrinogen. A second problem is the inability of "sham apheresis" to serve as a true placebo, as was recently pointed out at the Eighth Annual Apheresis Meeting by Sedar from the Boston VA Medical Center. Sedar (39) noted that for sham apheresis to meet appropriate criteria as a sham, no significant changes should occur in the extracorporeal circuit as the plasma circulates through the tubing and machine, and is returned to the patient untreated, leaving the patient in the status quo ante. However, data with sham alone show that significant changes may occur in platelet parameters (β-thromboglobulin and thromboxane A_2), clotting activation (fibrinopeptide A), and lymphocyte viability and subset composition, merely by passing blood through tubing and then separating and reconstituting it via a machine. This does not even include the effects of anticoagulant primers such as heparin. The solution to this problem may be to include concurrent "no-apheresis" groups or to alter the sham procedure to simply pass the blood behind a screen through a simple external circuit such as a roller pump.

A. Complications

Apheresis has become a relatively safe procedure (40–48) (see Table 2 for complications). One study of 181 patients treated with 1389 therapeutic plasma exchanges demonstrated complications in 1.6% and one unexpected death (40). The new generations of cell separators have sensitive alarms and measuring devices that decrease the risk of hemodynamic imbalance. One

Table 2 Apheresis Complications

- Procedure-related
    - Chills
    - Headache
    - Lightheadedness
    - Hypotension
    - Drug level alterations
    - Anemia
- Access-related
    - Infection
    - Thrombosis
    - Leakage/bleeding
- Related to replacement fluid/plasma protein anaphylaxis/hypersensitivity reaction
    - Hepatitis
    - Citrate toxicity
    - Electrolyte abnormality/arrhythmia
- Related to depletion of plasma constituents
    - Bleeding diathesis
    - Increase risk infection (?)
    - Thrombosis
- Cost-related
- Deaths—rare

area still in need of much improvement is vascular access. Technical complicatins often involve loss of access, clotting of access lines, or leakage of tubing.

Procedure-related complications include chills, headaches, lightheadedness/hypotension, therapeutic drug level alteration, congestive heart failure, and anemia. Chills are caused by replacement fluids given at temperatures lower than core body temperature and will respond to the use of blood warmers. Hypotension and, rarely, syncope are either vasovagal-mediated or due to fluid depletion. Disease exacerbation may occur if blood levels of drugs are radically altered. Congestive heart failure is usually due to fluid overload, and the very young and very old are the most susceptible. Anemia may be secondary to hemolysis in the extracorporeal circuit or may be a consequence of incomplete red blood cell separation, as can be seen in lymphoplasmapheresis.

Access-related problems depend on the access site and the device used. Prolonged cannulation with plastic tubing is associated with a 9% incidence of bacteria and infection of the cannulation site, and the bloodborne bacteria may be a problem thereafter. Thrombosis, bleeding, leakage, and dislodgement are additional problems.

Most problems relate either to replacement of fluid, plasma, or protein losses or depletion of plasma constituents. Replacement with fresh-frozen plasma is now done rarely (TTP) but has caused anaphylaxis (especially if severe IgA deficiency is present) as well as hypersensitivity reactions and hepatitis. Citrate toxicity is a common problem if replacement fluids are blood products anticoagulated with acid citrate dextrose (42) due to lowering plasma ionized calcium. Citrate toxicity may present with circumoral paresthesia, muscle twitching, tetany, nausea, vomiting, headache, chills, and syncope. Treatment is supplemental 10% calcium gluconate. A variety of other electrolyte problems may occur, and are more frequent and often more deleterious in patients with renal failure.

Removal of small amounts of plasma (1 to 1-½ liters) is usually uneventful and replacement may be done with physiological saline alone. However, removal of 2-4 liters requires albumin or fresh-frozen plasma replacement. Excessive depletion of fibrinogen is a complication of plasmapheresis (49), but clinically this manifests as a bleeding problem only if surgery is done immediately thereafter. Antithrombin III levels and factor VIII levels drop (49), but this does not completely explain the apparent predisposition to thrombosis in patients receiving apheresis. Both complement (C3, C4, and total hemolytic complement) and immunoglobulin levels drop, but an increased risk of infection probably is related more to underlying disease and drug therapy with corticosteroids and alkylating agents (30,49).

Apheresis is expensive, as much as $1500-$2000 dollars per treatment; however, new technical advances are lowering costs. For example, cryopheresis decreases protein losses substantially, thereby lowering the albumin replacement costs.

Complications of apheresis are reviewed in Table 2. Fatalities with apheresis are rare but they do occur. Europeans have in the past limited plasma depletion to 12.5 liters/year, but in the United States up to 60 liters or more is removed (43). The causes of death are difficult to determine because it is had to separate underlying disease and drug therapy complications from apheresis-associated problems. Thrombosis has occurred in rheumatic disease patients who received plasmapheresis (46) and may manifest as a pulmonary embolus, gangrene, or stroke. Death occurs from infection or arrhythmia and usually has as its cause disease-, drug-, and apheresis-related factors. Rare complications such as pulmonary artery occlusion with platelets and granulocytes (41) have also occurred.

IV. APHERESIS TREATMENT OF RHEUMATIC DISEASE

A. Rheumatoid Arthritis

Among the systemic rheumatic disorders, rheumatoid arthritis has the most severe articular manifestations and presents as a symmetrical polyarthritis involving both small and large joints (50). Diagnosis is based on the presence of prolonged morning stiffness, symmetrical joint pain and swelling, rheumatoid factor, rheumatoid nodules, and classic radiographic or histological changes (51). Extra-articular manifestations may include rheumatoid nodules, episcleritis, peripheral neuropathy, serositis, periungual infarcts, petechiae/palpable purpura, and skin ulcers. Many of these manifestations may originate with an immune complex-mediated vasculitis (52-54). Rheumatoid arthritis patients usually are treated initially with aspirin or nonsteroidal anti-inflammatory agents; next, if disease persists, with a disease-modifying antirheumatic drug (DMARDs, e.g., gold, *d*-penicillamine, antimalarial) (55-57); and, for 10% or more with intractable disease, immunosuppressive agents (58). DMARD-resistant intractable disease is treated with immunosuppression (58-61) using agents such as azathioprine, methotrexate (59), cyclphosphamide (60), or total lymphoid irradiation (61).

Evidence suggests that the stimulus for chronicity in rheumatoid arthritis may be deposition and persistence of antigenic material (62). Immune complexes containing immunoglobulin (including rheumatoid factor) and complement may be markers for persistent antigenic material (62). Rheumatoid synovium demonstrates a lymphocyte infiltrate with a high percentage of T lymphocytes (63). T-lymphocyte activation is thought to be a consequence of antigen presentation in association with major histocompatibility complex gene products by HLA-DR$^+$-coated interdigitating synovial cells (64).

Wagelius et al. and Paulus et al. depleted lymphocytes by means of thoracic duct drainage and demonstrated a clinical benefit to rheumatoid arthritis patients (2,21,65). The thoracic duct was cannulated in the neck just above the left subclavian vein. Lymph was collected in an iced sterile flask. The 24-hr collection of lymph, which ranged from 1 to 6 liters, was centrifuged once daily to remove the cells. The cell-free lymph was returned through a cannula inserted in the left external jugular vein. These procedures were done continuously for the duration of drainage (2,21,66,67).

From 10 to 46 X 109 cells were removed daily during the first few days of drainage, but the daily output rapidly decreased and was usually less than 5 X 109 after drainage had persisted for more than 3 weeks. There was considerable individual variation in the cumulative output of lymphocytes.

Substantial improvement was apparent within the first 10 days of drainage in subjects successfully cannulated, even though they were given no anti-inflammatory drugs. Similar improvement did not occur in the subjects who were not successfully cannulated. Rheumatoid nodules, when present prior to drainage, decreased in size or disappeared with treatment. Often profound immunosuppression occurred in patients drained for 30 days or more.

Eleven weeks of continuous thoracic duct drainage in a rheumatoid arthritis patient caused marked suppression of both cellular and humoral immunity as tested by skin graft, skin reactions to mumps, KLH, and DNCB, and antibody response to tetanus, *Salmonella*, and KLH (68,69). Some serum immunoglobulin concentrations were also decreased. The fall in lymphocyte output from the thoracic duct was accompanied by progressive peripheral blood lymphopenia. Early in drainage thoracic duct cells were almost all small, high-density lymphocytes as fractionated on a discontinuous density gradient. These responded to stimulation by purified phytohemagglutinin P, pokeweed mitogen, and concanavalin A with increased $[^3H]$TdR incorporation and lymphotoxin (cytotoxin) production. The lymphocytes in the late phase of drainage were larger, of low density, and responded poorly to mitogenic stimulation. The proportion of surface immunoglobulin-bearing cells remained constant at 20–30%. Clinically, the patient had significant improvement as measured by joint count and ring size. Thus, thoracic duct lymph contained both T- and B-type lymphocytes, and depletion of these by drainage led to marked changes in the density of cell populations. Immunological responses were depressed and clinical improvement occurred (68,69).

Intravenous reinfusions of 1 X 109 live autologous ^{51}Cr-labeled lymphocytes during clinical remission in several RA patients resulted in a generalized flare-up of the arthritis. Intra-articular injections of the lymphocytes resulted in flare-up in the injected joint (68). Relapse occurred within 2–12 weeks postdrainage with the longer remissions occurring in patients with longer drainage.

The most recent published evaluation of thoracic duct drainage described the treatment of four severe rheumatoid arthritis patients (70). Benefits were apparent in all patients during drainage, but duration of drainage and cumulative number of lymphocytes removed were not well correlated with degree of improvement. Ueo and associates (70) proposed that in addition to the effects of lymphocyte depletion, another hypothetical mechanism of action for thoracic duct drainage involved the accelerated migration of inflammatory cells from synovial tissues to the blood stream stimulated by dynamic changes of lymphocyte flow during thoracic duct drainage.

Thoracic duct drainage served its role as an investigational tool by highlighting the importance of lymphocytes and, most especially, T lymphocytes in the immunopathogenesis of rheumatoid arthritis. Unfortunately, the procedure itself is too expensive and difficult to be of practical use as a treatment modality. However, it did pave the way for the use of lymphocytapheresis and plasmapheresis as a treatment of rheumatoid arthritis (71).

The development of automated cell separators has allowed lymphocyte removal to be more easily accomplished by lymphocytapheresis and lymphoplasmapheresis. To do lymphocytapheresis, the blood from a large vein, arteriovenous shunt, or fistula is circulated through the cell separator and lymphocytes (and, to a lesser extent, monocytes and a few erythrocytes) are removed and the remainder of the blood infused back into the patient. Patients usually receive between nine and 21 treatments over 2-12 weeks. Controversy has arisen over the interpretation of results because of the difficulty in interpreting the additional benefits of rest, physical therapy, the placebo effect, and the risk/benefit and cost/benefit ratios.

Initial pilot studies with lymphocytapheresis and lymphoplasmapheresis demonstrated widely variable clinical benefits occurring early (three to six procedures) with duration of benefits lasting from a few weeks to up to a year (72-77). There was no clear correlation between the degree of clinical improvement and several factors, which included number of cells removed, degree of lymphopenia, serological parameters, immunological function as tested by investigators, decreases in Westergren sedimentation rate, or levels of rheumatoid factor, complement, immunoglobulin, and immune complexes (72-77). Side effects were few. Immunosuppression based on skin test reactivity to delayed hypersensitivity antigens or on the proportions of T or B lymphocytes was not required for therapy to be effective (76). One hypothesis to explain clinical benefits was that the broad range of clinical response reflected the broad spectrum of rheumatoid histopathology. Further, defining immunological subsets may be important as certain subsets are clearly more responsible. Also alteration of mononuclear cell function may be a significant beneficial factor in addition to immunosuppression (77).

Three controlled trials of patients with rheumatoid arthritis treated with lymphapheresis were carried out (78-80). At the National Institutes of Health, Karsh and associates studied lymphocytapheresis in 12 patients who were not treated concomitantly with an antirheumatic drug (78). Patients were randomized to receive lymphocytapheresis or to receive only a volume of plasma equal to that lost in the apheresis procedure. A statistically significant, albeit modest, antirheumatic effect was observed as evidenced by a decrease in the number of active joints, swollen joints, and the Ritchie articular index. A persistent lymphocytopenia was observed in the treated group but not in the control group. Any benefit attributable to hospitalization and bed rest was excluded by the study design. Wallace et al. studied 14 outpatients in a 3-week sham-controlled randomized study of lymphoplasmapheresis with a tapering schedule and with concurrent use of slow-acting antirheumatic drugs (73). Again there were significant improvements in the treatment group as compared to the control group. Improvements achieved statistical significance only in certain parameters but every index demonstrated the apheresis group to outperform the sham group (79). Verdickt and colleagues randomized 20 patients to either six lymphoplasmapheresis sessions or a control procedure (80). Benefits in terms of antirheumatic effect were modest and of short duration. T-cell subpopulations did not change nor did the use of lymphoplasmapheresis counteract the rebound effect noted with plasma exchange.

In summary, while lymphoplasmapheresis is an interesting research tool, clinical benefits are modest and of short duration. Additionally, lymphoplasmapheresis requires good cardiovascular function since a large extracorporeal volume is required (15% of total blood volume is out of the body at certain points of the procedure) and small numbers of red blood cells are removed with the lymphocytes, often worsening preexisting anemia.

Plasmapheresis is a simpler procedure requiring a smaller extracorporeal volume at any given time. Only plasma is removed and all cellular components are returned, avoiding the need for transfusion. Use of plasmapheresis for rheumatoid arthritis has been considered because rheumatoid arthritis patients have circulating rheumatoid factor and immune complexes (71).

Use of plasmapheresis to treat rheumatoid arthritis has resulted in only mild to moderate antirheumatic effects lasting only a short time and definitely not replacing standard treatment with gold, *d*-penicillamine, or azathioprine (5,71,81-84). Comparison of plasmapheresis with total lymphoid irradiation showed the benefits of plasmapheresis to be of a much shorter duration but the procedure to be much better tolerated (85). Its role in depleting immune complexes does not correlate with clinical benefit, and depletion of other mediators or improvement of reticuloendothelial function may be of greater importance. Numerous anecdotal reports suggest that plasmapheresis may be of benefit in the treatment of rheumatoid vasculitis (81,85-90). This benefit may be related to lowering plasma viscosity, removing cryoglobulin, or removing noncryoproteins, circulating rheumatoid factor, and immune complexes. Dwosh and associates studied 26 patients in a double-blind, crossover study of plasmapheresis therapy; they concluded that no clinically significant benefit should be attributed to plasmapheresis alone (91). Rothwell in a controlled study also found only marginal benefits from plasmapheresis once benefits of hospitalization and bed rest were taken into account (92).

Plasmapheresis has been reported to be much more effective as adjuvant therapy to cyclophosphamide and/or corticosteroids (93,94).

A limitation of the aforementioned apheresis treatments has been the high cost of replacement protein. Cryofiltration, a technique for on-line plasma separation and its treatment by cold filtration, enables selective removal of macromolecules and immune complexes from plasma while eliminating the high cost of protein replacement (95,96). While the technology is safe and the costs are lower, as with other apheresis approaches for rheumatoid arthritis, the clinical benefits are modest (95-97).

Wilder et al. (98) studied the variability in the responsiveness of rheumatoid arthritis patients to apheresis. He found that patients whose disease is characterized by a synovium densely infiltrated by lymphocytes, cutaneous anergy, and elevated levels of peripheral blood activated T cells seem to be apheresis-responsive. In contrast, a second group characterized by a fibrotic synovium, no anergy, and normal lymphocyte subpopulations seemed to be apheresis-unresponsivene. Further analysis of lymphocyte subpopulations may help to better clarify the apheresis responsive population of rheumatoid arthritis patients. Apheresis is an excellent tool for the study of rheumatoid arthritis. Subjective and objective benefits are well documented but improvement is short term. Apheresis is safe to use in rheumatoid arthritis so the risk/benefit ratio is favorable, but even with cryoapheresis the cost may be prohibitive. Perhaps apheresis techniques may be used to best advantage as adjunctive therapy in rheumatoid arthritis refractory to DMARDs or complicated by hyperviscosity syndrome or vasculitis. In the future, improved identification of apheresis-responsive subsets may improve the cost/benefit ratio and perhaps apheresis will find a place in combination therapy.

B. Systemic Lupus Erythematosus

Systemic lupus erythematosus (SLE) is a disorder of unknown etiology involving multiple organ systems with a variable course. The American Rheumatism Association has diagnostic criteria for SLE (99) which include malar rash, discoid lupus, polyarthralgias, photosensitivity, serositis, oral ulcers, neurological involvement, renal involvement, hematological involvement, positive antinuclear antibody test and biological fasle positive test for syphilis, anti-dsDNA or positive anti-Sm antibody. Polyarthralgias, hematological abnormalities, and skin abnormalities are the most common sensitive and specific findings (100). With the exception of patients with severe renal disease, 5-year survival exceeds 95% (101). Infection is the most common cause of death and corticosteroids increase the risk of death from infection (101, 102).

The specific etiology of SLE is unknown but current research suggests a major derangement of immunoregulation with production of an abundant variety of autoantibodies (103). Systemic lupus erythematosus may also be considered the prototype immune complex disorder (103,104). One view of the immunoregulatory defect in SLE is that there is a defect in suppressor T cells resulting in B-cell hyperactivity; this, then, results in autoantibody production including anti T-cell antibodies, thereby perpetuating the cycle (105). The B-cell hyperactivity is marked by hypergammaglobulinemia and autoantibody production (101-103). Activity of SLE seems to correlate with the number of circulating immunoglobulin-producing cells (106) and most of the clinical manifestations of SLE are attributable to immune complex deposition and consequent action of complement and other mediators of inflammation (104). One must consider whether potentially phlogistic immune complexes circulate or are formed in situ, although evidence from several sources suggests that at least some of the complexes circulate and then deposit (104,107,108).

Removal of circulating immune complexes and autoantibodies is one rationale for the use of apheresis in SLE (109). A second rationale is based on previously mentioned work on the mononuclear phagocytic system (reticuloendothelial system). The role of the mononuclear phagocytic system is to remove circulating immune complexes via Fc receptors on the immunoglobulin, and blockage of this system in SLE may be reversed by plasma exchange (110-113). A third hypothesis of why apheresis may be effective as a treatment of SLE was generated in a study of a patient unresponsive to conventional therapy who was noted to have a plasma factor that inhibited T-cell function, when assayed against IgG synthesis in vitro or against T-cell blastogenesis (114). After plasmapheresis therapy the anti-T-cell activity was no longer apparent.

Numerous reports of plasma exchange/plasmapheresis used alone or in combination with corticosteroids and/or cytotoxic drugs suggest short-term clinical benefits (109,111,112,114-123). Plasmapheresis has also been described as a beneficial treatment modality in a number of anecdotal reports of specific SLE manifestations including nephritis (124-126), pneumonitis (127,128), hematological abnormalities (127-129), deafness/cerebritis (130, 131), and vasculitis (132). One byproduct of this anecdotal experience was the realization that plasmapheresis used without concomitant cytotoxic therapy may have only short-lived benefits and a significant relapse rate (122). This understanding appears logical in the light of findings that while plasmapheresis does deplete circulating immune complexes or alter the equilibrium wherein they form, it may not be so effective if there is continuous antibody formation (133). In addition, following a plasmapheresis-induced depletion of circulating immune complexes, complement, and anti-DNA antibodies, depleted factor levels may subsequently rise *above* prepheresis levels, an antibody rebound phenomenon that may accompany a clinical disease relapse (134). One case report described what may be an exception to the aforementioned phenomena with a patient who had no circulating immune complexes, but in whom plasma exchange had rapid and striking effects on clinical symptoms and on serological abnormalities (135). One randomized trial with 20 patients either receiving six 4-liter plasma exchanges or a control procedure over a 2-week period showed the serological alterations to be short-lived (4 weeks), and there were no significant differences in clinical parameters between control and treatment groups (136).

Paulus and associates reported thoracic duct drainage to be beneficial in four SLE patients (137), suggesting possible benefits from depletion of certain lymphocyte subsets (137). Other apheresis approaches to SLE have included the use of extracorporeal immunoadsorption and filtration to extract either DNA (138) or other specific proteins (139). These approaches are in beginning developmental stages but appear promising. What may be the most promising approach to apheresis treatment of SLE is based on experimental and clinical data that suggest a feedback cycle which induces increased antibody synthesis after antibody depletion (antibody rebound) (31). Since increasing antibody levels are preceded by increased proliferation and, thus, vulnerability of pathogenic B-cell clones (34), the antibody rebound can be utilized for increased clonal depletion, if maximum pulse cyclophosphamide (36 mg/kg body weight) is applied shortly after initial large-volume plasmapheresis. This approach, termed synchronization therapy, was used in two SLE patients, both of whom had improvement in clinical symptoms and laboratory parameters including control of pneumonitis (140). Their conditions were stabilized 6 months later, by repeat synchronization therapy with plasmapheresis followed by cyclophosphamide therapy. The patients had not relapsed at a 14-month follow-up. Barr and associates reported that similar findings and benefits occurred in 26 SLE patients treated in the same fashion (141).

In summary, plasmapheresis alone seems not to be justified for the treatment of SLE. Plasmapheresis with cytotoxic agents may be a excellent induction therapy for various forms of lupus crisis (nephritis, hematological, pulmonary, CNS, vasculitis) and may be particularly effective when used in synchronization. However, further study is needed with well-designed controlled trials; research emphasis should be guided by the specific failures. Too little information is available in print to comment on lymphocyte depletion in SLE. Future treatment progress should parallel our understanding of pathogenic factors, since new immunoadsorbant columns will allow for selective filtrations and removal of phlogistic proteins.

C. Vasculitis

Vasculitis may be subdivided into diseases of small, medium, and large vessels (142). Small-vessel vasculitis involves venules, arterioles, and capillaries; is termed by pathologists leukocytoclastic vasculitis; and presents primarily with skin manifestations, i.e., palpable purpura. Medium-vessel vasculitis, a disease of small and medium-sized muscular arteries, is termed systemic necrotizing vasculitis. Polyarteritis nodosa is the classic model with morbidity and mortality related to ischemia of major organs. Large-vessel vasculitis is referred to as giant cell arteritis and primarily comprises temporal arteritis and Takayasu's arteritis.

Small-vessel vasculitis has been treated with plasma exchange and/or plasmapheresis, combined with steroids and/or cytotoxic drugs (143-149). The rationale for apheresis treatment of vasculitis includes removal of immune complexes and reversal of the blockade of the splenic component of the reticuloendothelial system (146). All case reports have been anecdotal and, as small-vessel vasculitis can be self-limiting, the benefits of apheresis are difficult to interpret. Cryoglobulinemia manifesting as a vasculitis will be discussed separately in Sec. IV.E.

Medium-vessel vasculitis is life threatening and standard treatment consists of cyclophosphamide or another alkylating agent and corticosteroids (146, 150,151). Classic polyarteritis nodosa has responded to plasma exchange/ plasmapheresis (150,151). Ouzan and associates have taken a unique approach to the treatment of polyarteritis nodosa occurring in association with persistent hepatitis B viremia; they treat by combining antiviral chemotherapy (vidarabin) with plasma exchange (152). Lockwood and associates found plasmapheresis to be of benefit in three cases of Wegener's granulomatosis (146), but three patients treated at UCLA with both plasmapheresis and lymphoplasmapheresis did not benefit (153).

In summary, few data and no controlled trials exist. Apheresis has occasionally been used as the sole treatment for vasculitis (150), but treatment with corticosteroids and immunosuppressives is still the standard and antiviral agents are considered experimental. Possible indications for apheresis treatment include situations when attempts to taper existing drug therapy result in recrudescence of disease. Apheresis may also be used in organ- or life-threatening vasculitis, in addition to alkylating agents and corticosteroids. Its use for small-vessel vasculitis should be primarily limited to study protocols or cryoglobulinemia.

D. Scleroderma

Scleroderma (PSS) is a multisystem disorder of unknown etiology (154). The skin changes in PSS are both dramatic and debilitating and have consequently received considerable attention (155). Pathological changes in PSS, however, are generalized; gastrointestinal, renal, cardiac, pulmonary, and other organ system involvements are major causes of both morbidity and mortality (156). Most cases of PSS have no clear etiology (157). Familial occurrence of PSS as well as association with histocompatibility antigens has been noted, but a definitive genetic basis remains unproven (158,159). Speculation as to the etiological and pathophysiological determinants of PSS has centered on explaining the vascular lesion which may link all facets of this multisystem disorder (160). The vascular lesion has inflammatory, proliferative, and indurative phases and may be linked to abnormal fibroblast activity (160, 161). The factors that trigger the vascular transformation and the messengers that relay information between endothelial cells and tissue fibroblasts remain to be determined.

Scleroderma is an uncommon disorder (162,163). Women are more commonly affected, and no racial predilection exists (164). Onset is in the third to fifth decades of life (165,166). Prognosis for survival is poor, with one study citing 50% of patients dead 7 years after initial diagnosis (167). Mortality increases with age, in males, and with renal, cardiac, and pulmonary involvement (168).

Currently, with the possible exception of scleroderma renal disease, treatment remains empirical and symptomatic (169). Trials of prednisone (170), dimethyl sulfoxide (171), *N*-acetylcysteine (172), *d*-penicillamine (173), and cytotoxic agents (174,175) have met with limited or no success.

Scleroderma, while still a disease of unknown etiology, has a wide range of associated immunological abnormalities. Because these abnormalities occur, PSS is believed to have either a significant association or a cause-effect relationship with immunological self-reactivity (157,176,177).

Raynaud's syndrome (RS) occurs in 95% or more cases of scleroderma (156,164). Raynaud's syndrome may occur in the absence of a known etiological factor—as Raynaud's disease; or, as Raynaud's phenomenon, in association with a large variety of disorders, including vibration or cold injuries, drugs, or connective tissue diseases.

Talpos and associates reported five cases of RS (two with PSS) in whom clinical benefits were obtained with plasmapheresis (179,180). Pain was diminished, digital ulcers healed, and the frequency of reported attacks decreased. Benefits lasted up to 6 months in this uncontrolled trial involving only five treatments. Cotton subsequently postulated that benefits may have been due to a decrease in serum viscosity, decreased platelet and red blood cell aggregation, and increased deformability of red blood cells (181). This same group next did a randomized comparison of plasma exchange, intermittent infusion of heparin, and oral placebo therapy in 27 patients with RS. No benefits were seen from heparin or oral placebo therapy but, again, improved symptoms and/or patency of digital arteries were seen with plasma exchange in seven of eight patients and the effects lasted 6 months (182). No patient had scleroderma. Evidence was presented that benefits may have derived from reduced serum viscosity, decreased circulating immune complexes, and increased red blood cell deformability in their RS patients treated with plasma exchange (180-184). Zahavi further elaborated on these studies, showing that in vivo platelet release reaction as measured by plasma β-thromboglobulin is enhanced in RS and decreases significantly and for prolonged periods of time after plasma exchange coincident with clinical improvements (185,186).

McCune and associates examined six women with scleroderma and severe RS (187). In a nonblinded fashion each patient received plasma exchanges or a placebo exchange (with return of the patient's own separated plasma). McCune et al. saw subjective improvement with decreased frequency of Raynaud's attacks and digital ulcer healing, but could show no objective improvement in occlusive digital arterial disease, having done only four plasma exchange treatments given at weekly intervals. A fascinating side note was that the *placebo* exchange resulted in at least transient changes in circulating serum proteins and digital circulation.

Scleroderma skin and gastrointestinal manifestations have responded to thoracic duct drainage in at least three of four cases (178). Dau in an uncontrolled clinical trial of plasmapheresis (4-52 exchanges over 1-24 months) combined with prednisone and cyclophosphamide showed clinical improvement in 14 of 15 scleroderma patients (188). Clinical improvement occurred, primarily with loosening of skin, relaxing of contractures, and healing of skin ulcers. Some, but not all, patients had decreases of gastrointestinal symptoms, reversal of inflammatory muscle disease, and occasional improvement of pulmonary and cardiac function (188). The fall in ANA titers was more than that of total IgG levels in six of nine patients with elevated titers. Increased levels of circulating immune complexes were found initially in only four patients, but 11 of 15 with increased levels of endothelial cell cytotoxic activity had significant reductions with therapy. Dau and associates treated 20 additional PSS patients with the same protocol over the next 2 years (189). Eighteen of 20 showed clinical benefits of which skin, muscle, and gastrointestinal improvement were most often cited. Several other anecdotal reports have cited clinical improvement with plasmapheresis (190-192); however, one report of seven patients had improvement in skin, articular, and muscle findings in three patients; and venous access was insufficient for apheresis therapy in three patients (193).

In 1987, we reported our preliminary findings from a prospective randomized controlled trial of apheresis treatment for PSS (194). Patients with PSS were randomized into control, plasmapheresis, or lymphoplasmapheresis groups. All patients had classic PSS and between 1 and 5 years of disease. Apheresis was done 21 times over 3 months and controls were untreated. Results, although preliminary (now with 23 patients), showed statistically significant improvement for treated groups over control in Rodnan skin scores, PT assessment tool, and both patient's global and physician's global assessment.

In summary, apheresis for PSS is still in the process of evaluation. Because the cost is high, use for Raynaud's disease/phenomenon should be restricted to patients with severe disease (nonhealing skin ulcers, impending gangrene) unresponsive to conventional therapy. Apheresis for PSS should be done on a research protocol if possible or for patients with worsening disease unresponsive to individual organ system therapy. Whether apheresis is better used for PSS with or without cytotoxic agents remains to be decided in future studies.

E. Cryoglobulinemia

Essential mixed cryoglobulinemia is an immune complex-mediated disorder with a cryoprecipitate containing 19S and 7S proteins (195-198). The clinical findings include leukocytoclastic vasculitis with palpable purpura, arthralgias/myalgias, constitutional symptoms, and renal involvement with glomerulonephritis (195,197). A mixed cryoglobulin implies at least two different immunoglobulin classes, including usually IgM with rheumatoid factor (anti-IgG) activity and IgG (196). Other laboratory findings include anemia, hypergammaglobulinemia, positive rheumatoid factor, hypocomplementemia, and in half the cases evidence of hepatitis B infection (195-197). Other clinical findings include hepatomegaly, splenomegaly, leg ulceration, digital gangrene, peripheral neuropathy, and central nervous system involvement (195,197). The worst prognostic factor is the development of glomerulonephritis which is associated with progression to renal failure in half the patients (198).

Plasma exchange and/or plasmapheresis has been used successfully (in anecdotal reports of xx patients) to treat the glomerulonephritis, nephrotic syndrome, and neurological manifestations of essential mixed cryoglobulinemia (199-201). Apheresis treatment is most often done in combination with corticosteroids and a cytotoxic agent—usually cyclophosphamide.

The mechanism of action of apheresis in mixed cryoglobulinemia is not completely explained by cryoprotein/immune complex removal and removal of noncryoprotein is also probably essential. Hamburger and associates found patients with essential cryoglobulinemia and glomerulonephritis to have defective reticuloendothelial system Fc receptor-mediated clearance of immune complexes (202). This defect was not found in patients with normal renal function. Perhaps plasma exchange/plasmapheresis reverses the blockade of the reticuloendothelial system, but this is unproven.

Apheresis is currently accepted as part of combination therapy for mixed cryoglobulinemia. Controlled trials are needed and consideration for apheresis therapy should include evaluation of the clinical course with special regard for renal function.

F. Poly/Dermatomyositis

Polymyositis is defined as the findings of three of the following: (1) proximal muscle weakness, (2) elevation of muscle enzymes, (3) characteristic electromyographic findings, (4) typical muscle histology (203-204). Dermatomyositis is defined by the same criteria but also requires a vasculitic skin rash. Childhood dermatomyositis fits all five of the above criteria but may have an antibody-mediated medium-vessel vasculitis as an additional finding (205). Etiology and pathogenesis remain unknown. However, autoantibodies have been characterized (206), and circulating immune complexes have been detected (207), as have circulating antibodies that mediate antibody-dependent cell-mediated cytotoxicity (208). T lymphocytes predominate in the inflammatory infiltrates (209,210) but B lymphocytes are also present (211) and the T4/T8 ratio is increased (212).

Polymyositis and dermatomyositis usually respond to corticosteroids, but immunosuppressive agents—methotrexate, chlorambucil, azathioprine, and cyclophosphamide—have also been used (203,204,213-215).

The histopathological findings in juvenile dermatomyositis include a vasculopathy wherein vessel wall deposits of IgM and a variable deposition of IgG and C3 are found in the muscle (216). These immune complexes, if not formed in situ, would suggest that the process might be amenable to plasmapheresis. Three anecdotal cases in the literature suggest that this may be true (217-219).

Uncontrolled trials in adult polymyositis and dermatomyositis suggest that plasmapheresis, combined with immunosuppressive drugs, and corticosteroids, results in improvement of clinical parameters (215) and may also benefit cases refractory to corticosteroids and/or cytotoxic agents (215,220), or cases inadequately controlled with steroids and/or cyclophosphamide or azathioprine (221). However most authors emphasize the need for concomitant immunosuppressive drug therapy (222). One alternative approach has been to use leukocytapheresis as a substitute for immunosuppressive therapy in combination with plasmapheresis (223).

In summary, only anecdotal reports have been published on the treatment of dermatomyositis/polymyositis and controlled trials are badly needed. Plasmapheresis and/or lymphocytapheresis has been used primarily in conjunction with corticosteroid therapy and/or immunosuppressive therapy for juvenile dermatomyositis, polymyositis, and dermatomyositis (224). Apheresis has also been used when drug therapy alone was unsuccessful. The number of cases reported is small and uncontrolled; however, apheresis should be considered if and when heroic measures are indicated.

G. Miscellaneous Syndromes

A large number of rheumatic disorders have been treated with apheresis. Uncontrolled anecdotal data can serve to stimulate future controlled studies. References for a small group of such reports include juvenile rheumatoid arthritis (5,225), psoriatic arthritis (5), Behçet's disease (226), scleromyxedema (227), and mixed connective tissue disease (228).

V. FUTURE DIRECTIONS

Apheresis therapy is very costly. Use of apheresis for even a small percentage of rheumatic disease patients would bankrupt the health care system and exhaust available supplies of protein replacement solutions. The costs may be decreased by the use of cryogelatin and membrane filtration, which allow immune complexes to be removed and the patient's plasma to be returned, and would minimize the cost for protein replacement (95-97). In addition, the identification before apheresis of subsets of rheumatic disease that are either apheresis-responsive or nonresponsive prior to treatment (as Wilder and associates did in a rheumatoid arthritis population) (98) can help decrease the overall costs of this therapy.

In addition, apheresis must be made more specific. This may be done by adsorption of plasma proteins during column perfusion. This process is more selective than plasma filtration and is already being developed. For example, "IMP" adsorption can remove rheumatoid factor and immune complexes, while "I-02" adsorption can remove rheumatoid factor, immune complexes, DNA antibodies, RNP antibodies, and Sm antibodies (22)9). Two such extracorporeal immunoadsorption and filtration systems have been successfully tried in SLE (138,139).

Also, apheresis technology will have to be used in combination with other treatment modalities. Synchronization therapy, whereby plasmapheresis induces proliferation of pathogenic clones which are then depleted by cytotoxic therapy, is just such an approach and has already been used to treat SLE (140,141).

Finally, apheresis technology will continue to be used as an investigational tool. Apheresis technology allows selective removal of circulating cell types, proteins, carbohydrates, and fats. Cells and proteins not accessible in the extravascular spaces are indirectly accessible if responsive to equilibration with intravascular contents. Thus an investigator with a relevant hypothesis on the complex immunopathogenesis of a rheumatic disease, if proven in animal models and suggested by clinical study, can try a relatively safe active intervention and then study the results. Such an experimental design is best exemplified by thoracic duct drainage done for rheumatoid arthritis patients, which resulted in dramatic clinical improvement, reduction of synovitis, and improvement of nodulosis. The study of thoracic duct drainage in RA established a role for circulating lymphocytes in the immunopathogenesis of rheumatoid arthritis. In the future more specific cytodepletion of clonal populations that are manufacturing pathogenic proteins, depletion of pathogenic proteins themselves, may be attempted. Extracorporeal treatment of cells with drugs or alteration of the genetic structure of a cell population prior to reinfusion may also be possible. The variations and permutations for deriving specific information via apheresis technology seem unlimited.

Currently several institutions are attempting "adoptive immunotherapy" for cancer patients. Lymphocytes are harvested by leukapheresis, activated by phytohemagglutinin, and the lymphokine-interleukin-2 producing "LAK" cells or lymphocyte-activated killer cells are reinfused to attack the tumor. These LAK cells and similar lymphokine-activated cells may be used to treat rheumatic diseases in the future, or perhaps other cell types will be harvested, activated, or altered, and then reinfused.

Above all, there is a need for definitive, prospective, randomized, controlled clinical trials that will allow meaningful decisions on the true value of apheresis in rheumatic disease.

REFERENCES

1. Klippel JH. Apheresis: biotechnology and the rheumatic diseases. Arth Rheum 1984; 27:1081-5.
2. Paulus HE, Machleder HI, Levine S, Yu DTY, MacDonald NS. Lymphocyte involvement in rheumatoid arthritis: studies during thoracic duct drainage. Arth Rheum 1977; 2):1249-62.
3. Jones JHV, Cumming RH, Buchnall RC. Plasmapheresis in the management of acute systemic lupus erythematosus. Lancet 1976; 1:709-11.
4. Lockwood CM, Rees AJ, Pearson TA, Evans DJ, Peters DK, Witson CB. Immunosuppression and plasma exchange in the treatment of Goodpasture's syndrome. Lancet 1976; 1:711-55.
5. Wallace DJ, Goldfinger D, Thompsen-Breton R, Martin V, Lowe CM, Bluestone R, Klinenberg JR. Advances in the use of therapeutic apheresis for the management of rheumatic diseases. Semin Arth Rheum 1989; 81-90.
6. Hamblin TJ. Update on plasmapheresis. Apheresis Bull 1983; 1:10-7.
7. Hamblin TJ. The apheresis register. Apheresis Bull 1983; 1145-51.
8. Hamblin TJ. Where now for therapeutic apheresis? Br Med J 1984; 289: 779-80.
9. Jones JV. Plasmapheresis: current research and success. Heart and Lung 1980; 9:671-4.
10. Lockwood CM, Peters DK. Plasma exchange in glomerulonephritis and related vasculitides. Ann Rev Med 1980; 31:167-79.
11. Cardella CJ. Plasma exchange: a new approach to immune modulation in rheumatic diseases. J Rheumatol 1979; 6:606-9.
12. Heden E. On the transfusion of pure red corpuscles in suspension in a artificial serum after hemorrhages. Arch Med Exp. 1902; 14:297-326.
13. Johnson J. A treatise on the medicinal leech. Longman, Hurst, Rees, Orme and Brown. 1816:4-9.
14. Hylland RG. Further evidence for plasmapheresis. Arth Rheum 1980; 23:129.
15. Waldenstrom JG. Plasmapheresis-blood letting revived and refined. Acta Med Scand 1989; 208:1-4.
16. Schmidt PJ. Therapeutic plasma exchange. N Engl J Med 1984; 310: 762-71.

17. Talbot CH. Medicine in medieval England. London: Oldbourne, 1967: 131.
18. Boyle R. Trials proposed to be made for the improvement of the experiment of transfusion blood out of one live animal into another. Philos Trans 1666; 22:385-8.
19. Abel JJ, Rowntree LG, Turner BB. Plasma removal with return of corpuscles (plasmapheresis). J Pharmacol Exp Ther 1914; 5:626-41.
20. Schwab PJ, Fahey JL. Treatment of Waldenstrom's macroglobulinemia by plasmapheresis. N Engl J Med 1969; 263:574-9.
21. Paulus HE, Machleder HI, Clements P. Prolonged thoracic duct drainage in rheumatoid arthritis and systemic lupus erythematosus. West J Med 1979; 130:209-324.
22. Ueo T, Tanaka S, Tominaga Y, Oganwa H, Sukurami T. The effect of thoracic duct drainage on lymphocyte dynamics and clinical symptoms in patients with rheumatoid arthritis. Arth Rheum 1979; 22:1405-12.
23. Nyman KE, Bangert R, Machleder H, Paulus HE. Thoracic duct drainage in SLE and cutaneous vasculitis: A case report. Arth Rheum 1977; 20: 1129-34.
24. Wallace DJ, Goldfinger D. Gatti R, Lowe C, Fan P, Bluestone R, Klinenberg JR. Plasmapheresis in the management of rheumatoid arthritis. Arth Rheum 1979; 22:703-10.
25. Shumak RH, Rock GA. Therapeutic plasma exchange. N Engl J Med 1984; 310:762-71.
26. Millward BL, Hoeltghe GA. The historical development of automated hemapheresis. J Clin Apheresis 1982; 1:25-32.
27. Flaum MA, Cuneo RA, Appelbaum FR. The hemostatic imbalance of plasma-exchange transfusion. Blood 1979; 54:694-702.
28. Barclay GR, Greiss MA, Urbaniak SJ. Adverse effect of plasma exchange on anti-D production in rhesus immunization owing to removal of inhibitory factors. Br Med J 1980; 1:1569-71.
29. Peters DK, Lockwood M. In Gurland, Heinze, Lee, eds. Therapeutic plasma exchange. Berlin: Springer-Verlag, 1981:139-46.
30. Friedman BA, Schork MA, Mocniak JL, Oberman HA. Short-term and long-term effects of plasmapheresis on serum proteins and immunoglobulins. Transfusion 1975; 15:467-72.
31. Jones JV. Plasmapheresis in SLE. In Hughes GRV, ed. Clinics in rheumatic disease. Vol 8. Systemic lupus erythematosus. Philadelphia: W.B. Saunders, 1982:243-60.
32. Rossen RD, Hersh EM, Sharp JT, McCredie KB, Gyorkey F, Suki WN, Eknoyan G, Reisberg MA. Effect of plasma exchange on circulating immune complexes and antibody formation in patients treated with cyclophosphamide and prednisone. Am J Med 1977; 63:674-82.

33. Euler HH, Krey U, Schroeder O, Loffler H. Membrane plasmapheresis technique in rats: confirmation of antibody rebound. J Immunol Meth 1985; 84:313–9.
34. Sturgill BC, Wofrzniak MJ. Stimulation of proliferation of 19S antibody-forming cells in the spleens of immunized guinea pigs after exchange transfusion. Nature 1970; 228:1304–5.
35. Schreiber AD. An experimental model of immune hemolytic anemia. In Frank MM, ed. Pathophysiology of immune hemolytic anemia. Ann Intern Med 1977; 87:210–22.
36. Haakenstad AD, Mannik M. Saturation of the reticuloendothelial system with soluble immune complexes. J Immunol 1974; 112:1939–48.
37. Berkman E. Issues in therapeutic aperhesis. N Engl J Med 1982; 306: 1418–20.
38. Orlin JB, Berkman EM. Partial plasma exchange using albumin replacement; removal and recovery of normal plasma constituents. Blood 1980; 56:1055–9.
39. Sedar RH. Alterations in blood components during plasmapheresis: in search of true "sham pheresis." American Society for Apheresis, Eighth Annual Apheresis Symposium, 4/87 Abstract.
40. Ziselman EM, Bongiovanni MB, Wurzel HA. The complications of therapeutic plasma exchnage. Vox Sanguin 1984; 46:270–6.
41. Rubenstein MD, Wall RT, Wood GS, Edwards MA. Complications of therapeutic apheresis, including a fatal case with pulmonary vascular occlusion. Am J Med 1983; 75:171–4.
42. Sutton DMC, Cardella CJ, Uldall PR, Deveber GA. Complications of intensive plasma exchange. Plasma Ther 1981; 2:19–24.
43. Plasmapheresis (273,3105): Fed Reg 38:19366 (No. 139, July 20, 1973).
44. Friedman BA, Schork MA, Mocniak JL, Oberman HA. Short and long term effects of plasmapheresis on serum proteins and immunoglobulins. Transfusion 1975; 15:467–72.
45. Sultan Y, Bussel A, Maisonneuve P, Paupevey M, Sitty X, Gajdos P. Potential danger of thrombosis after plasma exchanges in the treatment of patients with immune disease. Transfusion 1979; 19:588–98.
46. Doll NJ, Salvaggio JE. Stroke and gangrene: complications of therapeutic plasma exchange. Clin Exp Dialysis Apheresis 1981; 5:415–21.
47. Vangelista A, Frasca GM, Nanni-Costa A, Bonomini V. Effect of plasmapheresis on E-rosette receptors in SLE patients. J Clin Apheresis 1986; 3:100–2.
48. Bonomini V, Vangelista A, Frasca G, Nanni-Costa A, Borgnino LC. Effect of plasmapheresis on cellular immunity abnormalities in patients with systemic lupus erythematosus. Clin Nephrol 1984; 22:121–8.

49. Wood L, Jacobs P. The effect of serial therapeutic plasmapheresis on platelet count, coagulation factors, plasma immunoglobulin and complement levels. J Clin Apheresis 1986; 3:124-6.
50. Fleming A, Benn RT, Cerbett M, Wood PHN. Early rheumatoid disease. II. Patterns of joint involvement. Ann Rheum Dis 1976; 35:361-4.
51. Ropes MW, Bennet GA, Cobb A, Jacox R, Jessar RA. 1958 revision of diagnostic criteria for rheumatoid arthritis. Bull Rheum Dis 1958; 9: 175-6.
52. Cruickshank B. The arteritis of rheumatoid arthritis. Ann Rheum Dis 1954; 13:136-46.
53. Scott DGI, Bacon PA, Tribe CR> Systemic rheumatoid vasculitis. A clinical and laboratory study of 50 cases. Medicine 1981; 60:288-97.
54. Hart FW. Rheumatoid arthritis: extra-articular manifestations. II. Br Med J 1970; 2:747-52.
55. Urowitz MD, Gordon DA, Smythe HA, Pruzanski W, Ogryzlo MA. Azathioprine in rheumatoid arthritis: a double blind crossover study. Arth Rheum 1973; 16:411-8.
56. Curry HLF, Harris J, Mason RM. Comparison of azathioprine, cyclophosphamide and gold in the treatment of rheumatoid arthritis. Br Med J 1974; 3:763-6.
57. Paulus HE. Williams HJ, Ward JR. Azathioprine versus d-penicillamine in rheumatoid arthritis patients who have been treated unsuccessfully with gold. Arth Rheum 1984; 27:721-7.
58. Wilke WS, Krall PL. Resistant rheumatoid arthritis: what to do when conservative therapy doesn't work. Postgrad Med 1984; 75:69-77.
59. Hoffmeister RT. Methotrexate therapy in rheumatoid arthritis: 15 years experience. Am J Med 1983; 75:69-73.
60. Horslev-Petersen K, Beger JM, Nelin P. Intermittent cyclophosphamide in refractory RA. Br Med J 1983; 287:711-2.
61. Hanly JG, Hassan J, Moriarty M, Barry C, Molony J, Casey E, Whelan A, Feighery C, Bresninhan B. Lymphoid irradiation in intractable rheumatoid arthritis: a double blind, randomized study comparing 759-Rad treatment and 2000-Rad treatment. Arth Rheum 1986; 29:16-25.
62. Cook TDV, Hard ER, Jasin HE, Bienenstock J, Ziff M. Identification of immunoglobulin and complement in rheumatoid articular collagenous tissues. Arth Rheum 1975; 18:541-7.
63. Duke O, Panayi GS, Janossy G, Poulter LW, Tidman N. Analysis of T-cell subsets in the peripheral blood and synovial fluid of patients with rheumatoid arthritis by means of monoclonal antibodies. Ann Rheum Dis 1983; 42:357-61.
64. Janossy G, Duke O, Poulter LW, Panayi G, Bofell M, Goldstein G. Rheumatoid arthritis: a disease of T-lymphocyte/macrophage immunoregulation. Lancet 1981; 2:839-42.

65. Wegelius O, Laine V, Lindstrom B, Klockass M. Fistula of the thoracic duct as immunosuppressive treatment in rheumatoid arthritis. Acta Med Scand 1970; 187:539–44.
66. Paulus HE, Machleder HI, Bangert R, Stratten JA, Goldberg L, Whitehouse MW, Yu DTY, Pearson CM. A case report: thoracic duct lymphocyte drainage in rheumatoid arthritis. Clin Immunol Immunopathol 1973; 1:173–81.
67. Paulus HE, Machleder HI, Levine S. Yu DTY, MacDonald NS. Lymphocyte involvement in rheumatoid arthritis. Arth Rheum 1977; 20:1249–61.
68. Yu DTY, Paulus HE, Peter JB. Long-term thoracic duct drainage in a rheumatoid arthritis patient. In Kunze K, Desmedt JE, eds. Proceedings of the International Symposium, Giessen, 1973:191-5.
69. Yu DTY, Peter JB, Stratton JA. Lymphocyte dynamics: change in density profiles and response to phytohemagglutinin of human lymphocytes during prolonged thoracic duct drainage. Clin Immunol Immunopathol 1973; 1:456–62.
70. Ueo T, Tanaka S, Tominage Y, Ogauda H, Sakurami T. The effect of thoracic duct drainage on lymphocyte dynamics and clinical symptoms in patients with rheumatoid arthritis. Arth Rheum 1979; 22:1405–12.
71. Wallace J, Goldfinger D, Gatti R, Lowe C, Fan P, Bluestone R, Klinenberg JR. Plasmapheresis in the management of rheumatoid arthritis. Arth Rheum 1979; 22:703–10.
72. Karsh J, Wright DG, Klippel JH, Decker JL, Deisserath AB, Flye MW. Lymphocyte depletion of continuous flow cell centrifugation in rheumatoid arthritis. Arth Rheum 1979; 22:1055–9.
73. Hamburger MI, Gerardi EN, Fields TR. Lymphoplasmapheresis and reticuloendothelial system (RES) Fc receptor function in rheumatoid arthritis (RA). Arth Rheum 1981; 24:S98.
74. Tenenbaum J, Urowitz MB, Keystone EC. Leukapheresis in severe rheumatoid arthritis. Ann Rheum Dis 1979; 38:40–1.
75. Wright DG, Karsh J, Fauci AS. Lymphocyte depletion and immunosuppression with repeated leukapheresis by continuous flow cell centrifucation. Blood 1981; 58:451–8.
76. Karsh J, Yeadon C. Lymphapheresis in rheumatoid arthritis: the clinical and laboratory effects of a limited course of cell depletion. Clin Exp Rheumatol 1983; 1:119–24.
77. Wahl SM, Wilder RL, Katona IM, Wahl LM, ALlen JB, Scher I, Decker JL. Leukapheresis in rheumatoid arthritis: association of clinical improvement with reversal of anergy. Arth Rheum 1983; 26:1076–84.
78. Karsh J, Klippel JH, Plotz PH, Decker JL, Wright DG, Flye MW. Lymphapheresis in rheumatoid arthritis. Arth Rheum 1981; 24:867–73.

79. Wallace D, Goldfinger D, Lowe D. A double-blind controlled study of lymphoplasmapheresis (LP) in rheumatoid arthritis. N Engl J Med 1982; 306:1406–10.
80. Verdickt W, Dequeker J, Ceuppens JL, Stevens E, Gautama K, Vermylen C. Effect of lymphoplasmapheresis in clinical indices and T-cell subsets in rheumatoid arthritis: a double-blind controlled study. Arth Rheum 1983; 26:1419–28.
81. Brubaker DB, Winkelstein A. Plasma exchange in rheumatoid vasculitis. Vox Sang 1981;41:295–301.
82. Calabrese LM, Clough JD, Krakauer RS, Hoeltage GA. Plasmapheresis therapy of immunologic disease: report of nine cases and review of the literature. Cleveland Clin Quart 1980;47:53–72.
83. Dequeker J, Naesens M, Martens J, Picters R. The effect of plasma exchange in synovitis in rheumatoid arthritis. Scand J Rheumatol 1981; 10:273–9.
84. Wallace DJ, Goldfinger D, Klinenberg JR. Current status of therapeutic apheresis in rheumatoid arthritis. Artif Org 1981;5:297–8.
85. Scheinberg MA, Weltman E. Plasmapheresis vs. total lymphoid irradiation in the treatment of severe rheumatoid arthritis. Clin Exp Rheumatol 1985;3:127–30.
86. Scott DGI, Bacon PA, Bothamley JE, Allen C, Elson CJ, Wallington TB. Plasma exchange in rheumatoid vasculitis. J Rheumatol 1981;8:433–9.
87. Goldman JA, Casey HL, McIlwain H, Kirby J, Wilson CH, Miller SB. Limited plasmapheresis in rheumatoid arthritis with vasculitis. Arth Rheum 1979;22:1146–50.
88. Dequeker J, Walravens M, Leys A. Arteritis associated with hyperviscosity-like syndrome in rheumatoid arthritis treated by intermittent plasma exchange for 2.5 years. Rheumatol Rehabil 1981;20:203–7.
89. Bjelle A, Cedergren B, Wahlby L. Plasma exchange in two patients with rheumatoid vasculitis. Scand J Rheumatol 1981;11:58–62.
90. Orfonne J, Cassuto-Viginer E, Quaranta J, Lacour J, Ziegler G. Bullous and pustular rheumatoid vasculitis treatment by plasma exchange. Acta Derm Venereol 1983;63:125–7.
91. Dwosh IL, Giles AR, Ford PM, Pater JL, Anastassiades TP. Plasmapheresis therapy in rheumatoid arthritis: a controlled double-blind crossover study. N Engl J Med 1983;308:1124–9.
92. Rothwell RS, Davis P, Gordon PA, Dasguta MK, Hohny KV, Russel AS, Percy JS. A controlled study of plasma exchange in the treatment of severe rheumatoid arthritis. Arth Rheum 1980;23:785–90.
93. Van Wanghe P, Dequeker J. Effect of intravenous cyclophosphamide as an adjuvant to therapeutic plasma exchange in rheumatoid arthritis. Plasma Ther Transfus Technol 1982, 3:171–6.

94. Winkelstein A, Starz TW, Agarwal A. Efficacy of combined therapy with plasmapheresis and immunosuppressants in rheumatoid vasculitis. J Rheumatol 1984; 11:162-6.
95. Wallace DJ, Barnett EV, Nichols S, Hancock W, Vibert G, Curd J, Klinenberg JR, Goldfinger D. Immunologic dynamics in cryopheresis for rheumatoid arthritis. J Rheumatol 1983; 10:894-901.
96. Krakauer RJ, Wysenbeck AJ, Wallace DJ, Jones JV, Smith JW, Malchesky P, Greenstreet R, Goldfinger D, Klinenberg JR, McLeod B, Nose Y. Therapeutic trial of cryofiltration in patients with rheumatoid arthritis. Am J Med 1983; 74:951-5.
97. Abe Y, Katsume C, Mastsufara S, Ueno M, Matsugane T, Blastertig E, Smith JW, Malchesky PS, Nose Y. Selective removal of immune complexes by cryofiltration in rheumatoid arthritis. Trans Am Soc Artif Inter Organs 1983; 29:730-4.
98. Wilder RL, Yarboro CH, Decker JL. The effect of repeated leukapheresis in patients with severe refractory rheumatoid arthritis. Prog Clin Biol Res 1982; 106:49-60.
99. Tan EM, Cohen AS, Fries JF. The 1982 revised criteria for the classification of systemic lupus erythematosus. Arth Rheum 1982; 25:1271-7.
100. Estes D, Christian CL. The natural history of systemic lupus erythematosus by prospective analysis. Medicine 1971; 50:85-95.
101. Wallace DJ, Podell T, Weiner J. Systemic lupus erythematosus-survival patterns. JAMA 1981; 245:934-8.
102. Urowitz MB, Bookman AM, Koehler BE. The bimodal mortality pattern of systemic lupus erythematosus. Am J Med 1976; 60:221-5.
103. Sakane T, Steinberg AD, Green I. Studies of immune functions of patients with systemic lupus erythematosus. Arth Rheum 1980; 23: 225-31.
104. Brentjens J, Ossi E, Albini B. Disseminated immune deposits in lupus erythematosus. Arth Rheum 1977; 20:962-8.
105. Steinberg AD. Studies in immune regulation. In: Decker JL, ed. Systemic lupus erythematosus, evolving concepts. Ann Intern Med 1979; 91:587-604.
106. Grayson J, Blaese RM, Steinberg AD, Dooley NJ, Koski FR. Circulating immunoglobin secreting cells in patients with systemic lupus erythematosus. Clin Res 1979; 27:326A.
107. Nydegger VE, Lambert PH, Gerber H, Miescher PA. Circulating immune complexes in the serum in systemic lupus erythematosus and in carriers of hepatitis B antigen. Quantifications by binding to radiolabelled C1q. J Clin Invest 1974; 54:297-309.
108. Winfield JB, Koffler D, Kunkel HG. Specific concentration of polynucleotide immune complexes in cryoprecipitates of patients with systemic lupus erythematosus. J Clin Invest 1975; 56:563-70.

109. Jones JV, Bucknall RC, Cumming RH, Asplin CM, Fraser ID, Bothamley J, Davis P, Hamblin TJ. Plasmapheresis in the management of systemic lupus erythematosus? Lancet 1976; 1:709–11.
110. Frank MM, Hamburger MI, Lawlay TJ, Kimberly RIP, Plotz PH. Defective Fc-receptor function in lupus erythematosus. N Engl J Med 1979; 300:418-523.
111. Lockwood CM, Worlledge S, Nicholas A, Cotton C, Peters DK. Reversal of impaired splenic function by plasma exchange. N Engl J Med 1979; 300:524-30.
112. Hamburger MI, Gerardi TR, Fields RS. Reticuloendothelial system Fc receptor function and plasmapheresis in systemic lupus erythematosus: a preliminary report. J Artif Organs 1981; 2:264–9.
113. Hamburger MI, Lawley TJ, Kimberly RP. A serial study of reticuloendothelial system Fc receptor function in systemic lupus erythematosus. Arth Rheum 1981; 25:48–54.
114. Abdou NI, Lindsley HB, Pollock A. Plasmapheresis in active systemic lupus erythematosus: effects in clinical, serum and cellular abnormalities—case report. Clin Immunol Immunopathol 1981; 19: 44–54.
115. Kater L, Derksen RH, Houwert DA. Effect of plasmapheresis in active systemic lupus erythematosus. Neth J Med 1981; 24:209–16.
116. Jones JV, Robinson MR, Parciany RK. Therapeutic plasmapheresis in systemic lupus erythematosus Arth Rheum 1981; 24:1113-29.
117. Parry HF, Moran CJ, Snaith ML, Richards JDM, Goldstone AH, Nineham LJ, Hay FC, Morrow WJW, Roitt IM. Plasma exchnage in systemic lupus erythematosus. Ann Rheum Dis 1981; 40:224–8.
118. Moran CJ, Parry HF, Mowbray J, Richards JDM, Goldstone AH. Plasmapheresis in systemic lupus erythematosus. Br Med J 1977; 1: 1573–9.
119. Schilderman B, Dequeker J, Van de Putte I. Plasmapheresis combined with corticosteroids in uncontrolled active systemic lupus erythematosus. J Rheumatol 1979; 6:687–90.
120. Hamilton WAP, Vergani D, Bevis L. Plasma exchange in systemic lupus erythematosus. Lancet 1980; 1:1249.
121. Jones JV. Plasmapheresis in systemic lupus erythematosus. Clin Rheum Dis 1982; 8:243–60.
122. Schlansky R, DeHoratius RJ, Pincus T, Tung KSK. Plasmapheresis in sytemic lupus erythematosus: a cautionary note. Arth Rheum 1981; 24:49–53.
123. Young DW, Thompson RA, Mackie PH. Plasmapheresis in hereditary antioneurotic edema and systemic lupus erythematosus. Arch Intern Med 1980; 140:127–8.
124. Clark WF, Lindsay RM, Ulan RA. Chronic Plasma exchange therapy in SLE nephritis. Clin Nephrol 1981; 16:2–3.

125. Gipstein RM, Adams DA, Grabie MT, Peter JB. Response of lupus nephritis to plasmapheresis without demonstration of circulating immune complexes. Am J Med Sci 1982; 284:37–41.
126. Wallace DJ, Goldfinger D, Bluestone R, Klinenberg JR. Plasmapheresis in lupus nephritis with nephrotic syndrome: a long term followup. J Clin Apheresis 1982; 1:42–5.
127. Isbister JP, Ralston M, Wright R. Fulminant lupus pneumonitis with acute renal failure and RBC aplasia: successful management with plasmapheresis and immunosuppression. Arch Intern Med 1981; 141: 1981-3.
128. Millman RP,Cohen TB, Levinson AI. Systemic lupus erythematosus complicated by acute pulmonary hemorrhage: recovery following plasmapheresis nad cytotoxic therapy. J Rheumatol 1981; 8:1021-3.
129. Fitchen JJ, Cline MJ, Saxon A, Goldek DW. Serum inhibitors of hematopoiesis in a patient with aplastic anemia and systemic lupus erythematosus: recovery after exchange plasmapheresis. Am J Med 1979; 66:537–42.
130. Evans DT, Giles M, Horne DJ. Cerebral lupus erythematosus responding to plasmapheresis. Postrgrad Med J 1981; 57:247–51.
131. Hamblin TJ, Mufti GJ, Bracewell A. Severe deafness in systemic lupus erythematosus: its immediate relief by plasma exchange. Br Med J 1982; 284:1374.
132. Fruchter L, Gauthier B, Marino F. The use of plasmapheresis in a patient with systemic lupus erythematosus and necrotizing cutaneous ulcers. J Rheumatol 1983; 10:341-3.
133. Rossen RD, Hersh EM, Sharp JT, McCredie KB, Gyorkey F, Suki WN, Eknoyan G, Reisberg MA. Effect of plasma exchange on circulating immune complexes and antibody formation in patients treated with cyclophosphamide and prednisone. Am J Med 1977; 63:674–82.
134. Krapf F, Manger B, Koch B, Kraulledaf P, Kalden J. The estimation of circulating immune complexes, C3d and anti-ds DNA-antibody serum levels in the monitoring of therapeutic plasmapheresis in a patient with systemic lupus erythematosus: a case report. Clin Exp Rheumatol 1985; 3:159-62.
135. Passaleva A, Massai G, Emmi L, Stendardi L, Valesini G. Plasma exchange in the treatment of acute systemic lupus erythematosus without circulating immune complexes. Clin Exp Rheumatol 1985; 3:255-7.
136. Wei N, Huston DP, Lawley AD, Klippel JH, Hall RP, Balow JE, Decker JL. Randomized trial of plasma exchange in mild systemic lupus erythematosus. Lancet 1983; 1:17–22.
137. Nyman KE, Bangert R, Machleder H, Paulus HE. Thoracic duct drainage in systemic lupus erythematosus with cutaneous vasculitis. Arth Rheum 1977; 10:1129–34.

138. Terman DS, Buffaloe G, Cook G, Sullivan M, Mattioli C, Tillquist R, Ayus JC. Extracorporeal immunoadsorption: initial experience in human systemic lupus erythematosus. Lancet 1979; 2:824-7.
139. Moeda K, Shinzato T, Tsuruta Y, Usuda M, Sezaki R, Yoshida F, Yamada K, Ohbjayashi S, Narita S, Saito A, Ohta K, Yamawaki N, Furuta Inagaki K. Initial tratment of systemic lupus erythematosus with a new artificial reticuloendothelial system. Appl Biochem Biotechnol 1984; 10:193–6.
140. Schroeder JO, Euler HH, Loffler HG. Synchronization of plasmapheresis and pulse cyclophosphamide in severe systemic lupus erhtymatosus. Ann Intern Med 1997; 107:340-4.
141. Barr WG, Hubbel EA, Robinson JA. Plasmapheresis and pulse cyclophosphamide in systemic lupus erythematosus. Ann Intern Med 1988; 108:152–3.
142. Fauci AS, Haynes BF, Katz P. The spectrum of vasculitis. Ann Intern Med 1978; 87:660–7.
143. Valbonesi M, Garelli S, Montani F. Plasma exchange and immune complex disease: the predictability of immune complex removal to clinical response. Vox Sang 1982; 42:27–32.
144. Kauffman RH, Houwest DA. Plasmapheresis in rapidly progressive Henoch-Schonlein glomerulonephritis and the effect on circulating IgA immune complexes. Clin Nephrol 1981; 16:155–60.
145. Wysenbeek AJ, Calabrese LH, Mandel DR. Limited plasmapheresis in fulminant leukocytoclastic vasculitis. J Rheumatol 1982; 9:315–8.
146. Lockwood CM, Wooledge S, Nicholas A, Cotton C, Deters DK. Reversal of impaired splenic function in patients with nephritis or vasculitis (or both) by plasma exchange. N Engl J Med 1979; 300:524-30.
147. Cohen J, Lockwood CM, Calman CD. Plasma exchange in the treatment of leukocytoclastic vasculitis. J Roy Soc Med 1980; 73:458–80.
148. Valbonesi M, Garelli S, Mosconi G. Plasma exchange in the management of a patient with diffuse necrotizing cutaneous vasculitis. Vox Sang 1980; 39:241-5.
149. Kennedy C, Sanderson KV, Spey C. Painful bruising syndrome with vasculitis treated by plasmapheresis. Br J Dermatol 1970; suppl 14: 65-6.
150. Chalopin JM, Rifle G, Turc JM. Immunologic findings during successful treatment of HBeAg-associated polyarteritis nodosa by plasmapheresis alone. Br Med J 1980; 280:368.
151. Chenais F, Debru JL, Baret L. Plasma exchnage in the treatment of polyarteritis nodosa. In: Siederth MG, ed. Plasma exchange: plasmapheresis-plasma separation. Stuttgart: Schattauer Verlaz 1980: 285–8.
152. Ouzan D, Tremesi P, Strauss E, Chossegros P, Pasquier J, Zech P, Dujardin P, Delmont J, Trepo C. Superiority of plasma exchange

combined with vidarabin over classic therapy in the management of polyarteritis nodosa associated with hepatitis B virus. Plasma Ther Transfus Technol 1985; 6:487-92.

153. Weiner SR, Paulus HE. Treatment of Wegener's granulomatosis. Semin Resp Med. In press.
154. D'Angelo WA, Fries JF, Masi AT, Schulman LE. Pathological observations in systemic sclerosis (scleroderma): a study of fifty-eight autopsy cases and fifty-eight matched controls. Am J Med 1969; 46: 428-40.
155. Fisher ER, Rodnan G. Pathologic observations concerning the cutaneous lesion of progressive systemic sclerosis: an electron microscopic, histochemical and immunohistochemical study. Arth Rheum 1960; 3: 536-45.
156. Leinwant I, Duryee AW, Rivhter MN. Scleroderma based on a study of over 150 cases. Ann Intern Med 1954; 41:1003-41.
157. Haynes DC, Gershwin ME. The immunopathology of progressive systemic sclerosis (PSS). Semin Arth Rheum 1982; 11:331-51.
158. Greger RE. Familial progressive systemic scleroderma. Arch Dermatol 1975; 111:81-5.
159. Clements PJ, Opelz G, Terasaki PI, Liebling MR, Furst D. Association of HLA antigen A9 with progressive systemic sclerosis (scleroderma) tissue antigens. Tissue Antigens 1978; 11:357-61.
160. Campbell PM, LeRoy EC. Pathogenesis of systemic sclerosis: a vascular hypothesis. Semin Arth Rheum 1975; 4:351-68.
161. Fries JF. The microvascular pathogenesis of scleroderma: an hypothesis. Ann Intern Med 1979; 91:788-9.
162. Medsger T Jr, Masi AT. Epidemiology of systemic sclerosis (scleroderma). Ann Intern Med 1971; 74:714-21.
163. Kurland LT, Hauser WA, Ferguson RH. Epidemiologic features of diffuse connective tissue disorders in Rochester, Minn., 1951 through 1967, with special reference to systemic lupus erythematosus. Mayo Clinic Proc 1969; 44:649-55.
164. Rodnan GP. Progressive systemic sclerosis (diffuse scleroderma). In: Somber W, ed. Immunologic diseases. Boston: Little, Brown, 1971: 1052.
165. Medsger TA Jr, Masi AT. Epidemiology of progressive sclerosis. In: Rodnan GP, ed. Clinics in rheumatic diseases. London: W.B. Saunders, 1979:15.
166. Medsger TA Jr, Masi AT. The epidemiology of systemic sclerosis (scleroderma) among U.S. male veterans. J Chron Dis 1978; 31:73-85.
167. Medsger TA Jr, Masi AT, Rodnan GP, Benedek TG, Robinson H. Survival with systemic sclerosis (scleroderma): a live-table analysis of clinical and demographic factors in 309 patients. Ann Intern Med 1971; 75:369-78.

168. Rowell NR. The prognosis of systemic sclerosis. Br J Dermatol 1976; 95:57-60.
169. Cunningham PH, Andrews BS, Davis JS. Scleroderma: developments from Osler to the present. South Med J 1980; 73:770-4.
170. Thompson MD, Kim LK, Bentz RR, Alexander DK. Acute prednisone-induced disabling myalgias in scleroderma. Arth Rheum 1981; 24:639-40.
171. Binnick SA, Shore SS, Corman A, Fleischmaje R. Failure of dimethyl sulfoxide in the treatment of scleroderma. Arch Dermatol 1977; 111: 1393-8.
172. Furst DE, Clements PJ, Harris ER, Ross M, Levy J, Paulus HE. Measurement of clinical change in progressive systemic sclerosis: a 1 year double blind placebo controlled trial of nacetylcysteine. Ann Rheum Dis 1979; 38:356-61.
173. Bluestone R, Grahame R, Holloway V, Holt PJL. Treatment of sytemic sclerosis with D-penicillamine. A new method of observing the effects of treatment. Ann Rheum Dis 1970; 29:158-63.
174. Mackenzie AM. Prolonged alkylating drug therapy is beneficial in systemic scleroderma (PSS). Arth Rheum 1970; 13:334.
175. Steigerwald JC. Chlorambucil therapy in progressive systemic sclerosis. J Rheumatol (Suppl) 1974; 1:74.
176. Keysteone EC, Gladman DD, Baren M, Cane D, Poplonski L. Antigen-reactions in progressive systemic sclerosis. Arth Rheum 1982; 25:390-5.
177. Morse JH, Bodi BS. Autologous and allogenic mixed lymphocyte reactions in progressive systemic sclerosis. Arth Rheum 1982; 25:390-5.
178. Machleder HI, Paulus HE. Clinical and immunologic alterations observed in patients undergoing long-term thoracic duct drainage. Surgery 1978; 84:157-65.
179. Talpos G, White JM, Horrocks M, Cotton LT. Plasmapheresis in Raynaud's disease. Lancet 1972; II:416-7.
180. Talpos G, Cotton LT, White JM. Reply to letter to the editors. Lancet 1978; 1:672.
181. Cotton LT. Plasmapheresis in Raynaud's disease. Lancet 1978; 2:208.
182. O'Reilly MJG, Talpos G, Roberts VC. Controlled trial of plasma exchange in treatment of Raynaud's syndrome. Br Med J 1979; 1: 1113-5.
183. Hamilton WAP, O'Reilly MJG, Dodds AJ. Cited by Hamilton WAP, White JM, Cotton LT. Plasma exchange in Raynauds phenomenon (letter to the editor). Lancet 1980; 2:475.
184. Dodds AJ, O'Reilly MJG, Yates CJP. Hemorrheological response to plasma exchange in Raynauds syndrome. Br Med J 1979; 2:1186-7.
185. O'Reilly MJG, Zahavi J, Dubiel L. Plasmapheresis and platelet function in Raynaud's syndrome (abstract). Thromb Haemost 1979; 42:338.

186. Zahavi J, Hamilton WAP, O'Reilly MJG, Leyton J, Cotton LT, Kakkar VV. Plasma exchange and platelet function in Raynaud's phenomenon. Thromb Res 1980; 19:85-93.
187. McCune MA, Winkelman RK, Osmundsen PJ, Pineda AA. Plasma exchange: a controlled study of the effect in patients with scleroderma and Raynaud's phenomenon. J Clin Apheresis 1983; 1:206-14.
188. Dau PC, Kahaleh MB, Sagebriel RW. Plasmapheresis and immunosuppressive drug therapy in scleroderma. Arth Rheum 1981; 24:1128-36.
189. Dau PC. Therapeutic plasma exchange: dermatologic applications. In: Callen JP, ed. Dermatologic clinics. Vol. 1 Philadelphia: W.B. Saunders, 1983:571-89.
190. Glasson PH. Traitement de l'hypertension arterielle par plasmaphereses. Schweiz Med Wschr 1983; 113:189-91.
191. Richmond JM, D'Apice AJF, Muirden KD. Scleroderma crisis: response to therapy. Med J Aust 1980; 1:545-7.
192. Gouet D, Alcalay D, Thomas P. Traitement de la sclerodermie generalisee par echanges plasmatiques: a propos de 3 cas. Reve Med Interne 1982; 3:367-72.
193. Guillevin L, Leon A, Levy Y, Bletry O, Gayraud M, Andreu G, Godeau P. Treatment of progressive systemic sclerosis with plasma exchange. Seven cases: Int J Artif Organs 1983; 6:315-8.
194. Weiner SR, Kono DK, Osterman HA, Levy H, Paulus HE, Pitts W. Preliminary report of a trial of apheresis in the treatment of scleroderma. Arth Rheum 1987; 30: Supplement.
195. Gorevic PD, Kassab HJ, Levo Y. Mixed-cryoglobulinemia: Clinical aspects and long term followup of 40 patients. Am J Med 1980; 69: 287-308.
196. Cream JJ. Immune complexes in cryoprecipitates. Ann Rheum Dis 1977; 36 (Suppl 1):45-8.
197. Meltzer M, Franklin EC, Elias K, McClusky RT, Cooper N. Cryoglobulinemia: a clinical and laboratory study. Am J Med 1966; 40:837-42.
198. Balow JE, Austin HA, Tsokos GC. Plasmapheresis therapy in immunologically mediated rheumatic and renal diseases. Clin Immunol Rev 1984; 3:235-72.
199. Geltner D, Kohn RW, Grevic PD. The effect of combination therapy (steroids, immunosuppressives and plasmapheresis) on 5 mixed cryoglobulinemia patients with renal, neurologic and vascular involvement.
200. Berkman EM, Orlin JB. Use of plasmapheresis and partial plasma exchange in the management of patients with cryoglobulinemia. Transfusion 1980; 20:171-8.
201. Ginder PA, Middendorg DE, Abdou NI. Pancytopenia with mixed cryoglobulinemia: evidence for anti-precursor cell activity of cryoglobulin-effects of plasmapheresis. J Clin Immunol 1982; 2:55-8.

202. Hamburger, Mi, Gorevic PD, Lawley TJ. Mixed cryoglobulinemia: association of glomerulonephritis with defective reticuloendothelial system Fc receptor function. Trans Am Assoc Phys 1979; 91:104-12.
203. Bohan A, Peter JB, Bowman RL, Pearson CM. Computer-assisted analysis of 153 patients with polymyositis and dermatomyositis. Medicine 1977; 56:255-80.
204. Pearson CM, Bohan A. Spectrum of polymyositis and dermatomyositis. Med Clin N Am 1977; 61:439-57.
205. Sullivan DB, Cassidy JT, Petty RE. Dermatomyositis in the pediatric patient. Arth Rheum 1977; 20:327-31.
206. Wolfe JF, Adelstein E, Sharp GC. Antinuclear antibody with destined specificity for polymyositis. J Clin Invest 1977; 238:869-71.
207. Behan WMH, Barkas T, Behan PO. Detection of immune complexes in polymyositis. Acta Neurol Scand 1982; 65:320-34.
208. Iannaccone ST, Bowen D, Yarom A. In vitro study of cytotoxic factors against endothelium in childhood dermatomyositis. Arch Neurol 1984; 41:862-5.
209. Rowe DJ, Isenbert DA, McDougall J. Characterization of polymyositis infiltrates using monoclonal antibodies to human leucocyte antigens. Clin Exp Immunol 1981; 45:290-8.
210. Giorno R, Barden MT, Kohler PF. Immunohistochemical characterization of the mononuclear cells infiltrating muscle of patients with inflammatory and noninflammatory myopathies. Clin Immunol Immunopathol 1984; 30:405-12.
211. Fulthorpe JJ, Hudgson P. Immunocytochemical localization of immunoglobulins in the inflammatory lesions of polymyositis. J Neuroimmunol 1982; 2:145-54.
212. Behan WMH, Behan PO. Disturbance of regulatory lymphocyte subsets in polymyositis. Ann Neurol 1984; 15:112-4.
213. Henriksson KG, Sandstedt P. Polymyositis-treatment and prognosis: a study of 107 patients. Acta Neurol Scand 1982; 65:280-300.
214. Hoffman Gs, Franck WA, Raddatz DA. Presentation, treatment and prognosis of idiopathic inflammatory muscle disease in a rural hospital. Am J Med 1983; 75:433-8.
215. Dau PC, Miller RG, Denys EH. Experience with plasmapheresis in 153 neurologic patients. Int J Artif Organs 1982; 5:37-46.
216. Whitaker JN, Engel WK. Vascular deposits of immunoglobulin and complement in idiopathic inflammatory myopathy. N Engl J Med 1972; 286:333-8.
217. Dau PC, Bennington JL. Plasmapheresis in childhood dermatomyositis. J Pediatr 1981; 98:237-40.
218. Brewer EJ Jr, Giannini EH, Rossen RD. Plasma exchange therapy of a childhood onset dermatomyositis patient. Arth Rheum 1980; 23:509-13.

219. Anderson L, Ziter FA. Plasmapheresis via central catheter in dermatomyositis: a new method for selected pediatr patients. J Pediatr 1981; 198:240–1.
220. Dau PC. Plasmapheresis in idiopathic inflammatory myopathy: experience with 35 patients. Arch Neurol 1981; 38:544–52.
221. Reuther PA, Rohkamm R, Wiebecke D. Plasma exchange in idiopathic inflammatory myopathy. In: Nose Y, Malcechsky PS, Smith JW, eds. Plasmapheresis. New York: Raven Press, 1983:309–15.
222. Khatri BO, Luprecht G, Weiss SA. Plasmapheresis and immunosuppressive drug therapy in polymyositis. Muscles Nerve 1982; 5:568–9.
223. Cecere FA, Spiva DA. Combination plasmapheresis/leukocytapheresis for the treatment of dermatomyositis/polymyositis. Plasma Ther Transfus Technol 1982; 3:401–9.
224. Clymard JP, Schooneman F, Gerard A, You B, Legras B, Olive D, Glouquet J, Beurey J, Streiff F. Plasma exchange therapy in polymyositis and dermatomyositis: experience with nine patients. Plasma Ther Transfus Technol 1985; 6:493–7.
225. Brewere EJ Jr, Nickesen RW Jr, Rossen RD. Plasma exchange in selected patients with juvenile rheumatoid arthritis. J Pediatr 1981; 98:194–200.
226. Wechsler B, Du LTH, Hoang PL, Khalaf P, Piette JC, Rottembourg J, Toldeano D, Godeau P. Plasma exchange in Behcet's disease. Plasma Ther Transfus Technol 1985; 6:499–502.
227. Westheim AF, Lookingbill DP. Plasmapheresis in a patient with scleromyoxedema. Arch Dermatol 1987; 123:786–9.
228. Crapper RM, Dowling JP, Mackey FR, Whiteworth JA. Acute scleroderma in stable mixed connective tissue disease: treatment by plasmapheresis. Aust NZ J Med 1987; 17:327–9.
229. Samtleben W, Lysaght MJ, Gurland HJ. Therapeutic plasma exchange: achievements versus expectations. Contr Nephrol 1985; 44:223–35.

6

Total Lymphoid Irradiation

David E. Trentham
Harvard Medical School and Beth Israel Hospital, Boston, Massachusetts

I. RATIONALE

The extreme radiosensitivity of lymphocytes to ionizing irradiation led initially to the attempted use of this procedure for the induction of cellular immunosuppression that could prolong allograft survival in experimental animals. Single-dose irradiation regimens were evaluated initially but problems with bone marrow toxicity and cardiopulmonary inflammation led to their abandonment. In an effort to reduce the toxicity, an alternative approach was considered (1) whereby irradiation would be delivered in fractionated, incremental aliquots. In addition, radiation was administered by selective exposure of all major lymphoid regions of the body while nonlymphoid organs were shielded by lead blocks. This adaptation was termed fractionated total lymphoid irradiation (TLI) (2-7).

As an alternative to chemotherapy, TLI came into use as a method of depleting malignant lymphocytes in patients with Hodgkin's disease (2,8). During almost a quarter century of experience, well over 3000 patients with Hodgkin's disease have been treated solely with TLI and followed up for periods well in excess of 10 years (2,3,8,9). The efficacy of this treatment is widely recognized, and the incidence of leukemia or a second tumor arising in these patients within 10 years after treatment has been negligible. Most treated patients have remained in excellent health overall. Although Hodgkin's disease is well recognized as capable of inducing anergic defects in the cellular immune system, it is noteworthy that sustained cellular immunosuppression has been apparent in the successfully treated patients for a number of years following completion of TLI (2). This aspect prompted further consideration of the use of TLI in the treatment of immunologically mediated disease or as an adjunct in enhancing organ allograft survival.

II. PRECLINICAL EVALUATION

Dose-response studies in mice initially indicated that 3400 rads of TLI was capable of suppressing cellular immunity without untoward irradiation-induced consequences (1,10,11). This protocol was used to prolong allogeneic skin and bone marrow engraftment (1,10), aid the development of tolerance to foreign protein antigens (11), block the antibody response to a foreign antigen (12), and ameliorate autoimmune disease in the NZB/NZW (13,14) and MRL/1 (15) strains of mice. In rats, this dose of TLI was shown to expedite the induction of allograft acceptance (16), to decrease lymphocyte concentrations in the peripheral blood (17), and to partially suppress the adjuvant (18) and collagen (19) models of polyarthritis. Comprehensive evaluations of TLI for immunologically mediated arthritis were conducted in the collagen model (19). TLI completed 7 days before immunization with collagen was associated with a delay in the onset and a suppression of the arthritis in this disease. In contrast, TLI delivered during the initial stage of clinically evident arthritis did not affect the degree of joint inflammation or destruction. This outcome was reminiscent of early work showing that TLI combined with hindpaw irradiation was more effective than TLI alone in suppressing established adjuvant arthritis in rats (18). TLI administered either prior to immunization or during the early course of collagen arthritis decreased antibody responses to collagen significantly (19). Cellular immunity, measured by the incorporation of thymidine after in vitro stimulation with phytohemagglutinin, was abolished in rats 6 days after the end of TLI. Delayed hypersensitivity responses to collagen were decreased when measured in vivo 19–22 days after the end of TLI. However, these reactions returned to normal levels when tested 50 days after the end of TLI. These data indicated that recovery of at least some cellular immune functions had occurred in rats by 7 weeks after completion of TLI. These findings were similar to observations in mice that TLI could suppress antibody responses to primary immunization (12), as well as abnormal autoantibody levels present in the NZB (13,14) and MRL (15) strains. The cellular immunosuppression was similar to the impairment of T-cell functions in mice and rats observed after TLI by other laboratories (1,10,11,15,17). The temporary nature of the cellular immunosuppression produced by TLI was also consistent with observations that murine lymphocytes had regained the capacity to react to alloantigens in mixed-lymphocyte cultures by 70 days after TLI (1,10). A final comparison phase of the collagen arthritis study utilized cyclophosphamide administration (19). Although this immunosuppressive drug also suppressed the severity of arthritis and decreased antibody responses to collagen, there was no significant effect on the incidence of arthritis or on delayed-type hypersensitivity to collagen. Thus, TLI suppressed the incidence of arthritis and attenuated cellular immunity in rat collagen arthritis better than cylcophosphamide. These superiorities were considered to be potential treatment advantages in patients with rheumatoid arthritis.

Originally, it seemed logical that the mechanism accounting for TLI's cellular immunosuppression resided in specific elimination of T-lymphocyte populations. This concept was supported by the dose dependency of suppression achieved with TLI. It was highly surprising when evidence of a tolerogenic effect was obtained in mice given TLI (20). Mice inoculated with histoincompatible bone marrow cells following 3400 rads of TLI achieved a chimeric state and tolerance to donor alloantigens in the absence of graft-vs.-host disease (21-23). This outcome demonstrated that the host was tolerant of the graft and that the graft was incapable of eliciting a reaction in the host. This dual alteration was similar to that previously achieved in animals treated with antithymocyte globulin (6). These experiments imply that bone marrow cells are pivotal in the generation of the unresponsive state following TLI (6). The mechanism by which bone marrow cells contribute to this effect is unknown.

Additional studies of TLI in rodents indicated that the technique favored the generation of suppressor cells capable of abrogating both cellular and humoral responses. For example, suppressor cells arising after TLI are capable of dampening the mixed-lymphocyte reaction in an antigen-nonspecific manner (24). Histologically, these cells are large, immature mononuclear cells which are both cyclophosphamide- and radiation-resistant (24). The absence of phenotypic T-cell markers in these suppressor populations further favors the possibility that they derived from monocyte/macrophages (6).

In summary, basic work indicated that TLI results in marked depletion of mature T cells within lymphoid organs. The shielded bone marrow contains immunocompetent progenitor cells which then reconstitute and induce tolerance to either new protein antigens or introduced alloantigens. Thus, Slavin (6) proposed that TLI triggers conditions simulating the immature, tolerance-favoring neonatal immune system. Support for this concept is provided by the finding of similar suppression-inducing cells in fetal liver and neonatal spleen (24). The pathways by which these suppressor cells function after TLI are unknown (24-28). It is possible that the antigen-nonspecific suppressor cells abolish clonal expansion of antigen-responding cells leading to a state of immunosuppression. In addition, the tolerance studies are consistent with the possibility of antigen-specific suppressor cells leading to clonal depletion.

Subsequent work attempting to use TLI to induce permanent transplantation tolerance was relatively disappointing. Prolonged transplantation tolerance to organ allografts could not be readily established in dogs or primates exposed to TLI doses as high as 4000 rads (6,29). Similar experiments in humans have also not been consistently successful (6).

Although TLI was immunosuppressive in collagen arthritis, a paradoxical finding was encountered. Arthritis developed in 6% of immunized Sprague-Dawley rats that had received TLI (30). In these experiments, rats were given seventeen 200-rad fractions of TLI over a period that ranged between 30 and 45 days. The limbs and ears were outside the irradiation ports. Macroscopically evident arthritis developed within 3 weeks following completion of TLI and persistent until they were sacrificed 7-14 days later. The severity and pattern of joint inflammation were similar to that observed in rats with collagen or adjuvant arthritis. An additional rat developed a lesion of both external ears that resembled type II collagen-induced chondritis 6 days after completion of TLI (31). Joint radiographs in rats with post-TLI arthritis revealed periarticular bone destruction. Cartilage erosions and extensive degrees of pannus extending over the cartilage surface were found on light microscopy. Neovascularization and a large number of primarily mononuclear inflammatory cells were present in the synovial and subsynovial tissue. Deposits of immunoglobulin, complement, and fibrin were found within the synovium by immunofluorescence techniques. No overt or serological evidence of infection was present in the irradiated rats. Although the mechanism by which TLI triggers arthritis in this strain of rats is unknown, it is probable that TLI-mediated effects on the immune system are responsible for the phenomenon. One possibility is that an imbalance or perturbation in the immune system created by TLI allows clonal expansion of lymphoid cells which are capable of producing an autoimmune arthritis. Although unproven, this hypothesis is particularly provocative because of inferences it might have for the inception of autoimmune disease in humans.

III. DELIVERY OF TLI

Patients with rheumatoid arthritis entering trials of TLI have received two-field (32) or three-field (33) irradiation on an outpatient basis. To define radiation portals, patients are generally evaluated with a chest roentgenogram, an intravenous pyelogram, and a spleen scan. Bipedal lymphangiography may be helpful for patients with severe spinal deformity. A bone marrow biopsy is performed to assess hematopoiesis, and baseline thyroid function tests are conducted. Patients then begin a maintenance program of dental hygiene that continues for 1 year after completion of TLI treatment.

TLI is delivered by means of 4-MV photons from a linear accelerator. Additional ovarian shielding techniques, as used in patients with Hodgkin's disease, are used in premenopausal women (33). Radiation doses are calculated at midplane. Anteroposterior and posteroanterior fields are treated on alternate days. During radiation, patients are assessed by a complete blood count twice weekly.

Most patients have been treated with two fields (32–36). With this method, 2000 rads is delivered to the mantle portal and the inverted Y area, i.e., periaortic nodes, spleen, and pelvic nodes (32). Daily fractions are 160–180 rads. No break occurs between a change in treatment regions; this results in a total course of radiation therapy requiring approximately 5–6 weeks. Another initial study used a three-field technique (33). In this protocol a total of 3000 rads was delivered to the mantle, periaortic nodes and spleen, and pelvic nodes, using fractions of 160–180 rads. With treatment breaks, the treatment time was approximately 14–16 weeks (33).

IV. EFFICACY

Approximately 20% of adult patients with erosive rheumatoid arthritis who are followed regularly by a rheumatologist are refractory to currently available therapies. This impasse is attributable either to a lack of drug efficacy or to unacceptable side effects. Oral cyclophosphamide therapy has been used extensively in such patients but is now widely perceived to possess an extremely unfavorable risk/benefit ratio. Bone marrow toxicity, hemorrhagic cystitis, and induction of leukemia have largely led to an abandonment of this approach (5).

In contrast, it was recognized by 1975 that TLI treatment of Hodgkin's disease was associated with few serious long-term sequelae. For example, the sole complication noted in 70 patients with Hodgkin's disease treated with irradiation without chemotherapy during a period of 10 years at one institution was a single incidence of persistent thrombocytopenia (8). By this time, substantial evidence also had been obtained indicating that T cells participate in synovial inflammation in this disease. Short-term improvement in rheumatoid arthritis had been associated with lymphocyte depletion produced by thoracic duct drainage (37), extracorporeal irradiation of thoracic duct lymph (38), and blood leukapheresis (39).

These observations prompted investigators at Stanford University to conduct a pilot trial using 2000 rads of irradiation limited to the inverted y (pelvic) region in patients with refractory rheumatoid arthritis (40). This protocol produced profound blood lymphopenia with absolute lymphocyte counts of 400-500 cells/ml^3. Anti-inflammatory effects were also apparent. Unfortunately, the clinical improvement lasted only 4-6 months, and the flares in rheumatoid arthritis were accompanied by increasing lymphocyte counts.

In an attempt to sustain the lymphopenia and thereby prolong the clinical effects of irradiation therapy, investigative groups at Stanford (32) and Harvard Medical School (33) began open feasibility studies of TLI in patients with recalcitrant rheumatoid arthritis. The characteristics of the patients involved in both protocols were similar, and patients who had previously received therapy with cytotoxic drugs except azathioprine were excluded from the studies because there was a potential risk of bone marrow suppression or neoplasia. The TLI technique used at each institution reflected the manner in which Hodgkin's patients were routinely treated. At Stanford, a two-portal system was used in which the lymphoid regions were divided into those above and those below the diaphragm. At Harvard, a three-portal system consisting of a mantle portal, a paraaortic-splenic portal, and a pelvic portal was utilized. The infradiaphragmatic region was divided into two portals to decrease the severity of nausea or diarrhea during the irradiation period. A TLI dose of 2000 rads was delivered to the Stanford patients because this dose had produced demonstrable immunosuppression in mongrel dogs (29). In contrast, a higher dose of 3000 rads was delivered at Harvard because this dose was still appreciably lower than the 4000- to 4400-rad threshold at which irradiation-induced pneumonitis and pericarditis become frequent in Hodgkin's disease patients treated with TLI (2,8). In both institutions, patients received fractions of 150-200 rads 4-5 days a week. Thus, the patients finished the Stanford protocol in 5-7 weeks whereas a 4- to 16-week period was necessary to complete TLI at Harvard.

Degrees of clinical improvement that when patients were grouped attained statistical significance occurred in all studies. However, potentially important differences were manifested with these two protocols. The delivery of 2000 rads of TLI appeared not to lead to improvement until 1 or 2 months following completion of TLI (32). However, once it had been achieved, the improvement appeared to persist in an appreciable degree for 3-4 years following completion of radiotherapy (41). Perhaps not unexpectedly, the use of 3000 rads of TLI had a much more immediate impact on the disease (33). The data also suggested, through they did not prove, that a more substantial suppression of joint inflammation occurred in the patients treated with 3000 rads. Nonetheless, clear-cut evidence of partial disease recrudescence appeared approximately 8-12 months after completion of radiotherapy (33,42). Contrasting immunological outcomes also paralleled the clinical findings in each study. The 2000-rad, two-portal technique was associated with a persistent decline in the number and function of the CD4 T-cell subset (helper T cells) (32,41,43-46). Even during 2-3 years follow-up, no restoration in this profound deficit in the cellular immune system was evident (41). The three-portal approach also produced this specific immunological attenuation, but there was a restoration in the cellular immune system 8 and 12 months after completion of radiation (33). On the other hand, the normalization appeared to be only temporary because follow-up of the 3000 rad-treated patients 2-3 years later indicated significant blood lymphopenia and diminished numbers of CD4 cells (42). Of importance, neither study indicated that TLI had any effect on either autoantibody responses indicative of rheumatoid arthritis or the normal elements of the humoral immune and complement systems (32,33). When combined, the data from both studies indicated a major association between reduced CD4 activities and improvement in the articular manifestations of refractory rheumatoid arthritis.

In additional trials of 2000 rads of two-portal TLI in Ireland (36) and West Germany (34), substantial anti-inflammatory and cellular immunosuppressive effects were evident in similar patients with refractory rheumatoid arthritis. These effects persisted for at least 6-8 months after completion of the irradiation. Moreover, Strober and coworkers at Stanford demonstrated, in a randomized, double-blind, parallel group study, that the 2000-rad, two-portal technique produces a partial decrease in disease activity in most patients with rheumatoid arthritis (35). The changes in the immune status of the patients treated in the unblinded trials (32,33), along with the scientifically rigorous randomized study (35), provide objective evidence that a profound biological response to TLI occurs in patients with rheumatoid arthritis. In addition, the magnitude of change suggested in the Irish (36) and Stanford (35) studies that doses of 750 and 200 rads, respectively, were capable of conferring beneficial effects on recalcitrant rheumatoid arthritis. For example, patients treated with 200 rads in the Stanford study (35) experienced 50% of the reduction in joint swelling exhibited by the group receiving 2000 rads.

A subsequent trial of 2000 rads of TLI at Harvard (47) confirmed most of the observations reported in the initial studies. Approximately 60% of treated patients experienced measurable benefit that persisted for at least 6-8 months. At that time the return of partial disease activity became evident, but prompt improvement could be recreated by the administration of low-dose methotrexate, azathioprine, or even prednisone (47). CD4-specific immunosuppression was again strikingly apparent in these patients (47).

In summary, all investigative groups have concluded that radiotherapy produces a clinically important anti-inflammatory effect on the articular manifestations of rheumatoid arthritis and that this response is associated temporally with a preferential reduction in the CD4 subset. This shared finding demonstrates that cellular immunity is involved in the pathogenesis of rheumatoid arthritis. Interestingly, no effect on extra-articular manifestations of rheumatoid arthritis, except for a reduction in the size of the subcutaneous rheumatoid nodules, has occurred. This dissociation is consistent with the possibility that these manifestations are primarily antibody-mediated. Limited experience with 2000-rad, two-portal TLI in the treatment of severe systemic lupus erythematosus (48,49) and multiple sclerosis (50) also exists.

V. TOXICITY

Considerable liabilities as well as benefits accompany the use of TLI (5,7). In all studies (32-36,41,42,47-50) TLI is associated with a higher frequency of acute and long-term complications in patients with autoimmune disease than in patients with Hodgkin's disease. In the 2000-rad group in the randomized Stanford study (35), TLI was interrupted because of adverse reactions in four of the 13 patients; five developed temporary leukopenia, three had herpes zoster, and two were hospitalized because of treatment effects. Patient recruitment was suspended in our 2000-rad trial because five of the 13 patients developed herpes zoster (47). It is unclear whether increased age, duration of preexisting disease, or presence of earlier and intercurrent therapy explains this difference. Middle-aged patients with severe rheumatoid arthritis tolerate TLI poorly, with nausea, diarrhea, and/or fatigue being major problems for all patients. Temporary leukopenia interrupts TLI in 10-30% of patients. Of approximately 75 patients treated with TLI for rheumatoid arthritis, approximately 30% have developed self-limited herpes zoster infections. Higher than expected bacterial sepsis rates (four of 12) and mortality rates (four of 12) have further indicated that 3000-rad TLI may be hazardous for patients with rheumatoid arthritis (33). Approximately 10% of patients have developed hypothyroidism or complained of distressing degrees of xerostomia. Sterility and alopecia are also potential concerns.

In addition, 15-year follow-up data of Hodgkin's disease patients treated with TLI alone recently showed an 11-fold increased risk of leukemia (9). Although the number of cases used to derive this estimate is extremely small, the finding is particularly worrisome when considering any additional experimental studies of TLI in patients with nonneoplastic disease. Additional discussions of these issues can be found elsewhere (4-7,47).

VI. MISCELLANEOUS

It is now evident that future trials of TLI would impose a degree of hazard to patients with autoimmune disease. Hematological complications and the likelihood of the induction of sterility are major potential risks. It is also likely that the large amount of irradiation with TLI would compromise efforts to curtail future tumor growth by radiotherapy if a neoplasm developed.

If low doses of TLI are palliative (35,36), additional evaluations would be attractive. On the other hand, the use of reduced doses of irradiation may prove to be leukemogenic if they damage stem cell DNA without killing the cell. Trials of TLI with subsequent administration of methotrexate (47), cyclosporine, or anti-T-cell antibody (6) are being considered. Unfortunately, there are minimal data to appraise the safety of any sequential immunotherapy approach.

The dominant conclusion to be drawn from experiments with TLI in rheumatoid arthritis is that CD4 cells play a critical primary role in the pathogenesis of this disease. Although some experimental data led to a recent proposal that deficient T-cell activities within the joint contribute to rheumatoid inflammation (52), the immunological sequelae of TLI provide indirect evidence that the synovitis is mediated by a T-cell activation pathway. Lymphokine production would be an attractive but hypothetical way in which T cells might subserve this deleterious function.

The TLI experience also serves to direct future therapeutic approaches for patients with refractory rheumatoid arthritis. Preliminary findings indicated that the intravenous administration of monoclonal anti-CD4 for a 1-week period specifically attenuates CD4 cells and can abruptly ameliorate joint inflammation in patients with rheumatoid arthritis (53). The disease appears to remain partially quiescent for at least several months after completion of therapy. Similar results are evident when using polyclonal equine antithymocyte globulin in RA, although serum sickness prompted discontinuation of this study after three patients had been treated (R. H. Shmerling and D. E. Trentham, unpublished data). The outcome in both trials suggests that major consideration should be given to the use of monoclonal antibodies directed against T cells as an alternative to TLI in patients with refractory rheumatoid arthritis.

REFERENCES

1. Slavin S, Strober S, Fuks Z, Kaplan HS. Long-term survival of skin allografts in mice treated with fractionated total lymphoid irradiation. Science 1976; 193:1252–4.
2. Kaplan HS. Hodgkin's disease. 2d ed. Cambridge: Harvard University Press, 1980:366–441, 478–547.
3. Order SE. Clinical radiation research in rheumatoid arthritis: caution, progress and hope. Int J Radiat Oncol Biol Phys 1981; 7:129–30.
4. Strober S. Overview: effect of total lymphoid irradiation on autoimmune disease and transplantation immunity. J Immunol 1984; 132: 968–70.
5. Trentham DE, Weinblatt ME, Austen KF. Total lymphoid irradiation in tertiary care for rheumatoid arthritis. Ann Intern Med 1985; 102:544–5.
6. Slavin S. Total lymphoid irradiation. Immunol Today 1987; 8:88–92.
7. Zvaifler NJ. Fractionated total lymphoid irradiation: a promising new treatment for rheumatoid arthritis? Yes, no, maybe. Arth Rheum 1987; 30:109–14.
8. Hellman S, Mauch P, Goodman RL, Rosenthal DS, Moloney WC. The place of radiation therapy in the treatment of Hodgkin's disease. Cancer 1978; 42:971–8.
9. Tucker MA, Coleman CN, Cox RS, Varghese A, Rosenberg SA. Risk of second cancers after treatment for Hodgkin's disease. N Engl J Med 1988; 318:76–82.
10. Slavin S, Strober S, Fuks Z, Kaplan HS. Induction of specific tissue transplantation tolerance using fractionated total lymphoid irradiation in adult mice: long-term survival of allogeneic bone marrow and skin grafts. J Exp Med 1977; 146:34–48.
11. Zan-Bar I, Slavin S, Strober S. Induction and mechanism of tolerance to bovine serum albumin in mice given total lymphoid irradiation (TLI). J Immunol 1978; 121:1400–4.
12. Zan-Bar I, Slavin S, Strober S. Effect of total lymphoid irradiation (TLI) on the primary and secondary antibody response to sheep red blood cells. Cell Immunol 1979; 45:167–74.

13. Kotzin BL, Strober S. Reversal of NZB/NZW disease with total lymphoid irradiation. J Exp Med 1979; 150:371–8.
14. Slavin S. Successful treatment of autoimmune disease in (NZB/NZW)F_1 female mice by using fractionated total lymphoid irradiation. Proc Natl Acad Sci USA 1979; 76:5274–6.
15. Theofilopoulos AN, Balderas R, Shawler DL, Izui S, Kotzin BL, Strober S, Dixon FJ. Inhibition of T cell proliferation and SLE-like syndrome of MRL/1 mice by whole body or total lymphoid irradiation. J Immunol 1980; 125:2137–42.
16. Slavin S, Reitz B, Bieger CP, Kaplan HS, Strober S. Transplantation tolerance in adult rats using total lymphoid irradiation: permanent survival of skin, heart, and marrow allografts. J Exp Med 1978; 147: 700–7.
17. Strober S, Slavin S, Gottlieb M, Zan-Bar I, King DP, Hoppe RT, Fuks Z, Grumet FC, Kaplan HS. Allograft tolerance after total lymphoid irradiation (TLI). Immunol Rev 1979; 46:87–112.
18. Schurman DJ, Hirshman HP, Strober S. Total lymphoid and local joint irradiation in the treatment of adjuvant arthritis. Arth Rheum 1981; 24: 38–44.
19. McCune WJ, Buckley JA, Belli JA, Trentham DE. Immunosuppression by fractionated total lymphoid irradiation in collagen arthritis. Arth Rheum 1982; 25:532–9.
20. Zan-Bar I, Slavin S, Strober S. Induction and mechanism of tolerance to bovine serum albumin in mice given total lymphoid irradiation (TLI). J Immunol 1978; 121:1400–4.
21. Slavin S, Fuks Z, Kaplan HS, Strober S. Transplantation of allogeneic bone marrow without graft-versus-host disease using total lymphoid irradiation. J Exp Med 1978; 147:963–72.
22. Gottlieb M, Strober S, Kaplan HS. Cellular basis of graft versus host tolerance in chimeras prepared with total lymphoid irradiation. J Exp Med 1980; 152:736–41.
23. Slavin S, Yatziv S. Correction of enzyme deficiency in mice by allogeneic bone marrow transplantation with total lymphoid irradiation. Science 1980; 210:1150–2.
24. Weigensberg M, Morecki S, Weiss L, Fuks Z, Slavin S. Suppression of cell-mediated immune responses after total lymphoid irradiation (TLI) I. Characterization of suppressor cells of the mixed lymphocyte reaction. J Immunol 1984; 132:971–8.
25. Waer M, Ang KK, van der Schueren E, Vandeputte M. Influence of radiation field and fractionation schedule of total lymphoid irradiation (TLI) on the induction of suppressor cells and stable chimerism after bone marrow transplantation in mice. J Immunol 1984; 132:985–90.

26. Waer M, Ang KK, van der Schueren E, Vandeputte M. Allogeneic bone marrow transplantation in mice after total lymphoid irradiation: influence of breeding conditions and strain of recipient mice. J Immunol 1984; 132:991–6.
27. Lowry RP, Clark Forbes RD, Carpenter CB, Gurley KE, Merrill JP. Immune reactivity and immunosuppressive intervention in experimental nephritis. II. Effect of TLI on the course of two models of nephritis in the inbred rat. J Immunol 1984; 132:1007–12.
28. Myburgh JA, Smit JA, Stark JH, Browde S. Total lymphoid irradiation in kidney and liver transplantation in the baboon: prolonged graft survival and alterations in T cell subsets with low cumulative dose regimens. J Immunol 1984; 132:1019–25.
29. Strober S, Modry DL, Hoppe RT, Pennock JL, Bieber CP, Holm BI, Jamieson SW, Stinson EB, Schroder J, Suomalainen H, Kaplan HS. Induction of specific unresponsiveness to heart allografts in mongrel dogs treated with total lymphoid irradiation and antithymocyte globulin. J Immunol 1984; 132:1013–8.
30. Trentham DE, Brahn E, Williams W, McCune WJ, Belli JA. Connective tissue disease can develop in rats either spontaneously or after total lymphoid irradiation. J Rheumatol 1984; 11:410–2.
31. McCune WJ, Schiller AL, Dynesius-Trentham RA, Trentham DE. Type II collagen-induced auricular chondritis. Arth Rheum 1982; 25:266–73.
32. Kotzin BL, Strober S, Engleman EG, Calin A, Hoppe RT, Kansas GS, Terrell CP, Kaplan HS. Treatment of intractable rheumatoid arthritis with lymphoid irradiation. N Engl J Med 1981; 305:969–75.
33. Trentham DE, Belli JA, Anderson RJ, Buckley JA, Goetzl EJ, David JR, Austen KF. Clinical and immunologic effects of fractionated total lymphoid irradiation in refractory rheumatoid arthritis. N Engl J Med 1981; 305:976–82.
34. Nusslein HG, Herbst M, Manger BJ, Gramatzki M, Burmester GR, Fritz H, Sauer R, Kalden JR. Total lymphoid irradiation in patients with refractory rheumatoid arthritis. Arth Rheum 1985; 28:1205–10.
35. Strober S, Tanay A, Field E, Hoppe RT, Calin A, Engleman EG, Kotzin B, Brown BW, Kaplan HS. Efficacy of total lymphoid irradiation in intractable rheumatoid arthritis: a double-blind, randomized trial. Ann Intern Med 1985; 102:441–9.
36. Hanley JG, Hassan J, Moriarty M, Barry C, Molony J, Casey E, Whelan A, Feighery C, Bresnihan B. Lymphoid irradiation in intractable rheumatoid arthritis: a double-blind, randomized study comparing 750-rad treatment with 2,000-rad treatment. Arth Rheum 1986; 29:16–25.
37. Paulus HE, Machleder HI, Levine S, Yu DTY, MacDonald NS. Lymphocyte involvement in rheumatoid arthritis: studies during thoracic duct drainage. Arth Rheum 1977; 20:1249–62.

38. Edgren J, Klockars M, Weber T. Extracorporeal irradiation of thoracic duct lymph as immunosuppressive treatment in rheumatoid arthritis. Scand J Rheumatol 1976; 5:108-12.
39. Karsh J, Klippel JH, Plotz PH, Decker JL, Wright DG, Flye MW. Lymphapheresis in rheumatoid arthritis: a randomized trial. Arth Rheum 1981; 24:867-73.
40. Strober S, Kotzin BL, Hoppe RT, Kaplan HS. The treatment of intractable rheumatoid arthritis with lymphoid irradiation. Int J Radiat Oncol Biol Phys 1981; 7:1-7.
41. Field EH, Strober S, Hoppe RT, Calin A, Engleman EG, Kotzin BL, Tanay AS, Calin HJ, Terrell CP, Kaplan HS. Sustained improvement of intractable rheumatoid arthritis after total lymphoid irradiation. Arth Rheum 1983; 26:937-46.
42. Brahn E, Helfgott SM, Belli JA, Anderson RJ, Reinherz EL, Schlossman SF, Austen KF, Trentham DE. Total lymphoid irradiation therapy in refractory rheumatoid arthritis: fifteen- to forty-month followup. Arthritis Rheum 1984; 27:481-8.
43. Kotzin BL, Kansas GS, Engleman EG, Hoppe RT, Kaplan HS, Strober S. Changes in T-cell subsets in patients with rheumatoid arthritis treated with total lymphoid irradiation. Clin Immunol Immunopathol 1983; 27:250-60.
44. Kotzin BL, Strober S, Kansas GS, Terrell CP, Engleman EG. Suppression of pokeweed mitogen-stimulated immunoglobulin production in patients with rheumatoid arthritis after treatment with total lymphoid irradiation. J Immunol 1984; 132:1049-55.
45. Field EH, Engleman EG, Terrell CP, Strober S. Reduced in vitro immune responses of purified human Leu-3 (helper/inducer phenotype) cells after total lymphoid irradiation. J Immunol 1984; 132:1031-5.
46. Tanay A, Strober S, Logue GL, Schiffman G. Use of total lymphoid irradiation (TLI) in studies of the T cell dependence of autoantibody production in rheumatoid arthritis. J Immunol 1984; 132:1036-40.
47. Trentham DE, Belli JA, Bloomer WD, Anderson RJ, Lane H, Reinherz EL, Austen KF. 2,000-centigray total lymphoid irradiation for refractory rheumatoid arthritis. Arth Rheum 1987; 30:980-7.
48. Strober S, Field E, Hoppe RT, Kotzin BL, Shemesh O, Engleman E, Ross JC, Myers BD. Treatment of intractable lupus nephritis with total lymphoid irradiation. Ann Intern Med 1985; 102:450-8.
49. Ben-Chetrit E, Gross DJ, Braverman A, Weshler Z, Fuks Z, Slavin S, Eliakim M. Total lymphoid irradiation in refractory systemic lupus erythematosus. Ann Intern Med 1986; 105:58-60.
50. Cook SD, Devereux C, Troiano R, Hafstein MP, Zito G, Hernandex E, Lavenhar M, Vidaver R, Dowling PC. Effect of total lymphoid irradiation in chronic progressive multiple sclerosis. Lancet 1986; 1:1405-9.

51. de Sousa M, Lima Bastos A, Dynesius-Trentham R, Kerr S, Bernardo A, Gomes Duarte J, Trentham DE. Potential of indium-lll to measure inflammatory arthritis. J Rheumatol 1986; 13:6-16.
52. Firestein GS, Zvaifler NJ. The pathogenesis of rheumatoid arthritis: a critical assessment of the role of autologous stimulation in the perpetuation of rheumatoid synovitis. Rheum Dis Clin N Am 1987; 13:447-61.
53. Herzog Ch, Walker Ch, Pichler W, Aeschlimann A, Wassmer P, Stockinger H, Knapp W, Rieber P, Muller W. Monoclonal anti-CD4 in arthritis. Lancet 1987; 2:1461-2.

7

Gamma Interferon: Mechanism of Action and Use in Rheumatoid Arthritis

John D. Schindler
Biogen, Inc., Cambridge, Massachusetts

Douglas V. Faller
Harvard Medical School, The Children's Hospital, and Dana Farber Cancer Institute, Boston, Massachusetts

I. INTRODUCTION

Interferon is the name given by Isaacs and Lindenmann in 1957 to a substance produced by virally infected cells that caused "interference" with viral infection of uninfected cells (1). Interferon was subsequently shown to be produced by leukocytes (leukocyte interferon), fibroblasts (fibroblast interferon), and lymphocytes (immune interferon). Leukocyte and fibroblast interferons are acid-stable but immune interferon is inactivated at pH 2. These properties led to the classification nomenclature of type I interferons (leukocyte and fibroblast interferon) and type II interferon (immune interferon). In 1980, at an international meeting of the World Health Organization, the National Institute of Allergy and Infectious Disease reclassified the interferons based on antigenic properties as α-interferon (leukocytes), β-interferon (fibroblast), and γ-interferon (lymphocyte) (2). Subclasses of α-interferon were designated α_1, α_2, and so forth. Abbreviations established at that time were Mu for murine, Hu for human, r for recombinant, and IFN for interferon.

The ability of interferon to block viral infection led to the study of its ability to inhibit the growth of virally induced tumors. The success of interferon in blocking virally induced tumors was attributed to its antiviral activity (3). Some years later, in 1969, Gresser et al. showed that interferon could inhibit the growth of transplantable and carcinogen-induced tumors, thus showing that interferon had either intrinsic antitumor activity or induced an antitumor activity (4,5). Subsequent work revealed that the interferons have direct antiproliferative properties as well as indirect immune-mediated antitumor activities.

Leukocyte interferon was first tested clinically on osteosarcoma without success at the Karolinska Insitute in 1972 (6). However, preclinical work continued to indicate that interferon had antitumor activity, and interest and demand for clinical trials grew in the United States. In response, the National Cancer Institute (NCI) commissioned the production of natural leukocyte interferon by Kari Cantell and the Finnish Blood Transfusion Service. A series of "early" trials in various oncological disease processes was conducted with these preparations. Since the product contained only 1% α-interferon, consisting primarily of other lymphokines and the byproducts of production from leukocyte buffy coat preparations, the responses seen could not be directly attributed to interferon (7).

The molecular cloning of the gene for α-interferon, followed by the cloning of the genes for γ-interferon and β-interferon, with the subsequent production of large amounts of very pure (>98%) recombinant protein, has permitted careful studies of the clinical properties of the interferons (8,9). A large majority of the clinical trials with interferons have been conducted, primarily for historical reasons, in oncology. Interferons have not lived up to public expectations as anticancer agents. However, interferons, at least α-interferon, are a failure only in the context of the original expectation that interferons would be a panacea for all oncology indications. α-Interferon has been approved by the FDA for use in hairy cell leukemia (>90% response rate) and Kaposi's sarcoma. Significant antitumor activity has also been seen in melanoma, myeloma, lymphoma, and chronic myelogenous leukemia. More recently, both α- and γ-interferons have been tested with success against condylomata acuminata. Human papilloma virus, the causative agent of condylomata, is believed to be associated with cervical cancer. Interferon is now being tested in patients with cervical cancer. Thus, the cycle has now gone full circle to the original observations of Atanasiu and Chang, with interferon being tested in virally induced tumors.

The rest of this chapter will be devoted to γ-interferon, its preclinical and clinical properties, particularly as they relate to the clinical development of r-IFN-g in the treatment of rheumatoid arthritis (RA). Although the compound is not yet available commercially in the United States, it has been approved for use in RA in West Germany. The other clinical indications that look most likely to respond to therapy with r-IFN-g are condylomata acuminata, chronic granulomatous disease, and infectious diseases such as leishmaniasis and trypanosomiasis.

II. STRUCTURE OF γ-INTERFERON

Because of the propensity of γ-interferon to form nonconvalently linked dimers, it was originally believed to have a molecular weight of 50,000-70,000 (10). Work by Yip et al. revealed that molecules with molecular weights of 20,000 and 25,000 had γ-interferon activity. Later work revealed further heterogeneity in the molecular weight (11).

The gene for γ-interferon was molecularly cloned in 1982 by Gray et al. (12). Unlike α-interferon, which exists as a family of genes, there is only one gene encoding γ-interferon and it is located on chromosome 12 (13,14). The DNA sequence suggests that there is a 20-AA leader sequence that is cleaved during synthesis leaving a backbone of 146 AA. However, some forms of natural γ-interferon have a blocked N-terminal pyroglutamate, indicating that the N-terminal cys-tyr-cys is also cleaved from the molecule, thereby predicting a 143-AA chain (15). The carboxy terminus has also been found to be heterogeneous (16). The natural species of γ-interferon are cleaved at AA numbers 130, 131, 133, 135, 141, leaving molecules of 127 AA to 138 AA (assuming the loss of AAs 1-3, cys-tyr-cys). Variable glycosylation at positions 25 and 97 accounts for additional heterogeneity in the molecular weight of natural γ-interferon (17).

Once the gene encoding γ-interferon was cloned, it became possible to make large quantities of recombinant γ-interferon (r-IFN-g) for clinical testing. First, however, it was necessary to determine whether glycosylation and AA chain length were important to activity. Biogen chose to test a "full-length" unglycosylated molecule in preclinical tests. Genentech chose to test a "shortened" unglycosylated molecule with the three N-terminal AAs (cys-tyr-cys) deleted. Preclinical in vitro tests revealed no differences in activity between Biogen's r-IFN-g and natural γ-interferon. Published results using Genetech's r-IFN-g also revealed no differences. (These activities are reviewed later in this chapter). Although side-by-side comparisons of these two recombinant molecules have not been made, or at least published, it does appear that the in vitro properties, the in vivo pharmacokinetics, and the in vivo toxicities are similar. It has also been shown that lack of glycosylation does not affect the plasma half-life of r-IFN-g (18). Finally, r-IFN-g has important and significant in vivo biological effects.

III. PHYSIOLOGICAL SOURCES OF γ-INTERFERON

Before discussing the properties of γ-interferon in more detail, it is instructive to review which cells in the body produce γ-interferon and what stimuli induce γ-interferon synthesis and release. γ-Interferon can be induced in vitro by three categories of agents: (1) viruses and double-stranded nucleic acids; (2) mitogens and antigens; and (3) cytokines (19-22). It is likely that stimuli from all three categories play important roles in vivo. T lymphocytes were identified in 1974 as a cellular source of γ-interferon (23). Subsequent work demonstrated the CD4-positive subpopulation of T cells (helper T cells) to be the predominant source of γ-interferon, but CD8-positive cells (cytotoxic T cells) can also produce γ-interferon (24,25). Antibodies against the CD2 antigen and the hormone corticotropin (ACTH) can block induction of γ-interferon synthesis in T cells (26,27). Recently, large granular lymphocytes were also identified as producers of γ-interferon (28).

What induces the production of γ-interferon by T cells in vivo? Viral infection of T cells is able to induce γ-interferon by a direct mechanism. However, induction of γ-interferon by antigens and cytokines seems to involve a two-step process, i.e., two signals are needed. Thus, IL-1 or IL-2 in conjunction with an antigen or a mitogen can induce the production of γ-interferon (29-31).

γ-Interferon in turn induces production of IL-1, IL-2 receptors, IL-4 (B-cell growth factor), neopterin, and β_2-microglobulin; activates macrophages; and exerts functional control over several other cell types. The proteins induced by γ-interferon play a key role in the regulation of the cytokine network. This cytokine network is very complex with multiple stimulatory and regulatory loops as reviewed by Old (32). This complexity, which involves not only the activation but also the control of the immune network, helps to prevent detrimental hyperactivity of the immune system. After reviewing the activities of interferon and the proteins induced by γ-interferon, we will return to examine this complex network, albeit briefly, to see what predictions about the activity of γ-interferon in RA are possible.

IV. PRECLINICAL ACTIVITY OF γ-INTERFERON AS AN IMMUNE MODULATOR

As noted earlier, the interferons were originally discovered because of their antiviral properties. Antiproliferative activity and immunomodulatory properties were subsequently described. Early research was of necessity carried out with natural interferon preparations of variable purity. This lack of a pure preparation raised questions concerning the validity of the observed properties. However, most of the reported properties were verified as being truly due to interferon when recombinant products became available. Nevertheless, it has been suggested that the antiviral activity of the recombinant interferons is less than that of some of the natural products. Indeed, combinations of pure interferon preparations, e.g., type I and type II interferon, or type II and TNF, have shown synergistic activity similar to the natural products (33-36).

Establishment of the antiviral state in the cell by interferon is associated with the induction of many new proteins. The most important ones that play a role in antiviral activity are 2′5′-oligoadenylate synthetase (2′5′A), double-stranded RNA-dependent protein kinase, 2′5′A-dependent RNase, and the Mx protein (37-39).These enzymes lead to hydrolysis of viral mRNA and blockade of protein synthesis through inactivation of protein synthesis initiation factor.

Comparisons of both antiviral and antiproliferative activity between r-IFN-alpha and r-IFN-g have been conducted in in vitro models with purified recombinant material (40,41). Hu-r-IFN-*α* has been found to be less species-restricted in its activity than Hu-r-IFN-g. Hu-r-IFN-*α* has antiviral activity in pigs, cows, and monkeys (see Table 1) while Hu-r-IFN-g has no antiviral activity in any species tested except man. It is noteworthy that Hu-r-IFN-*α* is an effective treatment for shipping fever in cattle. r-IFN-*α* has more antiviral activity than r-IFN-g per antiviral unit as defined by the EMC virus/Wish cell test (see Table 2). Conversely, in most antiproliferative models, r-IFN-g has more antiproliferative activity than r-IFN-*α*. r-IFN-g not only has cystostatic activity but, unlike r-IFN-*α*, has cytocidal activity as well (see Table 3).

However, the most important differences between r-IFN-*α* and r-IFN-g may lie in their immunomodulatory properties. Both interferons activate NK cells. r-IFN-*α* does so in about 2 hr while r-IFN-g takes about 24 hr. The activation by r-IFN-g can be achieved by either a short exposure to a high concentration (1000 U/ml) of r-IFN-g or a long exposure to a low (10

Table 1 Activity of Recombinant Human *α*- and γ-Interferon When Cells of Various Species Are Challenged with VSV

Cell line	Species	r-IFN-α_2	r-IFN-g
L929	Mouse	0	0
Ratec	Rat	0	0
RK13	Rabbit	0	0
CRFK	Cat	0	0
MNCK	Dog	0	0
PK15	Pig	4+	0
NBL1	Cow	4+	0
Vero	Monkey	3+	0

0: no activity to 4+ highest activity.

Table 2 Concentration of Recombinant Human α- and γ-Interferon (U/ml) Necessary to Protect Hep-2 Cells Against Different Viruses

	Concentration of IFN (U/ml)	
Virus	r-IFN-α	r-IFN-γ
VSV	16	31
RSV	<1	62
HSV I	<1	250
HSV II	<1	62
Adeno	16	125
Vaccinia	125	250
CMV	>1000	1000
Pseudorabies	1	31

U/ml) concentration (42). Both interferons can also enhance antibody-dependent cell-mediated cytotoxicity (ADCC) (43-45). This enhanced ADCC occurs presumably because of the increase in Fc receptors on mononuclear cells in response to interferon. It is here, however, that the similarities in immunomodulatory actions between the two types of interferons cease.

Differences between type I and type II interferons related to immune enhancement are numerous. Many of these are related to macrophage activation. γ-Interferon is a "macrophage activation factor" (MAF) (46,47). It activates macrophages to be tumoricidal (48). It activates macrophages to kill parasites, in part by induction of intracellular oxygen radical synthesis (49). It increases DR (class II) MHC antigen expression, which is necessary to facilitate antigen presentation to lymphocytes by macrophages (50-52). γ-Interferon also increases the susceptibility of virally infected cells to antiviral cytotoxic lymphocytes (CTL) and of tumor cells to tumoricidal cells, in part by increasing class I and II MHC antigens on these targets (53–55).

In addition to enhancing macrophage phagocytosis, γ-interferon enhances polymorphonuclear (PMN) phagocytosis and oxidative burst, resulting in enhanced bactericidal activity (45). γ-Interferon also enhances PMN ADCC by increasing Fc receptor expression on PMNs (44).

γ-Interferon has a regulatory effect on B cells. Preexposure of resting B cells to 100 U/ml of γ-interferon has been reported to enhance their proliferative response to mitogens. In contrast, γ-interferon suppresses B-cell proliferation in response to B-cell stimulation factor-enhanced anti-Ig stimulation (56,57). γ-Interferon also regulates Ig isotype production in conjunction with IL-4 (B-cell-stimulating factor 1) (58). In vivo, γ-interferon acts as an adjuvant when administered with antigen to mice (59).

There is a specific cell membrane receptor for γ-interferon (60,61). This receptor is distinct from the receptor for type I interferons and it has been cloned (63). Evidence suggests that the receptor molecule is a protein kinase. There are high- and low-affinity receptors on monocytes (63,64). Both the N-terminal and C-terminal portion of the γ-interferon molecule have been shown to be critical for binding to the receptor and also for interferon activity (65,66). However, glycosylation does not appear to affect the binding of γ-interferon to its receptor, thus partially explaining the observed activity of recombinant nonglycosylated forms of γ-interferon (67). Interferon-resistant and nonresistant melanoma cells have been shown to be comparable in their ability to bind and internalize γ-interferon, suggesting that interferon resistance is not due to the loss of the interferon receptor (68).

In one study, at least 20 new cellular proteins were induced by treatment with γ-interferon (69). Certain proteins induced by γ-interferon are restricted to one or a few cell types, e.g., the induction of the IL-2 receptor, neopterin, and class II MHC antigen are restricted to lymphoid cells and production of β-globin in response to γ-interferon is restricted to erythroid cells (70). Other proteins seem to be induced in all γ-interferon-treated cells (e.g., class I MHC antigen molecules). γ-Interferon has been shown to increase tumor-associated antigens (TAA) such as carcinoembryonic antigen (CEA) and TAG 72 (71, 72). The induction of both class II molecules and TAA by γ-interferon has led to the recently initiated clinical trials of r-IFN-g and TAA directed monoclonal antibodies.

Does γ-interferon have as much activity in in vivo models as the in vitro results might suggest? The activities predicted from in vitro studies appear to

Table 3 Cytocidal Effects of Human Interferon on Hela Cells

IFN	Concentration (U/ml)	% Viability[a]	% Growth inhibition
r-IFN-g	1000	57	91
r-IFN-a_2	650	95	46

[a]The percent viability of HeLa cells receiving the buffer vehicles only (control cells) was 96%).

be born out in animal testing in rodents. Murine γ-interferon has been shown to be an effective agent against *Toxoplasma gondii* and *Listeria monocytogenes* infections in mice (73–76). γ-Interferon has also been shown to be an effective immunotherapeutic in metastatic disease (77–80). Both CTL and macrophage effector cells were found to be stimulated in their antitumor activity. A bell-shaped dose-response curve, with a peak at a relatively low dose of 1.5×10^6 U/kg, was observed. Higher doses, which would have greater antiproliferative effects, were not as effective. A similar bell-shaped dose-response curve for the number of immunoglobulin-secreting cells in response to antigen in animals treated with γ-interferon has been observed (59).

Xenografts of human tumors in nude mice provide a model to test antiproliferative properties of Hu-r-IFN-g. Untreated nude mice do not reject the human tumors and Hu-r-IFN-g because of its species specificity does not activate murine CTLs, macrophages, or PMNs. [Species specificity is due to the failure of the receptors to recognize the foreign interferon. The receptor can be bypassed by encapsulation of the interferon in liposomes, thus achieving "full activity" (81).] Such xenograft models, including the subrenal capsule assay, have shown γ-interferon to have direct anti-tumor antiproliferative activity in vivo (82).

In summary, γ-interferon, acting through its cell surface receptor, induces the production of many cellular proteins. Different proteins are induced in different cell types. Some of these proteins have been identified and their function is understood. The activation of macrophages, CTL, B cells, and PMNs has been well described.

In vivo animal models have demonstrated the antiproliferative activity of γ-interferon. They have also demonstrated both "low"-dose and "high"-dose antitumor activity. The low-dose activity has been shown to be due to activation of immune effector cells, CTLs, and macrophages. This bell-shaped dose-response curve has given rise to the concept of the optimal immunomodulatory dose (OID).

V. CLINICAL DEVELOPMENT OF γ-INTERFERON: ONCOLOGY AND IMMUNOMODULATORY STUDIES

The preclinical work thus revealed two possible strategies for development of Hu-r-IFN-g as a therapeutic agent in man: (1) a high-dose antiproliferative strategy such as was employed for testing of r-IFN-α in oncological diseases and (2) an immunological, or OID, lower dose approach. Both approaches have been used.

The maximum tolerated dose (MTD) (high-dose approach) is commonly used with antiproliferative agents in oncological indications. It was the antiproliferative activities of interferons that stimulated the interest of the NCI and the oncological medical community and motivated biotechnology companies to clone the interferons as some of their initial projects. Unfortunately, use of the MTD (1-3 mg/m^2 depending on schedule) of r-IFN-g has failed to demonstrate clinically meaningful, antitumor activity in a large variety of solid and hematological tumors.

The efficacy of the OID has not been extensively studied in phase II trials, although six phase I studies carefully examined immunomodulation by r-IFN-g. First, Nathan et al. studied macrophage activation using generation of H_2O_2 as a marker of activation (83). Doses of 0.1, 0.5, or 1.0 mg/m^2 (1 mg is roughly equal to 10^7 U) of r-IFN-g were given over 4 hr or 6 hr by intravenous (I.V.) infusion five times per week for 2 weeks or every other day for 2 weeks. All doses and both schedules produced statistically significant increases in macrophage H_2O_2 production over the first 5 days of therapy. Parameters of immune response during or just after the 2 weeks of therapy were not reported.

Kleinermann et al. looked at activation of macrophage tumoricidal properties in response to r-IFN-g (84). Peak activity was found at doses of 0.25 and 0.5 mg/m^2/day given by intramuscular (i.m.) injection. Doses of 0.1 and 1 mg/m^2 were, in general, inactive and 1.0 mg/m^2 occasionally downregulated the baseline activity. A 6-hr intravenous infusion of 0.25 mg/m^2 of r-IFN-g was also effective in increasing tumoricidal activity, while intravenous doses of 0.1 mg/m^2 were not. Activity was seen at day 4 and 7 of the 42-day dosing schedule, but response after day 7 was not studied.

Maluish et al. studied a range of r-IFN-g doses given intramuscularly for 15 days (85). Doses were 0.0001, 0.001, 0.01, 0.1, and 0.25 mg/m^2. A subcutaneous (s.c.) dose of 0.1 mg/m^2 was also studied. Parameters of immunological activation evaluated were natural killer (NK) cell activity, monocyte activation as judged by H_2O_2 production, number of Fc receptors on phagocytes, and amount of cell surface class II antigen expression on lymphocytes. The three highest intramuscular doses showed immunostimulatory activity. However, 0.01 mg/m^2 i.m. showed less activity than the 0.1 or 0.25 mg/m^2 i.m. and 0.25 mg/m^2 i.m. was both slightly toxic and less effective by day 15. The 0.1 mg/m^2 s.c. dose was judged better than the 0.1 mg/m^2 i.m. dose, the optimal intramuscular dose, because of ease of administration and more consistent activation of mononuclear cells. Daily administration of this dose for 15 days did not induce a tolerant or unresponsive condition. By 48 hr after the last dose, most immunological parameters had returned to baseline levels, indicating that dosing at least every other day may be required for maximal immunomodulation.

Aulitzky et al. studied 0.01, 0.10, 0.50 mg of r-IFN-g given subcutaneously once a week for 3 weeks (86). They studied neopterin levels and β_2-microglobulin levels. Both neopterin and β_2-microglobulin are macrophage products and indicators of macrophage activation. Both of these products, unlike NK and macrophage function, can be readily measured on a daily basis with commercially available assays.

Peak levels of these macrophage products occurred 2-3 days after injection of r-IFN-g and the magnitude of the response was correlated with the dose. Day 5 levels postinjection began to approach baseline levels. Weekly injections of 0.5 and 0.1 mg induced downregulation of the response.

Logan et al. studied the immunological effects of r-IFN-g given intravenously daily in a dose escalation trial (87). Three patients per group were treated. Dose levels of 0.003, 0.03, 0.30, and 1.0, and 3.0 mg/m^2 of r-IFN-g were given by 2-hr or 24-hr infusion. NK activity, 2′5′A-synthetase levels, and DR surface antigen levels were assessed on days 2, 5, and 12. The most immunologically active dose was 0.30 mg/m^2.

Murray et al. studied the activity of 0.03 and 0.50 mg/m^2 of r-IFN-g given once by 24-hr intravenous infusion (88). H_2O_2 generation and intracellular killing of *Toxoplasma gondii* and *Leshmania donovani* by macrophages were quantified. Macrophages showed significant increases in activity both immediately after infusion and 5-7 days after infusion.

In summary: (1) intramuscular and subcutaneous doses of r-IFN-g in the range of 0.1 mg/m^2 produced maximal immunomodulation; (2) intravenous doses of 0.25 mg/m^2 also produced maximal responses; (3) higher intramuscular and intravenous doses induced downregulation of the immune parameters studied after 1 or 2 weeks or at best no response at all; (4) response following a single dose was long-lived, (4-7 days), but once per week dosing predisposed patients to downregulation whereas dosing three to five times per week over 15 days did not. The antitumor activity of the OID in renal cell carcinoma has been reported by Otto et al. and confirmed by Aulitzky, but has not been reproduced in multicenter controlled trials (89,90).

Several studies have described the pharmacokinetics of r-IFN-g. Ernstoff et al. found a biphasic curve with a β half-life of 6-9 hr (91). Serum levels after a 0.3 mg/m^2 i.v. dose were below 55 pg/ml, the limit of the assay, but as reported above, this dose had maximal immunomodulatory activity in this study. Peak level following a dose of 3.0 mg/m^2 of r-IFN-g given over 2 hr was 8 ng/ml at 2 hr.

Toxicities of r-IFN-g are dose-related. High doses (above 1.0 mg i.v. or 0.5 mg i.m.) cause dose-limiting myelosuppression, hepatoxicity, or flulike syndrome (90). As with r-IFN-*α*, flulike symptoms consisting of fever, chills, nausea/vomiting, myalgia, and fatigue are frequently dose limiting for r-IFN-g.

At low doses, 0.1 mg or less, mild fever is often reported, but tolerance usually occurs with chronic dosing. Mild nausea, chills, and myalgia are sometimes reported as these lower doses, but myelosuppression is rare.

The astute reader will by now have noticed that no attempt has been made to predict how the in vitro and in vivo activities of γ-interferon would impact on RA. In fact, many of the activities of γ-interferon which are most relevant to potential mechanisms of therapeutic action in RA have not yet been mentioned. Therefore, before reviewing the clinical development of r-IFN-g in RA, the activities of γ-interferon that could influence the disease course of RA will be discussed.

VI. BIOCHEMICAL RATIONALE FOR THE USE OF γ-INTERFERON IN RHEUMATOID ARTHRITIS

Many of the activities attributed to γ-interferon in vivo and in vitro can be thought of as immunostimulatory. At first consideration, the concept of using an immunoadjuvant to treat a disease characterized by an already overactive immune or inflammatory reaction might be paradoxical. Indeed, a case could be made that γ-interferon might exacerbate the destructive processes in RA. For example, γ-interferon treatment will increase the proliferation of synovial fibroblasts in culture (92). As hyperplasia of the synovial tissue is thought to be intrinsic to disease progression, this activity of γ-interferon could theoretically be detrimental. In addition, γ-interferon activates vascular endothelial cells, facilitating the binding and extravasation of inflammatory mononculear cells, including granulocytes and monocytes (93,94). Furthermore, γ-interferon is a potent activator of monocytes and macrophages, stimulating the formation of toxic oxygen radicals, inducing the production of the inflammatory mediators IL-1 and TNF, and activating the monocyte to the capability of cellular cytotoxicity (95).

In view of these potentially disease-provoking activities, how was γ-interferon selected as a therapeutic agent for RA? Several observations suggested that despite the widespread inflammatory activity typical of RA, the levels of circulating and synovial γ-interferon in patients with RA were lower than those found in normal control subjects (96–100). Other investigators demonstrated a marked deficit in γ-interferon production by lymphocytes obtained from RA patients in response to infection or mitogenic stimuli (lectins) (96,101-103). Comparison of patients with active disease and those in remission demonstrated that recovery from disease was associated with increased γ-interferon levels (104). Finally, some of the slow-acting antirheumatoid agents like N-(2-carboxyphenyl)-4-chlorantrhonilic acid disodium (CCA), have been shown to stimulate production of γ-interferon from T lymphocytes (105).

Initial studies of γ-interferon in animal models of inflammation were encouraging. Interferon therapy reduced inflammation in the carrageenan-induced pleurisy model (106). Lipopolysaccharide-induced footpad swelling was also substantially reduced by administration of γ-interferon (107). As discussed below, recent clinical studies including multicenter, double-blind, placebo-controlled protocols also demonstrate clear efficacy of r-IFN-g in the treatment of RA.

What known actions of γ-interferon could explain this anti-inflammatory (or antirheumatoid) effect? There are five potential mechanisms and sites of γ-interferon action to explain these observations of clinical efficacy.

Despite the actions of γ-inteferon as a potent activator of the macrophage, interferons have also been demonstrated to suppress certain processes in monocytes. Monocytes play a key role in many inflammatory processes. In addition to being directly cytotoxic, they process and present antigen to lymphocytes, and they release potent local inflammatory mediators, such as IL-1, TNF, and eicosanoids. Interferons inhibit the release of inflammatory prostaglandins from human peripheral monocytes in response to exogenous IL-1 (108-111). Levels of metabolites from both the cyclooxygenase and lipoxygenase pathways of eicosanoid metabolism in monocytes, as well as the metabolism of arachidonic acid itself, are altered by γ-interferon (112,113). Thus, the apparent anti-inflammatory effects of interferon on monocytes may be partially responsible for its antirheumatic activity (114).

The observed ability of interferons to block the effects of the inflammatory mediator IL-1 extends to cells other than monocytes. IL-1 activates osteoclasts to resorb bone via the release of prostaglandins. γ-Interferon has been shown to block IL-1 induced osteoclast activation and prostaglandin release by bone (115,116).

Furthermore, interferons may be able to affect the balance of collagen and fibronectin synthesis and breakdown, normally controlled by cytokines and growth factors. Current studies suggest a model in which the synthesis of extracellular matrix and connective tissue (including collagen types I-IV and fibronectin) is stimulated by transforming growth factor γ (TGF-γ) and perhaps by IL-1 in mesenchymal and epithelial tissues, including synovium.

γ-Interferon will inhibit synthesis of collagen (types I and III) by synovial fibroblasts and type II collagen synthesis by chondrocytes (117–122). γ-Interferon has also been shown to prevent scar formation in vivo (123). Thus, it may influence the course of RA by inhibiting bone resorption and by influencing the synthesis of scar tissue and matrix repair (113).

γ-Interferon was recently demonstrated to block the proliferation of B lymphocytes, their expression of class II MHC antigen, and their secretion of IgG and IgG3 antibodies, in response to IL-4 (124,125). There are suggestions that this inhibition again is mediated by an action of γ-interferon on eicosanoid metabolism (126,127).

The ability of Epstein-Barr virus (EBV) to immortalize B cells by EBV is increased in patients with RA (128). Diminished regulation of EBV-induced B-cell proliferation is correlated with diminished production of γ-interferon in response to autologous stimulation (100). It is not known whether EBV is responsible for the decreased levels of γ-interferon observed in patients with RA, nor whether this then leads to EBV-induced B-cell proliferation, production of IgM/rheumatoid factor, and loss of control of immune response to "self." However, γ-interferon inhibits the proliferation of B lymphocytes and their elaboration of IgM in response to EBV infection, suggesting the potential for administration of γ-interferon to decrease the production of rheumatoid factor and restore normal response to self (102,129).

Finally, treatment with γ-interferon may restore or redirect the responsiveness of the dysfunctional immune system in RA. As mentioned previously, γ-interferon serum levels and production in vitro by stimulated lymphocytes (and presumably their own autocrine response to this lymphokine) is depressed in this disease (96,129). Although the etiology of RA is unknown, it may be caused by, or related to, an infectious agent that affects γ-interferon production. This etiological agent may be responsible for the induction of a nonspecific or a cross-reactive immune response that recognizes self antigens. Induction by exogenous γ-interferon of class I antigens presented in conjunction with a putative viral antigen might facilitate immune elimination of the infective agent (130). Alternatively, γ-interferon might suppress a nonspecific or cross-reactive immune response induced by a viral antigen but recognizing self antigens.

Thus, the pleotropic actions of γ-interferon on suppression of monocytes and monocyte inflammatory mediators, inhibition of bone resorption, inhibition of collagen and matrix synthesis, suppression of B-lymphocyte proliferation and antibody production, and potential stimulation of inhibited or misdirected T-lymphocyte function may all contribute to its observed antirheumatoid activity.

VII. CLINICAL STUDIES USING r-IFN-γ IN THE TREATMENT OF RHEUMATOID ARTHRITIS

To date, a number of clinical trials have employed r-IFN-g in the setting of active RA. In addition to safety assessment and dose-finding information, a number of efficacy parameters have been evaluated. These include performance status, joint swelling and tenderness, patient and physician perception of pain, grip strength, and laboratory measurements of inflammation. All of these studies utilized similar patient populations in terms of disease status and demographic criteria. The doses of r-IFN-g utilized and the length of treatment and follow-up differ, however, for each study. Table 4 summarizes these studies.

A. Zilly and Obert Study

The initial report of possible activity in RA was published in 1986 by Zilly and Obert (131). This study indicated that doses of 50–200 μg given subcutaneously might prove efficacious. This dose range is the same as that found to have maximum immunomodulatory activity in studies reviewed earlier in this chapter. These results led to a larger dose-finding study.

B. Lemmel Study

This study was carried out in Germany, based at the University of Ulm, and concluded in 1985 (132). r-IFN-g was administered for 20 days in an open, nonrandomized phase II trial in 49 patients with RA. Forty of these patients were available for statistical analysis. Fourteen of these patients received a single dose of 50 μg of r-IFN-g per day subcutaneously. The remaining 26 patients received 50 μg s.c. twice a day. Articular indices were evaluated throughout the study. The patients were classified as "responders" and "nonresponders" on the basis of changes in the Ritchie index or the Lansbury articular index. Patients were classified as responders if the Ritchie index improved between day 0 and day 20 by at least 30%. Patients were also classified as responders if either the Lansbury articular index or the Ritchie index improved by 25% over the 20 days, and if the other index improved by at least 15% over the same interval. Using these criteria for a therapeutic response, 10 of 14 patients receiving 50 μg of r-IFN-g per day were responders and 14 of 26 patients receiving 100 μg of r-IFN-g per day were responders. The investigators noted that a therapeutic response was achieved more slowly at the lower dose level, but there was a tendency for the response to be longer lived and of greater magnitude. Both doses of r-IFN-g were well

Table 4 List of RA Clinical Trials with r-IFN-g

Study	Duration	Investigator	No. of pts.	Findings
Pilot Several regimens	11/83–5/84	Zilly	46	Drug is well tolerated Drug seems to be effective in RA
Open phase II 50 or 100 μg daily × 20 days	5/84–10/85	Lemmel	49	60% response rate Optimal dose 50–100 μg
Open long-term 25–100 μg 2–3 ×/wk	5/84–1/88	Lemmel	120	Drug is effective in 41% of the patients for at least 1 year
Open phase II 10 or 100 μg 5×/wk × 4 weeks	7/85–8/85	Wolfe	33	Decrease in tender and swollen joints and in pain
Maintenance 10 or 100 μg 3×/wk	6/88–ongoing	Wolfe	17	Four pts on maintenance after 3 years
D.bl. ph II 100 μg or placebo 5×/wk × 1 wk then 2×/wk × 23 wk	8/85–12/87	Veys	26	Encouraging trends in efficacy parameters
D.bl., ph II 100 μg or placebo 5×/ × 12 weeks	12/85–6/86	Cannon	105	Improvements in tender and swollen joints, pain, and morning stiffness
Maintenance 100 μg 3–7 ×/wk	4/86–ongoing	Cannon	70	Nineteen pts on therapy with benefit after 2+ years
D.bl. phase III 50 μg or placebo daily × 20 days, then qod × 7 days	2/86–12/86	Lemmel	40	58% response rate; statistically significant superiority of r-IFN-g over placebo
Open study 50 μg 2×/wk	9/86–5/88	Lemmel	454	56% response rate; drug easily administered by MDs

tolerated. Adverse effects were mild and were characteristic of r-IFN-g administration, as noted in a variety of other clinical trials. Fever was reported in 11 of 40 patients. Other side effects recorded in at least 5% of the patients included headache, fatigue and weakness, flushing, nausea and vomiting. The lower dose regimen had a markedly lower incidence of side effects. Side effects and efficacy are summarized in Table 5. The conclusion from this study was that 50 μg of r-IFN-g given daily was better tolerated than, and as effective as, 100 μg of r-IFN-g given daily.

C. Wolfe Study

Concurrently, a single-blind (investigator-blind) dose-finding study was conducted by Dr. Wolfe at the Arthritis Center in Witchita, Kansas (133,134).

Table 5 Safety and Efficacy in the Phase II Lemmel Study

SAFETY	Total	Substudy A (1 X 50 μg)	Substudy B (2 X 50 μg)
Total no. of patients including those withdrawn	49	21	28
Number of patients with side effects	17	3	14
Types of side effects (possibly more than one per patient			
Fever (≥40°C)	14	2	12
Fatigue	2	1	1
Sweating	2	1	1
Flush	2		2
Headache	2		2
Chills	1		1
Hypotension	1		1
Local irritation	1		1
Total no. of side effects	25	4	21
EFFICACY			
Responders		10/14 (71%)	14/26 (54%)

Source: Ref. 132.

This study compared the safety and efficacy of 10 μg of r-IFN-g with 100 μg of r-IFN-g given subcutaneously five times per week for 4 weeks. Patients met the ARA criteria for RA and had active disease. They had been stabilized on NSAIDs for 1 month and/or SAARDs for at least 3 months. Prednisone up to 10 mg/day was allowed. Each joint was evaluated for tenderness and swelling on a scale of 0-3. Pain, morning stiffness, grip strength, physician and patient grading of disease severity, ESR, and patient disability as assessed by the Stanford Health Assessment questionnaire (HAQ) were evaluated weekly. Blood chemistry, hematology, and urinalysis were assessed weekly and all adverse experiences were recorded.

Thirty-three patients entered the study and 30 completed the 4-week treatment period. One patient withdrew for personal reasons, one withdrew for pyelonephritis (*E. coli*) unrelated to r-IFN-g, and one patient, also on auranofin, withdrew for proteinuria. In this last patient, both r-IFN-g and auranofin were stopped until resolution. Upon restarting auranofin, proteineuria recurred. As proteineuria is a recognized side effect of auranofin, the investigators concluded that this adverse experience was due wholly or in part to auranofin. A clinically unimportant fall in mean WBC (8.6 to 7.0) and a rise in mean SGPT (15.2 to 24.5) were seen in the 100-μg-dose group. As mentioned earlier, leukopenia and/or hepatotoxicity, as well as flulike syndrome, are the dose-limiting toxicities seen in oncology trials when high doses (3 mg/m^2) of r-IFN-g are given.

Patients in the 100-μg group experienced more improvement in all efficacy parameters than patients in the 10-μg group. These differences were not statistically significant because of the small number of patients in each group. In the 100-μg group, the mean number of tender joints decreased from 20.5 to 11.4 and the mean number of swollen joints decreased from 9.7 to 6.3. Clinically important improvement (CII) was defined as a fall of 30% or more in the tender or swollen joint score. In the 100 μg group, 81% of the patients experienced CII as judged by the tender joint score and 69% experienced CII as judged by the swollen joint score (see Table 6).

Of interest, three of five patients on penicillamine but zero of four on gold compounds showed clinically significant improvement (CSI) (≥50% decline in tender or swollen joint score).

The conclusion of this study was that r-IFN-g was safe when administered to patients with RA at 10 or 100 μg and that 100 μg was probably more efficacious than 10 μg.

D. Veys Study

In 1988, Veys reported the results of a third, dose-finding, phase II, prospective, single-center, randomized, double-blind, placebo-controlled trial of

Table 6 Number and Percentage of Patients with Clinically Important Improvement (⩾30% Decrease) in the Wolfe Study

		Clinially important improvement (⩾30% decrease)	
Dose (μg)	N	Tender joint score	Swollen joint score
10	14	9 (64%)	8 (57%)
100	16	13 (81%)	11 (69%)
Total	30	22 (73%)	19 (63%)

Source: Ref. 133.

r-IFN-g in patients with RA, carried out at the University of Ghent (135). This study was run concurrently with the two dose-finding studies reported above.

The study objectives were to (1) evaluate the safety and toxicity of r-IFN-g in patients with RA and (2) compare the efficacy of r-IFN-g to placebo in this population, although the small group size precluded statistical significance. There were two treatment groups of equal size. One group was treated with 100 μg of r-IFN-g 5 days/week by subcutaneous injections for the first week, followed by twice weekly dosing for the next 23 weeks. The control group was treated with placebo of the same volume and excipients and by the same schedule.

Patients selected for the trial were required to have classical or definite RA according to accepted criteria. Patients were required to have active disease, and functional classes of II or III, and could not be taking steroids or SAARDs.

Efficacy was assessed by both physician assessment of disease activity at regular intervals and patient assessment of disease activity. Safety was assessed from adverse experience reports, measurement of vital signs, clinical laboratory tests, physical examination, and electrocardiograms. Twenty-six patients with RA were enrolled in the study. Thirteen patients received r-IFN-g and 13 received placebo. The r-IFN-g and placebo groups did not differ with regard to demographic data, including age, gender, rheumatoid factor (RF) and antinuclear antibody (ANA) positivity, and past or present antirheumatoid drug use. In each group, 11 of 13 patients completed 24 weeks of treatment.

Because this was a dose-finding study with small numbers of patients in each group, statistical analysis of efficacy data between groups could not (and was not expected to) generate meaningful confidence limits. Analysis of the individual efficacy parameters over time within the r-IFN-g group showed statistically significant improvement in grip strength and in tender/painful joint scores compared to baseline. Comparison with the placebo group did not reach statistical significance for any efficacy parameters. The placebo group also demonstrated some improvement in disease activity over the course of the study.

There was clinically significant improvement (CSI) (defined as 50% or greater decrease) in the tender or painful joints score by week 24 in 36% of the patients in the r-IFN-g group as comapred to 20% of the placebo group. Similarly, by week 24, 36% of the patients in the r-IFN-g group demonstrated CSI in their swollen joint score. In comparison, 30% of the placebo-treated patients experienced CSI in this parameter at 24 weeks. The differences between groups did not reach statistical significance because of small number of patients.

The treatment with r-IFN-g was well tolerated. The only suspected adverse drug reaction reported by more than one patient in each group was pyrexia (six patients in the r-IFN-g group and two patients in the placebo group). Other reported reactions included fatigue, chills, edema, weight loss, headache, and gastritis. These reactions did not result in a change in treatment. The incidence of suspected adverse drug reactions was similar in the two groups. No significant abnormalities in hematological or clinical chemistry parameters occurred as a result of r-IFN-g therapy.

Four patients (two in each group) withdrew prior to completing 24 weeks of therapy. Two patients withdrew for lack of cooperation, and one patient for ineligibility. The fourth patient (r-IFN-g group) withdrew at week 4 because of a concomitant bacterial infection.

E. Conclusions from Dose-Finding Studies

The conclusions from these four dose-finding studies were as follows: (1) r-IFN-g was safe and well tolerated in patients with active RA; (2) 50 or 100 μg given daily for 3-4 weeks was the most efficacious regimen; (3) a 50-μg dose seemed to induce fewer episodes of fever than did 100 μg. However, patients receiving either dose quickly became tolerant to these adverse effects of r-IFN-g and did not report fevers after 7-10 days of treatment.

These conclusions led to the design of two double-blind studies of 4 and 12 weeks and several open label studies of a year or longer. These latter studies were designed to examine several regimens over 1 year in order to select the best long-term regimen.

F. Cannon Study

Recently, Cannon et al. presented the results of a prospective, multicenter, randomized, double-blind, placebo-controlled, 12-week trial of r-IFN-g in 105 patients with RA (136). The study objectives were to (1) compare the efficacy of r-IFN-g with placebo in patients with RA and (2) evaluate the safety and toxicity of r-IFN-g in this population. There were two treatment groups of equal size. One group was treated with 100 μg of r-IFN-g 5 days/week for 12 weeks by subcutaneous injection. The control group was treated with placebo of the same volume and excipients and by the same schedule.

Patients selected for the trial were required to have classical RA of at least 6 months duration according to ARA criteria. Patients were required to have active disease with disease stabilized by treatment with NSAIDs or steroids (equivalent to 10 mg prednisone per day or less) for 1 month or more, and/or treatment with a stable dose of a SAARD for 3 months or more. Efficacy was evaluated by both physician assessment of disease activity at regular intervals and patient assessment of disease activity. Safety was assessed from adverse experience reports, measurement of vital signs, clinical laboratory tests, physical examination, electrocardiograms, and chest X rays.

One hundred and five patients with RA were enrolled in the study. Fifty-four patients received r-IFN-g and 51 patients received placebo. The ages of the patients ranged from 20 to 74 years. The r-IFN-g and placebo groups did not differ with regard to demographic data, including age, gender, RF and ANA positivity, functional class, and past or present antirheumatoid drug use. Slightly more than 50% of the patients were receiving concomitant SAARDs. Forty-two patients in each group completed the 12-week trial.

There was CSI (defined as ⩾50% decrease) in joint tenderness score in 43% of patients after 8 and 12 weeks of r-IFN-g treatment. CSI in joint tenderness score in the placebo group occurred in 24% of the patients at 8 and 12 weeks (see Table 7). CSI in joint swelling scores during r-IFN-g treatment occurred in 38% of patients at 8 weeks and 29% of patients at 12 weeks. The CSI in joint swelling score in the placebo groups occurred in 12% of the patients at 8 weeks and 14% at 12 weeks.

The frequency of CSI in joint tenderness and swelling score was greater in patients receiving r-IFN-g than that seen in patients receiving placebo. This achieved statistical significance in the comparison of joint swelling scores at 4 and 8 weeks of therapy ($p < 0.05$). Statistical significance was lost by 12 weeks due to a combination of reasons. First, two patients in the r-IFN-g group experienced disease flare by week 12, due possibly to lack of disease stabilization at entry (intra-articular steroid treatment had been discontinued at 1 month prior to study entry). Second, the number of patients was too small.

Table 7 Number and Percentage of Patients with Clinically Signficant Improvement (CSI) (≥50% Decrease) in the Cannon Study

Parameter	Group	N	Week 4	P value[a]	Week 8	P value[a]	Week 12	P value[a]
Tender joint score	r-IFN-g	42	11 (26%)		18 (43%)		18 (43%)	
	Placebo	42	9 (21%)	0.798	11 (26%)	0.168	11 (26%)	0.168
Swollen joint score	r-IFN-g	42	9 (21%)		16 (38%)		12 (29%)	
	Placebo	42	2 (5%)	0.048	5 (12%)	0.011	6 (14%)	0.183

[a]P values from the Fischer's Exact T-test, $p < 0.05$ are considered significant.
Source: Ref. 136.

However, the most significant cause for the decrease in efficacy may have been a decrease in the immune response to r-IFN-g because of dosing that was too frequent. Too frequent dosing could lead to overstimulation and thus "burnout" of the γ-interferon specific immune response. Although phase I immunological studies did not investigate changes in immune parameters induced by r-IFN-g when administered for 15 days, clinical studies in RA have indicated a loss in response, when the frequency of administration of r-IFN-g is not reduced after 3–4 weeks (Obert, pers. commun.). Thus, the regimen used in this study was not optimal.

Nevertheless, the mean number of swollen joints decreased from 21 to 18 at 12 weeks in patients receiving r-IFN-g ($p < 0.03$). There was also a decrease in the number of swollen joints in patients receiving placebo from 20 to 19 at 12 weeks ($p = 0.20$). The intergroup comparison was not statistically significant at 12 weeks ($p = 0.23$). A similar pattern was seen with joint swelling score.

Morning stiffness of patients after 12 weeks of treatment with r-IFN-g was statistically less than that reported before treatment ($p = 0.01$). No intragroup differences were seen in the placebo patients. For morning stiffness, pain assessment on a visual analog scale, and grip strength, there was a trend for greater improvement in the r-IFN-g group compared to the placebo group, but this difference did not achieve statistical significance. The Stanford Health Assessment Questionnaire (HAQ) score decreased from 1.8 to 1.6 in patient receiving r-IFN-g whereas no change was seen in patients receiving placebo. The difference in changes in HAQ score was statistically significant when r-IFN-g and placebo groups were compared ($p < 0.03$).

This study confirmed the beneficial effect of receiving penicillamine and r-IFN-g (statistically significant association) and the lack of improvement when receiving gold and r-IFN-g (nearly statistically significant). Table 8 shows the changes in tender and swollen joint scores for patients receiving r-IFN-g and either penicillamine or gold.

Suspected adverse drug reactions reported by at least 10% of the patients were fever, chills, nausea, headache, dizziness, vasodilation, injection site reaction, fatigue, and diarrhea. In the majority of cases these reactions did not result in a change in treatment. Fever ($p < 0.05$), often with chills, and local injection site reactions ($p < 0.01$) were more common in the r-IFN-g-treated group than in the placebo-treated patients. Otherwise, the incidence of suspected adverse drug reactions was similar in the two groups.

Twenty-one patients (12 r-IFN-g and nine placebo) withdrew before completing 12 weeks of therapy. The numbers of patients withdrawn from the r-IFN-g and placebo groups were not statistically different ($p = 0.63$). Six patients in the r-IFN-g and four patients in the placebo groups were withdrawn because of lack of efficacy. Two patients in the r-IFN-g dose

Table 8 Effect of Concomitant Gold or Penicillamine on Response to r-IFN-g in the Cannon Study

	Mean change in tender/painful joint score at week 12			Mean change in swollen joint score at week 12		
Concomitant drug	r-IFN-g (N)	Placebo (N)	P value[a]	r-IFN-g (N)	Placebo (N)	P value[a]
Concomitant gold			0.7192			0.0643
Yes	0.5 (14)	- 2.1 (16)		- 0.6 (14)	-3.8 (16)	
No	-10.4 (28)	- 9.7 (26)		- 9.8 (28)	-1.4 (26)	
Concomitant penicillamine			0.3110			0.0495
Yes	-26.5 (4)	-13.6 (7)		-20.3 (4)	0.1 (7)	
No	- 4.7 (38)	- 6.5 (35)		- 5.3 (38)	-3.4 (35)	

[a]P values are obtained from covariate analysis, p values < 0.05 are considered significant.

Source: Ref. 136.

group and three in the placebo group withdrew because of adverse experiences. The two patients in the r-IFN-g group withdrew for (1) leukopenia which resolved after stopping treatment, and (2) proteinuria. The patient with proteinuria stopped both r-IFN-g and gold. The proteinuria resolved, but recurred upon challenge with gold. This event was therefore most likely due to the treatment with gold. The remaining patients in both groups who discontinued treatment withdrew consent or (in one case) discontinued required antirheumatic medication.

There were no medically important changes in the mean values of any laboratory parameters. However, there was a statistically significant fall in mean WBC count from 8.3 to 6.6 in patients receiving r-IFN-g ($p < 0.001$) and an increase in WBC count from 8.5 to 8.6 in patients receiving placebo. A decrease of PMN count from 5.8 to 4.7 at 12 weeks in the r-IFN-g-treated patients was statistically different from the small PMN increase from 6.2 to 6.4 seen in patients receiving placebo ($p < 0.001$).

Overall, the investigators found that some clinical improvement occurred in both r-IFN-g-treated and placebo-treated groups of patients. Although the improvement with r-IFN-g was greater than that with placebo, the differences were generally not statistically significant. r-IFN-g was well tolerated in this group of patients with RA.

G. Second Lemmel Study

One multicenter, placebo-controlled, double-blind, randomized clinical study was reported by Lemmel in 1988 (137). Ninety-one patients with RA were treated for 28 days with r-IFN-g or placebo, with 50 μg/day being administered for the first 20 days, followed by 50 μg every other day for the next 8 days, delivered subcutaneously. Seventy-nine of these patients were evaluable, 40 of whom had received r-IFN-g. Demographic criteria and disease status were comparable between the two groups. Patients were allowed into the study if receiving NSAIDs or SAARDs, providing they had been receiving treatment long enough to be stabilized. Twenty percent of the patients were receiving SAARDs.

In this study, the criteria for being classified as a responder were improvement in the Ritchie or Lansbury index by at least 30% at day 28. Twenty-three of the 40 patients in the r-IFN-g group (58%) were responders whereas only 11 of the 39 placebo-treated patients (28%) were responders. These results were significant with a probability of error of less than 1% (Table 9).

The side effects of therapy occurred with equal frequency in the two arms of the study, and included nausea, fatigue, headache, and diaphoresis. Daily maximum body temperature was slightly higher in the interferon-treated

Table 9 Number and Percentage of Responders (≥30% Improvement in Ritchie or Lansbury Index) in the Second Lemmel Study

Group	N	Responders	P value[a]
r-IFN-g	40	23 (58%)	<0.01
Placebo	39	11 (28%)	

[a]P value from χ^2 test
Source: Ref. 137.

group. The only patient who discontinued treatment because of adverse experience in the r-IFN-g group did so because of a local skin reaction, with erythema and induration at the injection site.

This study again indicated that r-IFN-g was safe in RA and showed with statistical significance that r-IFN-g was efficacious in RA.

H. Juvenile Rheumatoid Arthritis

Pernice et al. reported the results of a small trial employing r-IFN-g in the treatment of children with severe, refractory juvenile RA (138). Eight patients with systemic onset juvenile RA were treated with 0.5 μg r-IFN-g per kilogram daily for 3 weeks, and treatment was then continued for several months on an individually adapted scheme of decreasing frequency. Six of eight patients showed improvement in morning stiffness, pain on movement, and general well-being. Laboratory signs of inflammation, including C-reactive protein and ESR, improved in all eight patients. No adverse effects were reported. Thirteen patients with other forms of juvenile RA did not respond to r-IFN-g treatment.

I. Long-Term Open Label Trials

Patients in the studies reported by Wolfe and Cannon were allowed to receive open label treatment with r-IFN-g following the 4 weeks or 12 weeks, respectively, of controlled treatment. Frequency of injection was reduced to three times per week in the Wolfe study and could be 3, 5, or 7 days/week, depending on patient and investigator evaluation in the Cannon study.

Seventeen of the 30 patients completing the Wolfe study entered the long-term maintenance phase of that study. Eight patients received more than 1 year of treatment. Seven of these patients were still on treatment after 2 years, and five patients were on treatment after 3 years. All discontinuations of treatment were due to loss of efficacy, except for one patient. This patent, after 1 year without flulike symptoms, began to experience fever (102°F), nausea, aching, and chills. This patient did not have detectable antibodies to r-IFN-g.

The losses of efficacy did not occur in the articular indices of tender and swollen joint scores, but rather in the evaluation of pain, stiffness, and fatigue. CSI (⩾50% decrease in tender or swollen joint score) was seen in all 13 patients at 3 months, 11 of 12 patients at 6 months, and thereafter in all patients including those who stopped for loss of efficacy as discussed above. It is possible that the increase in pain, myalgia, and fatigue was due to the r-IFN-g therapy rather than disease activity.

Figure 1 shows the kinetics of response to the two dose levels of r-IFN-g used in the Wolfe study for patients who continued treatment for at least 6 months. It can be seen that the majority of the improvement occurred within the first 4 weeks of five times per week dosing with 100 μg of r-IFN-g, but it took 16 weeks to achieve maximum response if the dose was only 10 μg. Since response was maintained after reduction at week 4 from five times per week to three times per week in the 100-μg group, this study supported the rationale for lowering the frequency of administration after 3–4 weeks of 100 μg of r-IFN-g as advocated by Lemmel and colleagues. Additional support

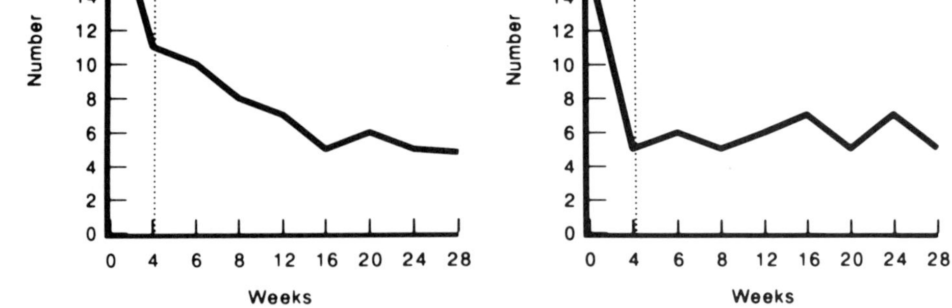

Figure 1 Response to two dose levels of r-IFN-g: mean number of tender joints.

comes from the loss of efficacy in the swollen joint score between week 8 and week 12 in the Cannon study, in which dosing was continued at five times per week for the full 12 weeks (136).

Seventy of the 84 patients who completed the 12-week double-blind Cannon trial were enrolled in the long-term prospective trial of r-IFN-g in RA (139,140). After the first 12 weeks of dosing at 100 μg/day, 5 days/week, r-IFN-g injections were given three to seven times per week and adjusted individually.

Forty-three patients (61%) after 1 year and 24 patients (34%) after 2 years continued the drug with sustained clinical benefit. Over 2 years, r-IFN-g was discontinued in 46 patients. Twenty-one withdrew for loss of efficacy, with three experiencing a "flare-up" of disease. Two patients discontinued r-IFN-g for suspected adverse drug reactions, which consisted of (1) gastrointestinal distress and (2) flulike symptoms. Several patients also developed local reactions at the site of injections of r-IFN-g.

Long-term treatment of RA with r-IFN-g was generally well tolerated and associated with sustained clinical improvement in RA patients.

Two open-label, long-term studies have been conducted in West Germany by Lemmel and Obert (pers. commun.). These studies are ongoing and have enrolled 120 and 454 patients, respectively. Preliminary results support the safety and efficacy of long-term treatment with r-IFN-g.

J. Summary of Clinical Trials

To summarize all the evaluable clinical studies of r-IFN-g in patients with RA: (1) The drug is well-tolerated. (2) There is a consistent tendency toward improvement in tender and swollen joint scores as evaluated using various criteria, in the patients treated with r-IFN-g. (3) The well-recognized placebo effect, and the waxing and waning course typical of RA, make placebo-controlled trials imperative but serve to obscure the statistical significance of responses to r-IFN-g, except in the largest trials. (4) Individual patients in each of the studies have had remarkable responses. This may define a subpopulation of patients with RA which is sensitive to r-IFN-g therapy. The challenge will be to find parameters to prospectively identify such a subpopulation if it exists. (5) There seem to be additive or synergistic effects between r-IFN-g and penicillamine. Although a synergistic effect of r-IFN-g and penicillamine has not been evaluated in vitro, many other combinations of antirheumatic drugs, including r-IFN-g, have shown synergy. The lower efficacy of r-IFN-g when given concomitantly with gold, which has been reported to have effects on macrophages, may be due to the inability of macrophage function to be further altered after initiation of therapy with r-IFN-g. This may indicate that r-IFN-g efficacy in RA is effected at least in part through its effects on macrophages.

Future double-blind trials and long-term follow-up with larger groups are required to further define the potential efficacy of and tolerance for r-IFN-g in RA.

REFERENCES

1. Issacs A, Lindenmann J. Virus interference: I. The interferon. Proc R Soc Ser B 1957; 147:258–67.
2. Interferon nomenclature. Nature 1978; 286:110.
3. Atanasiu P, Chany C. Action d'un interferon provenant de cellules malignes sur l'infection experimentale du hamster nouveau-ne par le virus du polyome. CR Acad Sci 1960; 251:1687-9.
4. Gresser I, Bourali C, Levy JP. Increased survival in mice inoculated with tumor cells and treated with interferon preparations. Proc Natl Acad Sci USA 1969; 63:51-6.
5. Gresser I, Bourali C. Antitumor effects of interferon preparations in mice. J Natl Cancer Inst 1970. 45:365–75.
6. Galvani D, Griffiths SD, Cawley JC. Interferon for treatment: the dust settles. Br Med J 1988; 296:1554-6.
7. Krown SE. Editorial: Interferon in 1987: the half full glass. J Cancer Res Clin Oncol 1987; 113:503–6.
8. Streuli M, Nagata S, Weissmann C. At least three human type alpha interferons: structure of alpha 2. Science 1980; 209:1343-7.
9. Nagata S, Taira H, Hall A, Johnsrud L, Streuli M, Escodi J, Boll W, Cantell K, Weissman C. Synthesis in *E. coli* of a polypeptide with human leukocyte interferon activity. Nature 1980; 284:316-20.
10. Yip YK, Pang RHL, Urban C, Vilcek J. Partial purification and characterization of human gamma (immune) interferon. Proc Natl Acad Sci USA 1981; 78:1601-5.
11. Yip YK, Barrowclough BS, Urban C, Vilcek J. Molecular weight of human gamma interferon is similar to that of other human interferons. Science 1982; 215:411-13.
12. Gray PW, Leung DW, Pennica D, Yelverton E, Najarian R, Simonsen CC, Derynck R, Sherwood PJ, Wallace DM, Berger SL, Levinson AD, Goeddel DV. Expression of human immune interferon cDNA in E. coli and monkey cells. Nature 1982; 295:503–8.
13. Feinstein SI, Mory Y, Chernajovsky Y, Maroteaux L, Nir U, Lavie V, Revel M. Family of human alpha interferon like sequences. Mol Cell Biol 1985; 5:510-17.
14. Gray PW, Goeddel DV. Structure of the human immune interferon gene. Nature 1982; 298:859–63.

15. Kelker HC, Le J, Rubin BY, Yip YK, Nagler C, Vilcek J. Three molecular weight forms of natural human interferon gamma revealed by immunoprecipitation with monoclonal antibody. J Biol Chem 1984; 259: 4301–4.
16. Pan Y-CE, Stern AS, Familletti PC, Khan FR, Chizzonite R. Structural characterization of human interferon gamma—Heterogeneity of the carboxyl terminus. Eur J Biochem 1987; 166:145–9.
17. Adolf GR. Structure and effects of interferon-gamma. Oncology 1985 suppl 1; 42:33–40.
18. Bose S, Hickman J. Role of the carbohydrate moiety in determining the survival of interferon in the circulation. J Biol Chem 1977; 252:8336–7.
19. Isaacs A. Interferon. In: Smith DM, Lauffer MA, eds. Advances in virus research. Vol. 10. New York: Academic Press, 1963:1–35.
20. Field AK, Tytell AA, Lampson GP, Hilleman MR. Inducers of interferon and host resistance. II. Multistranded synthetic polynucleotide complexes. Proc Natl Acad Sci USA 1967; 58:1004–10.
21. Wheelock EF. Interferon-like virus-inhibitor induced in human leukocytes by phytohemagglutinin. Science 1965; 149:310–1.
22. Green JA, Cooperband SR, Kilbrick S. Immune specific induction of interferon production in cultures of human blood lymphocytes. Science 1969; 164:1415–7.
23. Stobo J, Green I, Jackson L, Baron S. Identification of a subpopulation of mouse lymphoid cells required for interferon production after stimulation with mitogens. J Immunol 1974; 112:1589–93.
24. Martinez-Maza O, Andersson U, Andersson J, Britton S, DeLey M. Spontaneous production of interferon gamma in adult and newborn humans. J Immunol 1984; 132:251–5.
25. Archer DL, Smith BG, Ulrich JT, Johnson HM. Immune interferon induction by T-cell mitogens involves different T-cell subpopulations. Cell Immunol 1979; 48:420–6.
26. Wilkinson M, Morris A. The E receptor regulates interferon-gamma production: four-receptor model for human lymphocyte activation. Eur J Immunol 1984; 14:708–13.
27. Johnson HM, Torres BA, Smith EM, Dion LD, Blalock JE. Regulation of lymphokine (gamma interferon) production by corticotropin. J Immunol 1984; 132:246–50.
28. Young HA, Ortaldo JR. One-signal requirement for interferon gamma production by human large granular lymphocytes. J Immunol 1987; 139:724–7.
29. Kasahara T, Hooks JJ, Dougherty SF, Oppenheim JJ. Interleukin-2 mediated immune interferon (IFN-gamma) production by human T cells and T cell subsets. J Immunol 1983; 130:1784.
30. Wikocil R, Weiss A, Imboden J, Kamin-Lewis R, Stobo J. Activation of a human T cell line: a two-stimulus requirement in the pretranslational

events involved in the coordinate expression of interleukin 2 and interferon gamma genes. J Immunol 1985; 134:1599.
31. Grabstein K, Dower S, Gillis S, Urdal D, Larsen A. Expression of interleukin 2, interferon gamma, and the IL-2 receptor by human peripheral blood lymphocytes. J Immunol 1985; 136:4503.
32. Old LJ. Polypeptide mediator network. Nature 1987; 326:330-1.
33. Fleischmann WR Jr, Newton RC, Fleischmann CM, Colburn NH, Brysk MM. Discrimination between non-malignant and malignant cells by combinations of IFN-gamma and IFN-alpha/beta. J Biol Response Modif 1984; 3:397-405.
34. Czarniecki CW, Fennie CW, Powers DB, Estell DA. Synergistic antiviral and antiproliferative activities of *E. coli* derived human alpha, beta, and gamma interferons. J Virol 1984; 49:490-6.
35. Ueno M. Interleukin 2 induced cytotoxicity on renal cell carcinoma. 2. Synergistic effects of interleukin 2 and interferon gamma. Keio J Med 1986; 35:90-100.
36. Wong GHW, Krowka JF, Stites DP, Goeddel DV. In vitro anti-human immunodeficiency virus activities of tumor necrosis factor-alpha and interferon gamma. J Immunol 1988; 140:120-4.
37. Friedman RM, Vogel SN. Interferons with special emphasis on the immune system. In: Advances in immunology. Vol. 34. Academic Press, 1983:97-140.
38. Silverman RH, Jung D, Dieffenbach CW, Sengupta DN, Nolan NL. Purification and analysis of 2-5A-dependent RNase, the 80,000 dalton 2-5A-binding protein. Abstract. ISIR Meeting November 2-6, 1987, Washington, D.C.
39. Haller O, Grob R, Staeheli P. IFN-activated Mx gene: natural selection of alleles in wild mice. Abstract. ISIR Meeting November 2-6, 1987, Washington, D.C.
40. Rubin BY, Gupta SL. Differential efficacies of human type I and type II interferons as antiviral and antiproliferative agents. Proc Natl Acad Sci USA 1980; 77:5928-32.
41. Harada M, Matsumoto M. Preclinical studies of recombinant human interferon gamma: effects on NK and ADCC activities of human peripheral blood lymphocytes. 1983. Shionogi Research Laboratories, Fukashima-Ku, Osaka, Japan.
42. Herberman RB, Ortaldo JR, Riccardi C, et al. Interferon and NK cells. In: Hadden JW, ed. Advances in immunopharmacology. New York: Pergamon Press, 1983:147-52.
43. Itoh K, Inoue M, Kataoka S, Kumagai K. Differential effect of interferon expression of IgG- and IgM-Fc receptors on human lymphocytes. J Immunol 1980; 124:2589-95.
44. Perussia B, Kobayashi M, Rossi ME, Anegon I, Trinchieri G. Immune interferon enhances functional properties of human granulocytes: role

of Fc receptors and effect of lymphotoxin, tumor necrosis factor and granulocyte-macrophage colony-stimulating factor. J Immunol 1987; 138:765–74.
45. Matsumoto S, Takei M, Moriyama M, Imanishi H. Augmentation of antibody-dependent cellular cytotoxicity of polymorphonuclear leukocytes by interferon-gamma: mechanism dependent on enhancement of Fc receptor expression and increased release of activated oxygens. Chem Pharm Bull 1987; 35:1571–8.
46. Murray HW. Intereron-gamma, the activated macrophage, and host defense against microbial challenge. Ann Intern Med 1988; 108:595–608.
47. Bancroft GJ, Schreiber RD, Bosma GC, Bosma MJ, Unanue ER. A T cell-independent mechanism of macrophage activation by interferon gamma. J Immunol 1987; 139:1104–7.
48. Mentzer SJ, Burakoff SJ, Faller DV. CDw18 regulation of phorbol ester-induced human monocyte-mediated cytotoxicity. Cell Immunol 1988; 115:66–77.
49. Kemmerich B, Rossing TH, Pennington JE. Comparative oxidative microbicidal activity of human blood monocytes and alveolar macrophages and activation by recombinant gamma interferon. Am Rev Respir Dis 1987; 136:266–70.
50. Kelley VE, Fiers W, Strom TB. Cloned human interferon gamma, but not interferon beta or alpha, induces expression of HLA-DR determinants by fetal monocytes and myeloid leukemic cell lines. J Immunol 1984; 132:240–5.
51. Sonnenfeld G, Meruelo D, McDevitt HO, Merigan TC. Effect of type-I and type-II interferons on murine thymocyte surface antigen expression: induction or selection? Cell Immunol 1981; 57:427–39.
52. Pober JS, Collins T, Gimbrone MA Jr, Cotran RS, Gitlin JD, Fiers W, Clayberger C, Krensky AM, Burakoff SJ, Reiss CS. Lymphocytes recognize human vascular endothelial and dermal fibroblast Ia antigens induced by recombinant immune interferon. Nature 1983; 305:726–9.
53. Flyer DC, Burakoff SJ, Faller DV. Retrovirus-induced changes in major histocompatibility complex antigen expression influence susceptibility to lysis by cytotoxic T lymphocytes. J Immunol 135:2287–92.
54. Bukowski JF, Welsh RM. Interferon enhances the susceptibility of virus-infected fibroblasts to cytotoxic T cells. J Exp Med 1985; 161:257–62.
55. Saito T, Berens ME, Welander EC. Characterization of the indirect antitumor effect of gamma-interferon using ascites-associated macrophages in a human tumor clonogenic assay. Cancer Res 1987; 47:673–9.
56. Boyd AW, Tedder TF, Griffin JD, Freedman AS, Fisher DC, Daley J, Nadler LM. Preexposure of resting B cells to interferon gamma enhances proliferative response to subsequent activation signals. Cell Immunol 1987; 106:355–65.

57. Mond JJ, Finkelman FD, Sarma C, Ohara J, Serrate S. Recombinant interferon gamma inhibits the B cell proliferative response stimulated by soluble but not by Sepharose-bound anti-immunoglobulin antibody. J Immunol 1985; 135:2513–7.
58. Snapper CM, Paul WE. Interferon gamma and B cell stimulatory factor-1 reciprocally regulate Ig isotype production. Science 1987; 236:944–7.
59. Nakamura M, Manser T, Pearson GDN, Daley MJ, Gefter ML. Effect of IFN-gamma on the immune response in vivo and on gene expression in vitro. Nature 1984; 307:381–2.
60. Celada A. The interferon gamma receptor. Lymphokine Res 1988; 7: 61–73.
61. Branca A. Interferon receptors. In Vitro Cell Dev Biol 1988; 24:155–65.
62. Novick D, Orchansky P, Revel M, Rubinstein M. The human interferon gamma receptor. J Biol Chem 1987; 262:8483–7.
63. Fischer DG, Novick D, Orchansky P, Rubinstein M. Two molecular forms of the human interferon gamma receptor. J Biol Chem 1988; 263: 2632–7.
64. Aiyer RA, Serrano LE, Jones PP. Interferon gamma binds to high and two affinity receptor components on murine macrophages. J Immunol 1986; 136:3329–34.
65. Magazine HI, Carter MJ, Russell JK, Torres BA, Dunn BM, Johnson HM. Use of synthetic peptides to identify an N-terminal epitope on mouse gamma interferon that may be involved in function. Proc Natl Acad Sci USA 1988; 85:1237–41.
66. Leinikki PO, Calderon J, Luquette MH, Schreiber RD. Reduced receptor binding by a human interferon gamma fragment lacking 11 carboxyl-terminal amino acids. J Immunol 1987; 139:3360–6.
67. Littman SJ, Devos R, Baglioni C. Binding of unglycosylated and glycosylated human recombinant interferon gamma to cellular receptors. J Interferon Res 1985; 5:471–6.
68. Gomi K, Akinaga S, Oka T, Morimoto M. Analysis of receptors, cell surface antigens, and proteins in human melanoma cell lines resistent to human recombinant beta or gamma interferon. Cancer Res 1986; 46: 6211–6.
69. Weil J, Epstein CJ, Epstein LB, Sedmak JJ, Sabran JL, Grosberg SE. A unique set of polypeptides is induced by gamma interferon in addition to those induced in common with alpha and beta interferons. Nature 1983; 301:437–9.
70. Miller BA, Perrine SP, Antognetti G, Perlmutter D, Emerson SG, Sieff C, Faller DV. Recombinant gamma interferon: a regulator of fetal hemoglobin production by cord blood BFU-E derived erythroblasts. Blood 1987; 69:1674–81.
71. Ucer U, Bartsch H, Scheurich P, Pfizenmaier K. Biological effects of gamma interferon on human tumor cells: quantity and affinity of cell

membrane receptors for gamma interferon in relation to growth inhibition and induction of HLA-DR expression. Int J Cancer 1985; 36:103–8.

72. Greiner JW, Hand PH, Noguchi P, Fisher PB, Pestka S, Schlom J. Enhanced expression of surface tumor associated antigens on human breast and colon tumor cells after recombinant human leukocyte α-interferon treatment. Cancer Res 1984; 44:3208–14.
73. Kierszenbaum F, Sonnenfeld G. Characterization of the antiviral activity produced during *Trypanosoma cruzi* infection and protective effects of exogenous interferon against experimental Chagas' disease. J Parasitol 1982; 68:194–8.
74. Herman R, Baron S. Effects of interferon inducers on the intracellular growth of the protozoan parasite, *Leismania donovani*. Nature 1970; 226:168–9.
75. Koga T, Mitsuyama M, Handa T, Watanabe Y, Nomoto K. Gamma interferon-mediated increase in the number of Ia-bearing macrophages during infection with listeria monocytogenes. Infect Immun 1987; 55: 2300–3.
76. Buchmeier NA, Schreiber RD. Requirement of endogenous interferon gamma production for resolution of *Listeria monocytogenes* infection. Proc Natl Acad Sci USA 1985; 82:7404–8.
77. Talmadge JE, Tribble HR, Pennington W, Phillips H, Wiltrout RH. Immunomodulatory and immunotherapeutic properties of recombinant gamma interferon and recombinant tumor necrosis factor in mice. Cancer Res 1987; 47:2563–70.
78. Giri SN, Hyde SM, Marafino J Jr. Ameliorating effect of murine interferon gamma on bleomycin-induced lung collagen fibrosis in mice. Biochem Med Metab Biol 1986; 36:194–7.
79. Black PL, Phillips H, Tribble HR, Pennington R, Schneider M, Talmadge JE. Correlation of immunomodulatory and therapeutic activities of interferon and interferon inducers in metastatic disease. J Cell Biochem 1988; 36:377–92.
80. Silagi S, Dutkowski R, Schaefer A. Eradication of mouse melanoma by combined treatment with recombinant human interleukin 2 and recombinant murine interferon-gamma. Int J Cancer 1988; 41:315–22.
81. Fidler IJ, Fogler WE, Kleinerman ES, Saiki I. Abrogation of species specificity for activation of tumoricidal properties in macrophages by recombinant mouse or human interferon gamma encpasulated in liposomes. J Immunol 1985; 135:4289–96.
82. Twentyman PR, Workman P, Wright KA, Bleehen NM. The effects of alpha and gamma interferons on human lung cancer cells grown in vitro or as xenografts in nude mice. Br J Cancer 1985; 52:21–9.
83. Nathan CF, Horowitz CR, De La Harpe J, Vadhan-Raj S, Sherwin SA, Oettgen HF, Krown SE. Administration of recombinant interferon

gamma to cancer patients enhances monocyte secretion of hydrogen peroxide. Proc Natl Acad Sci USA 1985; 82:8686–90.
84. Kleinerman ES, Kurzrock R, Wyatt D, Quesada JR, Gutterman JU, Fidler IJ. Activation of suppression of the tumoricidal properties of monocytes from cancer patients following treatment with human recombinant gamma-interferon. Cancer Res 1986; 46:5401–5.
85. Maluish AE, Urba WJ, Longo DL, Overton R, Coggin D, Crisp ER, Williams R, Sherwin SA, Gordon K, Steis RG. The determination of an immunologically active dose of interferon-gamma in patients with melanoma. J Clin Oncol 1988; 6:434–45.
86. Aulitzky W, Gastl G, Aulitzky WE, Nachbaur K, Lanske B, Kemmler G, Flener R, Frick J, Huber C. Interferon gamma for the treatment of metastatic renal cancer: dose-dependent stimulation and downregulation of beta-2 microglobulin and neopterin responses. Immunobiol 1987; 176:85–95.
87. Logan TF, Ernstoff MS, Kirkwood JM, Gerich B, Friberg D, Whiteside T, Eddy B, Witman P, Schindler J, Herberman RB, Reich S. Changes in natural killer cell (NK) phenotype in peripheral blood (PB) of patients (PT) with renal cell carcinoma and melanoma treated with recombinant interferon gamma. Abstract, Annual Meeting AACR, 1987.
88. Murray HW, Scavuzzo D, Jacobs JL, Kaplan MH, Libby DM, Schindler J, Roberts RB. In vitro and in vivo activation of human mononuclear phagocytes by interferon gamma. J Immunol 1987; 138:2457–62.
89. Otto U, Conrad S, Schneider AW, Klosterhalfen H. Recombinant interferon gamma in the treatment of metastatic renal cell carcinoma. Results of a phase II trial. Arzeneimittelforschung (W. Germany) 1988; 11: 1658–60.
90. Huber C, Autlizky W, Gastl G, Aulitzky WE, Herold M, Frick J. Treatment of metastasizing renal cell carcinoma with an optimum biological response modifying dose of rIFN-gamma. Abstract of poster presentation. Society for biological therapy annual meeting Nov. 6–9, 1988; Berkeley, California.
91. Ernstoff MS, Trautman T, Davis CA, Reich SD, Witman P, Balser J, Rudnick S, Kirkwood JM. A randomized phase I/II study of continuous versus intermittent intravenous interferon gamma in patients with metastatic melanoma. J Clin Oncol 1987; 5:1804–10.
92. Brinckerhoff CE, Guyre PM. Increased proliferation of human synovial fibroblasts treated with recombinant immune interferon. J Immunol 1985; 134:3142–6.
93. Mentzer SJ, Burakoff SJ, Faller DV. Interferon gamma induction of LFA-1 mediated homotypic adhesion of human monocytes. J Immunol 1986; 137:108–13.

94. Arnaout MA, Lanier LL, Faller DV. Relative contribution of the leukocyte molecules Mol. LFA-1, and p150,95 (leuM5) in adhesion of granulocytes and monocytes to vascular endothelium is tissue- and stimulus-specific. J Cell Physiol 1988; 137:305–9.
95. Mentzer SJ, Crimmins MAV, Burakoff SJ, Faller DV. Alpha and beta subunits of the LFA-1 membrane molecule are involved in human monocyte-endothelial cell adhesion. J Cell Physiol 1987; 130:410–5.
96. Malaise MG, Franchimont P. Defective in vitro gamma interferon production in rheumatoid arthritis. Arth Rheum 1987; 30:230–1.
97. Firestein GS, Zvaifler NJ. Peripheral blood and synovial fluid monocyte activation in inflammatory arthritis. II. Low levels of synovial fluid and synovial tissue interferon suggest that gamma interferon is not the primary macrophage activating factor. Arth Rheum 1987; 30: 864–71.
98. Malaise MG, Bastings M, Reuter AM, Vrindts-Gevaert Y, Bernier J, Sondag D, Frere MC, Goldstein G, Franchimont P. In vitro effects of thymopentin on the gamma-interferon production by peripheral blood mononculear cells from normal subjects and from patients with rheumatoid arthritis. Immunol Lett 1987; 4:323–7.
99. Husby G, Williams RC Jr. Immunohistochemical studies of interleukin-2 and gamma interferon in rheumatoid arthritis. Arth Rheum 1985; 28:174–81.
100. Hasler F, Bluestein HG, Zvaifler NJ, Epstein LB. Analysis of the defects responsible for the impaired regulation of EBV-induced B cell proliferation by rheumatoid arthritis lymphocytes. II. Role of monocytes and the increased sensitivity of rheumatoid arthritis lymphocytes to prostaglandin E. J Immunol 1983; 131:768–72.
101. Lotz M, Tsoukas CD, Fong S, Dinarello CA, Carson DA, Vaughan JH. Release of lymphokines after infection with Epstein-Barr virus in vitro. II. A monocyte-dependent inhibitor of interleukin 1 downregulates the production of interleukin 2 and interferon alpha in rheumatoid arthritis. J Immunol 1986; 136:3643–8.
102. Lotz M, Tsoukas CD, Curd JG, Carson DA, Vaughan JH. Effects of recombinant human interferons on rheumatoid arthritis B lymphocytes activated by Epstein-Barr virus. J Rheumatol 1987; 14:42–5.
103. Combe B, Pope RM, Fischbach M, Darnell B, Baron S, Talal N. Interleukin-2 in rheumatoid arthritis: production of and response to interleukin-2 in rheumatoid synovial fluid, synovial tissue and peripheral blood. Clin Exp Immunol 1985; 59:520–8.
104. Cheetham B, Hertzog P, Emery P, McMullen G, Marzuki S, Chambers P, Linnane A. Increased interferon (IFN) activity associated with recovery from rheumatoid arthritis (RA). J Interferon Res 1987; 6:804.

105. Ohara M, Igarashi S, Kobashi C, Nanmiya M, Yoshida H, Kasukawa R. The effects of the antirheumatic agents N-(2-carboxyphenyl)-4-chloroanthranilic acid disodium (CCA) and D-penicillamine on the NK and ADCC activities and interferon production of lymphocytes. J Immunopharmacol 1984; 6:163-72.
106. Ghiara P, Baralini M, Tagliabue A, Boraschi D. Anti-inflammatory activity of IFN-beta in carrageenan-induced pleurisy in the mouse. Clin Exp Immunol 1986; 66:606-14.
107. Heremans H, Dijkmans R, Sobis H, Vandekerckhove F, Billiau A. Regulation by interferons of the local inflammatory response to bacterial lipopolysaccharide. J Immunol 1987; 138:4175-4179.
108. Dore-Duffy P, Perry W, Kuo HH. Interferon-mediated inhibition of prostaglandin synthesis in human mononuclear leukocytes. Cell Immunol 1983; 79:232-9.
109. Rachmilewitz D, Karmeli F, Panet A. Interferon inhibits prostaglandin E2 synthesis and stimulates (2′-5′) oligoadenylate synthetase activity in peripheral blood mononuclear cells of inflammatory bowel disease patients. J Interferon Res 1985; 5:629-35.
110. Browning JL, Ribolini A. Interferon blocks interleukin 1-induced prostaglandin release from human peripheral monocyte. J Immunol 1987; 138:2857-63.
111. Dore-Duffy P, Perry W, Kuo H-H. Macrophages release arachidonic acid prostaglandin E_2, and thromboxane in response to late complement components. J Immunol 1983; 133:2145-50.
112. Boraschi D, Censini S, Baralini M, Ghiara P, DiSimplicio P, Tagliabue A. Interferons inhibit LTC4 production in murine macrophages. J Immunol 1987; 138:4341-6.
113. Boraschi D, Censini S, Baralini M, Tagliabue A. Regulation of arachidonic acid metabolism in macrophages by immune and nonimmune interferons. J Immunol 1985; 135:502-5.
114. Browning J. Interferons and rheumatoid arthritis: insight into interferon biology? Immunol Today 1987; 8:372-3.
115. Gowen M, Nedwin GE, Mundy GR. Preferential inhibition of cytokine-stimulated bone resorption by recombinant interferon gamma. J Bone Miner Res 1986; 1:469-74.
116. Hoffmann O, Klaushofer K, Gleispach H, Leis HJ, Luger T, Koller K. Peterlik M. Gamma interferon inhibits basal and interleukin 1-induced prostaglandin production and bone resorption in neonatal mouse calvaria. Biochem Biophys Res Commun 1987; 143:38-43.
117. Kahari VM, Heino J, Vuorio T, Vuorio E. Interferon alpha and interferon gamma reduce excessive collagen synthesis and procollagen mRNA levels of scleroderma fibroblasts in culture. Biochim Biophys Acta 1988; 968:45-50.

118. Amento EP, Bhan AK,McCullagh KG, Krane SM. Influences of gamma interferon on synovial fibroblastlike cells. J Clin Invest 1985; 76:837-48.
119. Duncan MR, Berman R. Gamma interferon is the lymphokine and beta interferon the monokine responsible for inhibition of fibroblast collagen production and late but not early fibroblast proliferation. J Exp Med 1985; 162:516-27.
120. Stephenson ML, Krane SM, Amento EP, McCroskery PA, Byrne M. Immune interferon inhibits collagen synthesis by rheumatoid synovial cells associated with decreased levels of the procollagen mRNAs. FEBS Lett 1985; 180:43-50.
121. Goldring MB, Sandell LJ, Stephanson ML, Krane SM. Immune interferon suppresses levels of procollagen mRNA and type II collagen synthesis in cultured human articular and costal chondrocytes. J Biol Chem 1986; 261:9049-56.
122. Freundlich B, Bomalski JS, Neilson E, Jimenez SA. Regulation of fibroblast proliferation and collagen synthesis by cytokines. Immunol Today 1986; 7:303-6.
123. Granstein RD, Murphy GF, Margolis RJ, Byrne MH, Amento EP. Gamma-interferon inhibits collagen synthesis in vivo in the mouse. J Clin Invest 1987; 79:1254-8.
124. Coffman RL, Carty J. A T-cell activity that enhances polyclonal IgE production and its inhibition by interferon-gamma. J Immunol 1986; 136:949-54.
125. Mond JJ, Carmen J, Sarma C, Ohara J, Finkelman FD. Interferon gamma suppresses B cell stimulation factor (BSF-1) induction of class II MHC determinants on B cells. J Immunol 1986; 137:3534-7.
126. Goodman M. Regulation of B cell activation by prostaglandins: cell cycle-specific effects on activation by anti-immunoglobulin and 8-mercaptoguanosine. J Immunol 1986; 137:3753-7.
127. Straite ND, Panayi GS. Prostaglandin regulation of B lymphocyte function. Immunol Today 1984; 5:175-7.
128. Vaughan JH. Immune system in rheumatoid arthritis: possible implications in neoplasms. Am J Med 1985; 78:6-11.
129. Lotz M, Tsoukas CD, Robinson CA, Dinarello CA, Carson DA. Basis for defective responses of rheumatoid arthritis synovial fluid lymphocytes to anti-CD3 (T3) antibodies. J Clin Invest 1986; 78: 713-21.
130. Mentzer SJ, Rothelin R, Springer TA, Faller DV. Cell surface structures involved in the cytotoxic T lymphocyte response to human synovial cells. J Cell Physiol 1988; 137:173-8.
131. Zilly A, Obert HJ. Therapie der chronischen polyarthritis. Morbid Mortal Week 1986; 128:87-9.

132. Lemmel EM, Franke M, Gaus W, Hartl PW, Hofschneider PH, Miehlke K, Machalke K, Obert HJ. Results of a phase II clinical trial on treatment of rheumatoid arthritis with recombinant interferon gamma. Rheumatology 1987; 7:127–32.
133. Schindler J, Kennedy SM, Wolfe F. Potential of gamma interferon in rheumatoid arthritis. Adv Inflamm Res 1988; 12:305–11.
134. Wolfe F, Cathey MA, Hawley DJ, Balser JP, Schindler JD. Clinical trial with r-IFN-g in rheumatoid arthritis. In: Pincus SH, ed. Biologically based immunomodulator in the therapy of rheumatic diseases. 1st ed. New York, 1986:379–96.
135. Veys EM, Mielants H, Verburgen G, Grosclaude J-P, Meyer W, Galazka A, Schindler J. Interferon gamma in rheumatoid arthritis–a double blind study comparing human recombinant interferon gamma with placebo. J Rheumatol 1988; 15:570–4.
136. Cannon GW, Pincus SH, Emkey RD, Denes A, Cohen SA, Wolfe F, Saway PA, Jaffer AM, Weaver AL, Cogen L, Schindler JD. Double-blind trial of recombinant interferon gamma versus placebo in rheumatoid arthritis. Arth Rheum. 1989; 32:964-73
137. Lemmel EM, Brackertz D, Franke M, Gaus W, Hartl PW, Machalke K, Mielke H, Obert HJ, Peter HH, Sieper J, Sprekeler R, Stierle H. Results of a multicenter placebo-controlled double-blind randomized phase III clinical study of treatment of rheumatoid arthritis with recombinant interferon-gamma. Rheumatol Int 1988; 8:87–93.
138. Pernice W, Schuchmann L, Dippell J, Suschke J, Vogel P, Truckenbrodt H, Schindera F, Humburg C, Brzoska J. Therapy of systemic juvenile rheumatoid arthritis with gamma interferon. A pilot study in nine patients. Arth Rheum 1989; 32:643–6.
139. Cannon GW, Schindler JD, Kennedy SM, Emkey RD, Denes A, Cohen SA, Wolfe F, Saway PA, Jaffer AM, Weaver AL, Cogen L. Long-term follow-up of recombinant interferon gamma in rheumatoid arthritis. 52nd Annual Meeting of the ARA, Houston, 1988.
140. Cannon GW, Emkey RD, Denes A, Cohen SA, Wolfe F, Jaffer AM, Weaver AL, Cogen L, Gulinello J, Kennedy SM, Schindler JD. Prospective two year followup of r-IFN-g in RA. J Rheumatol. In press.

8

Future Approaches to the Diagnosis and Therapy of Rheumatoid Arthritis

Robert I. Fox, Charles A. Robinson, Gary W. Williams, John G. Curd, and Clifford W. Colwell, Jr.
Scripps Clinic and Research Foundation, La Jolla, California

Thomas F. Bumol
Lilly Research Laboratories, Indianapolis, Indiana

I. ABSTRACT

Long-term studies of rheumatoid arthritis (RA) patients have shown that current therapies are not satisfactory, as evidenced by the significant proportion of patients who progress with erosive deforming disease. Therefore, new approaches to diagnosis and treatment need to be considered.

In the area of diagnosis, new methods of recombinant DNA technology in combination with serological studies might be used to identify specific subgroups of RA patients. In view of the broad variability of treatment response among different patients, specific immunogenetic markers should be sought that have prognostic value. For example, polymorphisms that encode the histocompatibility antigens (especially the HLA-D loci), T-cell antigen receptor, and immunoglobulin genes may provide a genetic profile for each patient. The recent development of rapid methods for detection of these DNA polymorphisms by a method called "polymerase chain reaction" (PCR) may allow for these tests to be performed in a cost-efficient manner. Taken together with currently available serological data (including rheumatoid factor titer, acute phase reactants such as ESR and fibronectin, and perhaps circulating cytokine levels), we may be able to use our present medications more effectively either as single agents or in combinations. The increased cost of initial diagnosis would be balanced by our more effective use of slow-acting antirheumatic drugs.

In order to develop novel methods of future therapy for RA, we present a model of pathogenesis based around the generation of type A (macrophage-like) presynoviocytes in the bone marrow, their subsequent migration to the inflamed joint via the high endothelial venules, and the terminal differentiation of the type A synoviocyte within the RA synovial membrane. The synovial hyperplasia that characterizes erosive RA is attributed to a "paracrine" interaction between type A synoviocytes and type B (fibroblast-like) synoviocytes. As a result of mutual interdependent stimulation of these cells in the RA synovium, a series of cytokines (particularly interleukin-1 and interleukin-6) are liberated that further perpetuate the inflammatory process and affect adjacent vascular cells, lymphoid cells, and osteoclasts. This model differs significantly from previously described models of RA pathogenesis that are centered around T-cell immune responses against autoantigens. We propose that new remittive therapies may be developed based on their ability to interrupt the generation of presynoviocytes in the bone marrow and their subsequent differentiation into type A synoviocytes.

In addition to "systemic therapy," new approaches to intra-articular therapy should be considered. For example, a pharmacological agent could be coupled to a specific cytokine and infused intra-articularly. The ligand would be chosen for its ability to bind to a cell surface receptor on type A synoviocytes, so that the ligand-drug complex would be internalized and the pharmacological agent delivered in high concentration to the relevant cells. Alternatively, liposomes could be used to coat pharmacological agents, since type A synovial cells have phagocytic properties for liposomes and thus the drug could be delivered intracytoplasmically in high concentration. These methods can target drugs to a particular cell type. Another approach is to direct pharmacological agents to an important "region" of the RA joint, such as the interface of the pannus eroding into adjacent bone. For example, particular components of the extracellular matrix in this region (such as fibronectins) may provide a target for a specific monoclonal antibody coupled to a pharmacological agent. Novel linkers between the antibody and drug can be created such that the drug is only liberated in critical amounts when a second signal (such as external ultrasound) is administered. In a general sense, the use of intra-articular infusion of pharmacological agents might proceed in parallel to methods currently being developed for therapy of certain solid tumors, since the great expense of joint replacement may make these treatments cost-effective.

Ultimately, the specific diagnosis and treatment of RA will be determined by identification of the environmental agent(s) that initiate this disorder. However, at the present time these factors remain unknown and efforts must be made to better utilize our existing therapies. The high frequency of disease progression with current therapies suggests that new pharmacological approaches are justified, including a more aggressive approach to intra-articular therapy.

II. INTRODUCTION

Rheumatoid arthritis (RA) is a common disease that affects 2-3 million people in the United States alone (1,2). A substantial proportion of affected individuals will develop erosive joint disease and require surgical joint replacement despite therapies including disease-modifying antirheumatic drugs (DMARDs) such as gold, penicillamine, antimalarials, and methotrexate (3,4). Taken together, clinical studies have suggested that DMARD therapy may at best delay the development of erosive lesions in a substantial proportion of RA patients (5). In some patients with intractable RA, immunosuppressive agents including azathioprine, methotrexate, cyclophosphamide, and combinations of these drugs have proven beneficial (6). However, the potential side effects, including bone marrow toxicity and neoplasia, have limited their frequency of use and the dose that is given (7).

Synovectomy by surgical methods has received extensive study (8). Although there may be transient benefit in selected RA patients, the general consensus is that the synovial proliferations returns within several years, the procedure is relatively expensive, and complete removal of synovial tissue frequently is not technically possible. Radionuclide synovectomy has been studied by Sledge (9,10) and others (11). These results have been promising but are potentially limited by the recurrence of synovitis and the reluctance of physicians to repeatedly administer radiation in proximity to bone marrow elements. However, the success of "radioactive synovectomy" has suggested the possibility that specific pharmacological agents might be used intra-articularly against the proliferating synoviocytes.

In this chapter, we will first review evidence that suggests that the type A synoviocyte plays a central role in the pathogenesis of RA. Next, lymphokines, cytokines, and growth factors that may play a role in RA pathogenesis will be briefly discussed. Finally, new approaches to diagnosis and therapy will be presented.

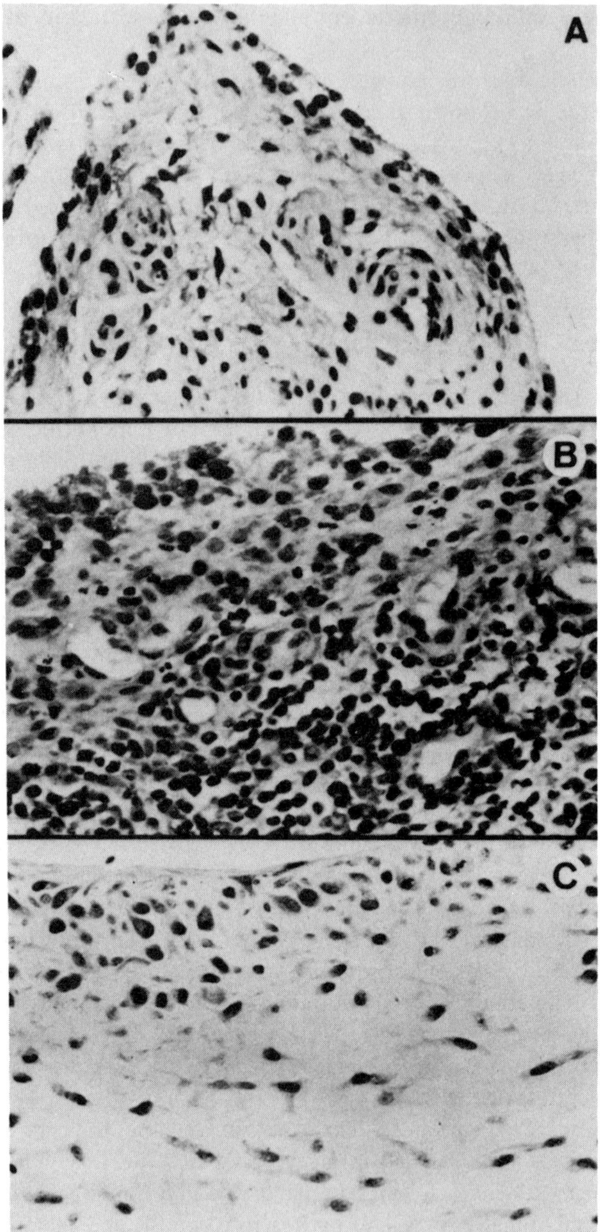
A
B
C

III. BACKGROUND

A. Importance of the Synoviocyte in Rheumatoid Arthritis

Synovial joints are lined by cells that normally function to secrete lubricating substances for the bony surfaces and to remove cellular debris from the synovial cavity (12). The lining cell layer is normally only one to two cells in thickness (Fig. 1, frame A). In RA, the synovial lining becomes markedly thickened due to an increased number of synovial cells and increased size of the individual synoviocytes (Fig. 1, frames B and C). In most RA patients with longstanding disease, there is a lymphocyte infiltrate (Fig. 1, frame B) that is located in the layer below the proliferating synoviocytes. However, in some RA patients (Fig. 1, frame C), the synoviocyte hyperplasia occurs in the absence of significant lymphocyte infiltrates (12). The types of synoviocytes in normal joints and their alterations in RA will be more fully discussed below. Briefly, synoviocytes have been subdivided into macrophage-like (type A) and fibroblast-like (type B) cells. The interactions of synovial lining cells with each other and with other cell types in the joint (i.e., lymphocytes, endothelial cells, osteoblasts, osteoclasts, etc.) represent the fundamental "abnormalities" responsible for the pathogenesis of RA. Any model of RA must explain the histological observations of cell-cell interaction that occur within the synovial tissue. Since the pathology of RA has been extensively described (13,14), it will be the task of immunology and cell biology research to define in molecular terms the signals that occur between these cells in normal and disease states.

Several lines of evidence argue that the macrophage-like (type A) synoviocyte plays the pivotal role in the pathogenesis of RA. First, arthroscopic synovial membrane biopsies obtained early in the course of RA show that the initial pathogenetic events involve proliferation of the synovial lining cell and vascular angiogenesis (15-17). These events may be closely related since stimulated macrophage-like cells (including type A synoviocytes) (18) release an angiogenesis-stimulating factor that is probably identical to tumor necrosis

---

Figure 1 Histology of normal and rheumatoid arthritic joints. (A) The normal synovial lining layer is one to three cells thick. The subsynovial tissue consists of fibrocytes, blood vessels, and a few histiocytes, all between collagen bundles. (B) A biopsy of rheumatoid arthritis synovial membrane has hyperplasia and lymphocytic infiltration. (C) A synovial biopsy from a different rheumatoid patient shows thickening of the synovial membrane associated with proliferation of synoviocytes but with few infiltrating lymphocytes.

factor α (TNF) (19). Lymphocytic infiltration into the synovial membrane only occurs later (15,20), possibly in response to factors released from the synoviocytes. Second, the critical feature of RA is the erosion of bone by the advancing synovial tissue. The interface of synovium and bone (termed the pannus) contains predominantly synoviocytes and is relatively devoid of lymphocytes or granulocytes (13,21-23). The invasive and "tumor-like" properties of synoviocytes from the rheumatoid pannus can be reproduced in vitro (24). The bone erosion probably results from release of interleukin-1 (IL-1) by type A synovial cells that subsequently regulate adjacent bone osteoclasts (25). Finally, some RA patients with progressive erosive disease have synovial membrane biopsies with marked synoviocyte hyperplasia and little lymphocytic infiltration (26). Taken together these results suggest that synoviocytes (particularly the macrophage-like type A synoviocyte) may play a critical role in RA from the earliest stages of disease. However, the specific signals actually released by the synoviocytes in situ (particularly early in the course of disease) remain unknown. The hyperproduction of specific cytokines or failure to respond to normal differentiation signals may provide clues to therapy. Since it is the type A synoviocyte that migrates to the synovial tissue and interacts with the resident type B synoviocyte, we will initially review the origin and possible regulatory controls of type A synovial cells.

B. The Type A Synoviocyte

Historically, synovial lining cells were subdivided into type A (macrophage-like) and type B (fibroblast-like) based on their electron microscopic appearance (27). Additional cell types that are less abundant have also been reported (14,28). In normal or osteoarthritic joints, the type B (fibroblastic) synoviocyte predominates (29,30). In contrast, the RA synovium is characterized by a marked increase in the proportion of type A (macrophage-like synoviocytes (27).

The use of immunohistological methods to detect specific enzymes (31, 32) and monoclonal antibodies (26) to detect "monocyte-like" antigens has supported the concept that type A cells in RA synovial membrane are phenotypically and functionally related to monocytes. For example, the synovial membrane shows a large number of lining cells that react with the "T200 antigen," a marker that is shared among cells of hematopoietic lineage but is absent from mesenchymal cells. In particular, these cells react with monoclonal antibody Leu-M5 (MoAb Leu-M5) that detects the monocyte-associated form of T200 (Fig. 2, frame A). Type B synoviocytes, which contain procollagen in their cytoplasm, can be detected by immunohistological methods (frame B); comparison of serial sections from the same RA patient's synovial biopsy (frames A and B) show that the type A and type B cells appear to have extensive cell-cell contacts. Of importance, the type A cell does not appear to expand clonally in a manner that excludes its adjacent type B cells. Both type A and type B synoviocytes express cell surface HLA-DR molecules (Fig. 2, frame C). These class II histocompatibility antigens may participate in pathogenesis by either presenting antigens to immune cells (either autoantigens or exogenous antigens) or by serving directly as targets for immune attack (33). In comparison to RA biopsies, few cells expressing the macrophage-associated marker Leu-M5 were found in the osteoarthritic joint (Fig. 2, frame D).

Further support for the bone marrow-derived origin of type A synoviocytes comes from the elegant studies of Edwards and Willoughby (34). They irradiated mice lethally and reconstituted them with bone marrow stem cells from a donor mouse strain (the beige mouse) that contained "giant mitochondria." After several months, the joints of the irradiated reconstituted mice showed synovial lining type A cells with giant mitochondria (i.e., donor origin), while the type B synoviocytes contained small mitochondria (i.e., recipient host origin). Although other interpretations of these data are possible (13,35), it seems likely that synovial type A cells are derived from a bone marrow stem cell. Similar observations have been made in man after bone marrow transplantation, where alveolar macrophages (36) and Kupffer's cells in the liver (37) have the sex karyotype of the donor. In these latter patients, the host macrophages disappear soon after chemotherapy (used for preparation of the patient for bone marrow transplant) and the donor macrophages begin to reappear in the tissues approximately 3 months after transplantation (37). Although synoviocytes and Kupffer's cells each arise from bone marrow-derived cells, it remains unknown whether commitment to a specific tissue (e.g., to a pulmonary alveolar macrophage, synoviocyte, Kupffer's cell) occurs while still in the bone marrow or whether a circulating precursor undergoes terminal differentiation in response to the specific tissue microenvironment. This issue will be discussed in further detail later in this chapter, since therapeutic strategies to eliminate presynoviocytes (e.g., in the marrow or circulation) may lead to significant side effects if presynoviocytes are also precursors for other crucial cell lineages.

In contrast to type A synoviocytes, type B synoviocytes probably arise from the differentiation of resident tissue fibroblasts (34). During the 10th week of embryologic development a fluid-filled space develops in the limb bud at the position of the future joint and local fibroblasts assume a type B synoviocyte morphology to line this cavity; type A synoviocytes do not

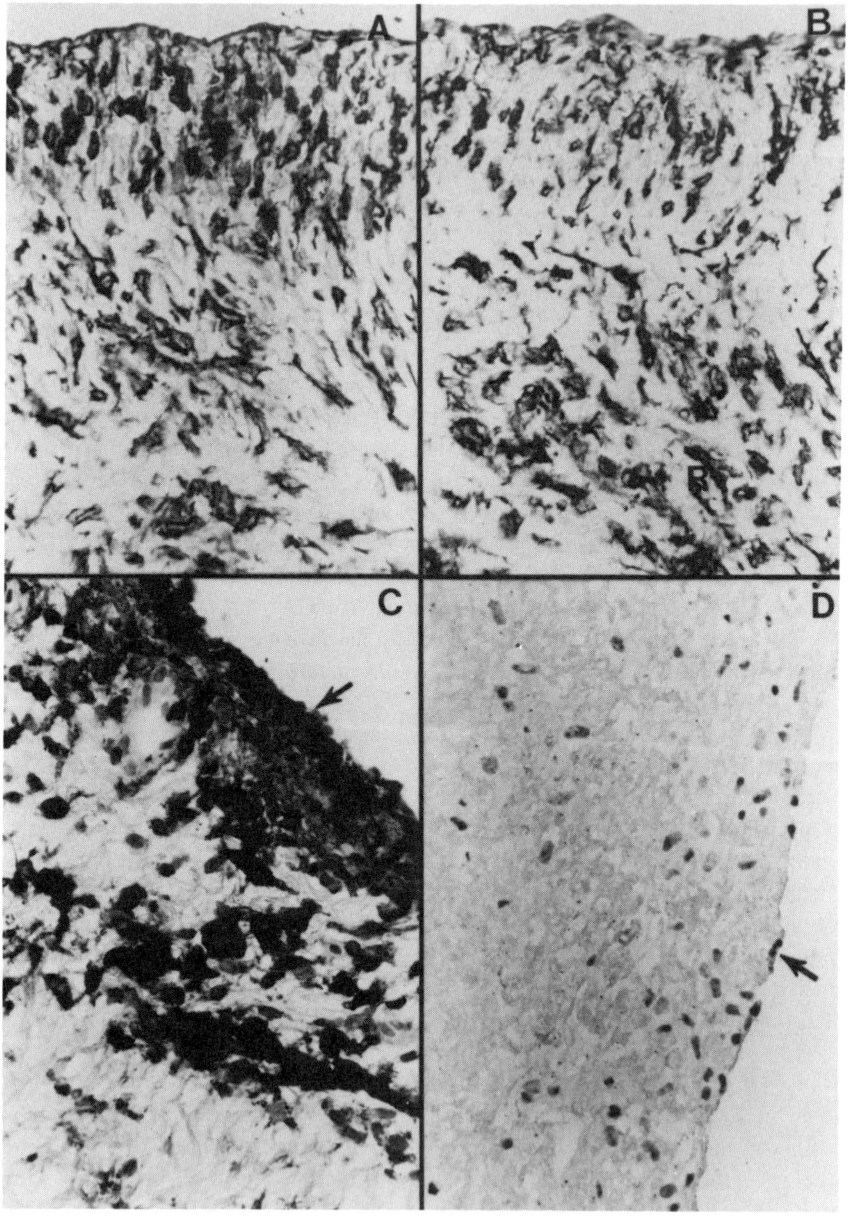
A
B
C
D

migrate to this site until later, when hematopoietic precursors that have developed in the fetal liver migrate to the future joint cavity (38). In adult animals, a "synovial lined cavity" can be reproduced by air injection into the subdeltoid tissues to create a cell-free space, and this microenvironment induces the "differentiation" of type B synoviocytes (39). Presumably, with time or appropriate antigenic stimulation, type A synovicocytes will subsequently migrate to this cavity. Such a model holds great potential promise for understanding the differentiation signals that regulate synovial cell traffic during embryogenesis or pathogenesis of arthritis.

In summary, the RA synovium initially develops as an interdependent proliferation of type A and type B synoviocytes, with lymphocytes arriving in the joint later. The type A cells originate in bone marrow, migrate through the bloodstream to the synovial membrane where they probably recognize a specific receptor on the high endothelial venule (40–42), and exit into the joint. This is shown schematically in Fig. 3. The type A synoviocyte then becomes intercalated into an architecture provided by the type B synoviocytes, including specific components of the extracellular matrix such as fibronectin (43–45). It is important to emphasize that our knowledge of type A and type B synovial cells remains extremely limited. Type A synoviocytes have not been adapted to long-term tissue culture suitable for biochemical analysis. Long-term cultures of fibroblast-like cells (type B synoviocytes) indicate that in vitro passage may alter their biochemical, morphological, and immunochemical properties (32,46–48). Therefore, it will be necessary to carefully identify the specific gene products expressed by the synoviocytes within the microenvironment of the RA synovium and to determine the in vitro culture conditions that most closely reproduce these properties.

Figure 2 Immunohistology of synovial lining cells in normal and rheumatoid joints using monoclonal antibodies. (A) A synovial biopsy from an RA patients contains cells with monocyte-like antigens detected by monoclonal antibody Leu-M5. This antigen is present on bone marrow-derived cells and is a member of the "T200" supergene family. (B) RA synovial biopsy stained to detect type B synoviocytes containing precollagen C. (C) A synovial biopsy from an RA patient stained for histocompatibility antigen HLA-DR. (D) A synovial tissue from a patient with osteoarthritis, stained with monoclonal antibody Leu-M5.

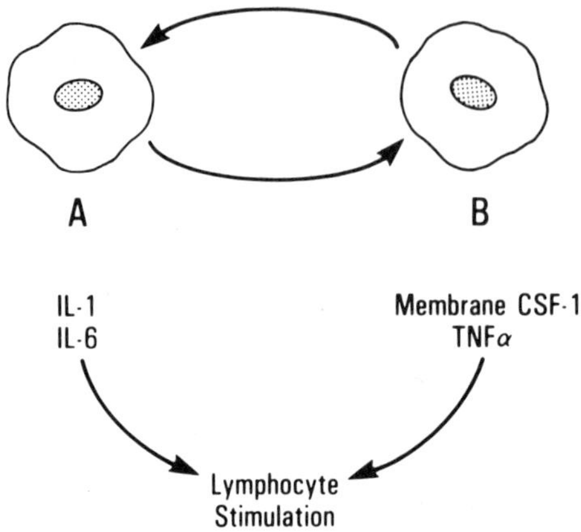

Figure 3 A model of pathogenesis for rheumatoid arthritis. A schematic model based on "paracrine" interaction of type A (labeled as cell A) and type B synoviocytes (labeled as cell B) is presented. The macrophage-like type A synoviocyte may express specific receptors (i.e., the *fms* oncogene product) for the growth factor CSF-1. The fibroblast-like type B synoviocyte may express the CSF-1 growth factor on its cell surface. As a result of the stimulation of the type A synoviocyte, certain factors (including IL-1 and IL-6) would be released that could stimulate the type B synoviocyte. This reciprocal stimulation is termed a paracrine interaction. The factors released from the synoviocytes (IL-1, IL-6, and TNF) could interact with other cells within the synovial tissues including lymphocytes and high endothelial venules.

C. Lymphokines and Growth Factors

Since the functional properties of synoviocytes are influenced by lymphokines and other growth factors, a brief review of the complex field will be presented. The reader is referred to several excellent reviews of this rapidly changing field (25,49–51). Several lymphokines that may play a role in RA are listed in Table 1.

Gene cloning revealed two distinct interleukin-1-like molecules (termed IL-1α and IL-1β) that share only about 26% sequence homology yet have many similar biological effects. IL-1 plays an important role in T-cell activation, since stimulated macrophages release this cytokine (or present membrane associated IL-1) to specific receptor(s) on T cells. IL-1 may also play an important role in B-cell activation. In addition to these effects on the immune system, these cytokines affect other cell types that play a role in RA.

Table 1 Cytokines of Potential Importance Rheumatology

Lymphokine	Source	Activates or induces
A. Interleukin-1α Interleukin-1β	Monocytes Synoviocytes Endothelial cells Keratinocytes	T cells Acute phase reactant Prostaglandin E_2 Fever Bone and cartilage resorption High endothelial cell adhesion Collagenase production CSF-1 and GM-CSF IL-6 synthesis Hematopoiesis
B. Interleukin-2	T cells	T-cell and B-cell growth Macrophage and natural killer cells
C. Interleukin-3	T cells	Differentiation of bone marrow stem cells and mast cells
D. Interleukin-4	T cells	T-cell, B-cell; and mast cell growth B-cell differentiation (IgE)
E. Interleukin-5	T cells	B-cell differentiation (IgA)
F. Interleukin-6	Macrophages Fibroblasts Synoviocytes Endothelial cells T cells	B-cell differentiation Plasmacytoma growth factor, some activities similar to those of IL-1
G. GM-CSF	T cells Monocytes	Monocyte production Monocyte adhesiveness Inhibits neutrophil migration
H. TNF-α TNF-β	Macrophages T cells	Some activities similar to those of IL-1 Angiogenesis stimulation Inhibits transformed cell growth Cachexia
I. Interferon-γ	T cells Natural killer cells	Monocyte cytokine production HLA–D expression Natural killer activity

Fibroblasts are stimulated to proliferate and release collagenase (52,53). Bone resorption is facilitated by IL-1 binding to osteoblast/osteoclast receptors (25). IL-1 increases the ability of endothelial cells to transform into "high endothelial cells" and bind circulating lymphocytes (49). Other actions include the elevation of acute phase reactants (due to binding on receptors of hepatocytes) and fever (due to binding on receptors in the brain). Each of these activities can be correlated with clinical/pathological features in the RA patient. However, the effects in vivo may be complex. For example, low levels of IL-1 stimulate osteoblasts, but in higher doses the osteoblasts are suppressed (25). Further, IL-1 has synergistic interactions with other factors (especially tumor necrosis factor and prostaglandin E_2) that may alter its activities on bone remodeling at a particular dose (25,54). These multiple activities and interactions may represent a tremendous problem in designing therapies that depend on antagonist or agonist strategies for a single cytokine.

A variety of different cell types are able to produce IL-1, although the major source for RA patients in vivo may be monocytes and type A synoviocytes (53,55,56). Of interest, IL-1 can promote the production of additional monocytes by stimulating fibroblastic cells to produce macrophage-stimulating factor (CSF-1) and granulocyte-macrophage-stimulating factor (GM–CSF) (57). Not all monocytes produce equal amounts of IL-1 (58,59); increased production may be associated with differentiation of a promonocyte into a tissue monocyte (60). Allison (49) proposed that an important mechanism of action for antirheumatic drugs is the interference with the differentiation of promonocytes into synoviocytes (i.e., their ability to produce large amounts of IL-1).

In addition to IL-1, a large number of other cytokines and growth factors probably play an important role in TA (Tables 1 and 2). In view of the high proportion of T cells expressing activation antigens such as HLA-DR (61-63), it was initially expected that synovial tissues would produce large amounts of IL-2 (IL-2). However, most investigators have been unable to detect IL-2 in RA synovial fluid or tissue extracts (56,64–66). Other products of activated T cells are interferon-γ (IFNγ) and interleukin-3 (IL-3); however, only a small proportion of RA synovial fluid samples have detectable levels of these lymphokines (56,67).

Recently, several new lymphokines including IL-4, IL-5, and IL-6 have been cloned (Table 1). Their specific role in RA pathogenesis remains unknown. IL-4 has a wide variety of functions including activation of T cells, B cells (especially specific isotypes of IgG and IgE production), and stimulation of myelomonocytic precursors [reviewed in (68)]. IL-4 induces monocytes to become multinucleated giant cells (69); such giant cells are occasionally

Table 2 Peptide Growth Factors Are Multifunctional

Growth factor	Proliferative effects	Antiproliferative effects	Effects unrelated to proliferation
Epidermal growth factor	Keratinocytes, fibroblasts	Hair follicle cells, squamous carcinoma cells	Suppression of gastric acid secretion
Fibroblast growth factor (basic)	Many mesenchymal cells, especially endothelial cells	Ewing's sarcoma cells, other tumor cells	Regulation of pituitary and ovarian cell function
Tumor necrosis factor-α	Diploid fibroblasts, epithelial cells	Many tumor cells	Inhibition of lipoprotein lipase, stimulation of collagen
Transforming growth factor-β	Fibroblasts, osteoblasts	Fibroblasts, epithelial cells, T lymphocytes, osteoblasts	Suppression of immunoglobulin secretion and adrenal steroidogenesis
Interleukin-1	Lymphocytes, keratinocytes, fibroblasts	Breast cancer cells	Endogenous pyrogen, bone resorption
Interleukin-2	T and B lymphocytes, oligodendrocytes	T lymphocytes, oligodendrocytes	Increased cytotoxic activity of monocytes
Interleukin-6	Hybridoma, plasmacytoma cell lines	Breast cancer cells	Increased expression of cell surface antigens and secretion of immunoglobulins

Source: Ref. 73.

seen in RA synovial tissues (13,14) and may reflect the in vivo action of this lymphokine.

Recently, particular attention has been focused on interleukin-6 (Table 1). This factor has been found in increased amounts in synovial fluid, probably due to its production in vivo by synovial lining cells and plasma cells (70). IL-6 can induce B-cell differentiation, plasmacytoma growth, and can stimulate hepatocyte production of acute phase reactants by the liver (71-73). Since IL-1 is a potent inducer of IL-6, it remains unclear whether some of the biological effects of IL-1 are mediated by subsequent induction of IL-6 (51).

In addition to cytokines, a series of growth factors (Table 2) have recently been cloned and have equally complex interactions (74). For example, transforming growth factor β stimulates fibroblast growth in the presence of platelet-derived growth factor but inhibits fibroblast growth if epidermal growth factor is present (75). Another important interaction may be that of IL-4 and TNF, since IL-4 can either enhance or antagonize hematopoiesis, depending on the prsence of IL-3 (76). These results emphasize that lymphokines and growth peptides are not limited to a single physiological activity in vivo. Rather, cells probably respond to pattern of regulatory signals (74). From a therapeutic point of view, these complex interactions and redundancy of effects by different factors will greatly limit our ability to manipulate the synoviocyte by addition of a single growth factor.

In summary, inflammatory events in the RA synovium are mediated by a complex interaction of cytokines, growth factors, and products of arachidonic acid metabolism. Of particular importance, cytokines such as IL-1, IL-6, and TNF that may be produced by synoviocytes have been found in RA synovial fluid. In contrast, factors associated with activated T-cells such as IL-2, IL-3, or interferon-γ are infrequently detected in the RA joint. This suggests that pharmacological destruction of synoviocytes producing these cytokines (i.e., IL-1, IL-6, TNF) should be a specific goal in developing new therapies for RA.

D. A Model of RA Based on Paracrine Stimulation of Type A and Type B Synoviocytes

The growth and differentiation of synoviocyte type A cells is likely to be influenced by its interactions with adjacent cells, including "autocrine," "paracrine," and "endocrine" interactions. Autocrine growth stimulation (as occurs in certain solid tumors) refers to the ability of a cell to facilitate its own growth by releasing factors that bind to its own cell surface receptors

(77). Paracrine stimulation refers to one cell generating a signal that stimulates an adjacent cell; in turn, the original cell receives a stimulatory signal from the second cell. Finally, endocrine stimulation occurs when one cell secretes a soluble factor that stimulates a second cell over a spatial distance that requires the "hormone" to diffuse to its specific receptor. Examination of RA synovial tissues provides some clues to the mechanisms that may be involved. If an autocrine mechanism were predominantly responsible, then a "clonal" type of proliferation of type A synovial cells would be expected. However, the hypertrophied synovial lining consists of the mutual expansion of both type A and type B synoviocytes (Figs. 1 and 2). Therefore, it is likely that some type of paracrine stimulation between these cell types is occurring that requires their cell-cell contact. The presence of lymphocytes in the deeper layers of the synovial tissues in most patients suggests that the lymphocytes may secrete factors that diffuse to synovial lining layer (i.e., an endocrine mechanism). Of course, it remains possible (and perhaps likely) that stimulated type A synoviocytes release factors that serve as cofactors to stimulate their own growth or metabolic activity. However, the close cell-to-cell contacts between type A and type B synoviocytes noted on immunohistological examination of RA synovial tissues suggests that paracrine interactions are the limiting factor.

A model of RA synovial proliferation is shown schematically in Fig. 3. The growth factor CSF-1 is probably expressed on the surface of type B synoviocytes, since it is present on the cell membrane of normal and neoplastic cells of fibroblastic origin (78). It is possible that cell surface CSF-1 is a more potent stimulus for macrophage stimulation than soluble CSF-1. This may explain the need for close cell-cell interaction between the type A and type B synoviocytes in the RA joints. The type A synoviocytes probably express the receptor for the factor CSF-1 (i.e., the *fms* oncogene) since this marker is present on macrophage-like cells. In a reciprocal fashion, the type A synoviocyte secretes IL-1 (79,80) that stimulates fibroblast growth, as well as their production of collagenase and IL-6 (53,81,82). An attractive feature of this model is that the growth factors CSF-1 (83), GM-CSF (84), and TNF (85) were recently reported to be present in RA synovial fluid (86).

Factors liberated from type A synoviocytes such as IL-1 (87), IL-6 (88), lysosomal enzymes, oxygen metabolites, and cytolytic proteinases all activate lymphocytes. The lymphocytes in turn will release factors including interferon-γ, lymphotoxin, and interleukins that further stimulate the type A synoviocytes and reperpetuate the cyle.

Another important interaction is that factor including interferon-γ will induce increased histocompatibility antigens HLA-DR and HLA-DQ on macrophages. These induced histocompatibility antigens may further stimulate lymphocytes. In this manner, a positive feedback circuit is developed that leads to continued recruitment and metabolic activity of synoviocytes and lymphocytes. This is shown schematically in Fig. 3. In summary, the interactions of type A synoviocytes with other cells and soluble factors within the synovial membrane are likely to be quite complex.

Several other models have been proposed for the pathogenesis of RA. The large number of $CD4^+$ T cells found in RA synovial tissues has suggested that RA develops as an autoimmune response against a particular exogenous agent (such as a viral antigen localized in the joint) or an autoantigen (such as collagen). Each of these models is supported by animal models of arthritis or the finding of an exogenous agent in the synovial tissues of patients with conditions resembling RA (e.g., spirochete antigens in Lyme arthritis). Our proposed model for RA differs from these models since the T lymphocyte (or B lymphocyte) does not occupy the central role in pathogenesis. The relative absence of lymphocytes in the earliest stage of RA synovitis, the relative paucity of lymphocytes in some RA synovial biopsies late in disease, and the absence of T-lymphocyte-related interleukins in synovial fluid have suggested a secondary role for the T cells in RA joint destruction. It remains important to search for infectious agents that may trigger RA, perhaps by infecting type A synoviocytes or their precursors in a manner that alters their interactions with other synovial cells. However, these infectious agents may vanish soon after initiating the RA synovitis, leaving behind a self-perpetuating process of synovial hyperplasia.

IV. NOVEL APPROACHES TO THERAPY

A. Better Use of our Existing Medications: Early Diagnosis and Early Treatment

Many years ago when describing the limitations of cancer therapy, Dr. Paul Erlich noted that if we did not have "better bullets," then we must learn to aim better. It is likely that our present failure to frequently alter the relentless progression of erosive disease derives in part from therapy "too little, too late." We generally await the appearance of erosive lesions on joint X-ray prior to institution of remittive agents such as gold, penicillamine, or methotrexate. We then give a medication (such as gold) for up to 6 months, hoping that the patient will respond and not have toxic side reactions. If the initial treatment is not successful (either nonresponse or toxic side effects), then the entire process is repeated with another remittive agent. A substantial number of RA patients will undergo progressive joint erosions and deformity during the interval of waiting (and hoping) for therapeutic response. From a prognostic point of view, it is reasonable to consider RA as a series of closely related diseases that may be divided into subgroups that differ in their response to specific therapies.

One immediate goal for the future is to use currently available clinical and laboratory data to identify specific variables that predict prognosis (89) or therapy/toxicity response to specific agents. For example, autoantibody production, specific histocompatibility genes (90,91), acute phase reactants (89), or specific histological patterns on synovial biopsy (26,56,92,93) may aid in predicting joint destruction.

This is shown schematically in Table 3, where a group of patients (labeled A, B, C, D, etc.) are initially subdivided based on the presence of a routine clinical laboratory parameter such as rheumatoid factor titer or acute phase reactants (i.e., ESR, fibrinogen, CRP, etc.). They would then be further subdivided on the basis of a genetic marker, such as the presence of histocompatibility antigen HLA-DR4 (94,95). Further subgroups could be based on specific DNA markers such as the recently recognized high frequency of a specific DNA sequence that defines a subset of HLA-DR4 patients at high risk for RA (96). A newly developed diagnostic technique termed "polymerase chain reaction" (PCR) aplication seems particularly well suited for inexpensive rapid determination of DNA-encoded markers (97) such as histocompatibility (HLA) genes. It is easy to imagine this technology adapted to a multichannel analyzer for DNA analysis (98), analogous to the multichannel analyzer routinely used for electrolytes or liver function tests. As an example, consider the determination of histocompatibility genes in a given patient. A small sample of blood is used as a source of each patient's DNA. A segment of the particular gene of interest (i.e., HLA-D) first is enzymatically amplified. The amplified histocompatibility gene sequence is checked for the

Table 3 Subclassification of Patients with Symmetric Erosive Polyarthritis

Patients with RA	A	B	C	D
Autoantibody (i.e., rheumatoid factor)	+	+	+	-
Histocompatibility Antigen (i.e., DR4)	+	+	-	-
Histocompatibility subtype (i.e., DR4 epitope)	+	-	-	-

presence or absence of specific alleles (i.e., HLA-DR1, DR2, DR3, DR4, etc.) using a nonradioactive, colorimetric probe. In this manner, patients with a histocompatibility antigen suggestive of poor long-term prognosis might be more rapidly advanced to remittive agents such as gold or methotrexate. The choice of the specific therapeutic agents might also be more rationally predicted using a pattern of genetic markers correlated with susceptibility/toxicity. This earlier initiation of a specific therapy may allow treatment of RA at a stage when the disease process was still susceptible to complete remission. This approach would be equivalent to cancer treatment while the disease was still in situ or the "tumor burden" was still low.

In addition to HLA-D genetic loci, other genes important in immune response can be detected at the DNA level. For example, the T-cell antigen receptor (TCAR) consists of two chains, termed TCAR-α and TCAR-β. Each chain consists of a variable region and a constant region, in addition to "diversity" or "joining" segments. There are "alleles" (i.e., different DNA sequences that are inherited in a Mendelian manner) for both the variable region and constant region segments; these alleles can currently be detected by a technique called "restriction length polymorphism." However, it is likely that these alleles can be detected by the use of PCR and serve as an additional marker to define a "genetic profile" for each patient. The determination of both HLA and TCAR genetics may prove particularly important, since studies in mice recently showed that particular combinations of alleles of these genes predispose to autoimmune disease. Finally, the immunoglobulin genes have genetic varability that is referred to as "allotype." Since it technically difficult to detect allotype by serological methods, it may be possible to use PCR for this purpose (since the molecular basis for different allotypes resides in their amino acid sequence and thus should be detected at the DNA level). In summary, a wide variety of genetic markers are available to define subsets of RA patients and the molecular biological techniques are currently available. The key factor in these studies will be the careful clinical characteriziation of a large number of RA patients who have received adequate trials of remittive therapies and can serve as prototypes to determine which (if any) combination of genetic markers provide prognostic information.

B. Preventing the Generation of Presynoviocytes in the Bone Marrow

In developing new strategies of treatment, it seems reasonable to concentrate on the type A synoviocyte. As demonstrated by Edwards and Willoughby (34), these cells probably originate in bone marrow (illustrated in Fig. 4).

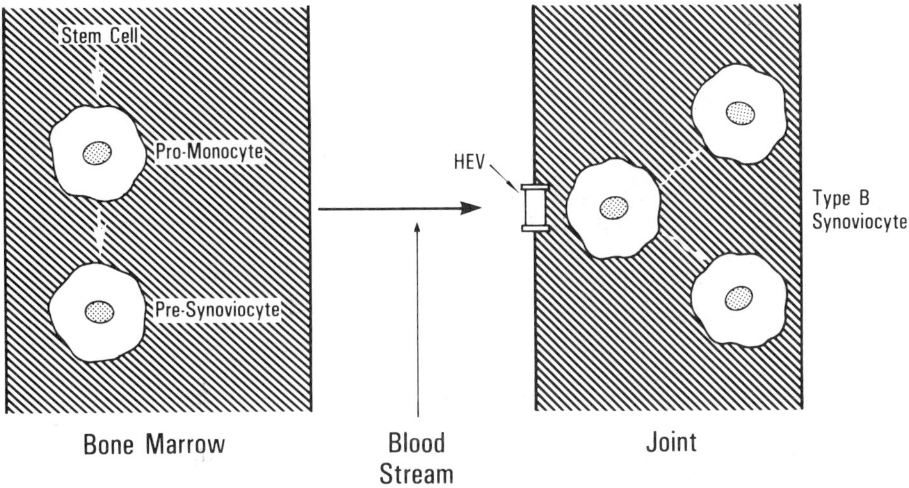

Figure 4 Precursors of type A synoviocytes are generated within the bone marrow and migrate through the circulation to the synovial tissues. The circulating presynoviocytes probably bind to and enter the synovium through specialized vascular endothelial cells termed high endothelial venules (HEV).

However, little is known about the specific precursors of type A synoviocytes in man. For example, the synoviocyte may arise from the circulating monocyte (Fig. 5), frame A). Alternatively, the stem cell may undergo partial differentiation into a synoviocyte precursor within the bone marrow (Fig. 5, frame B). Since pluripotential stem cells circulate in man (50), it is possible that circulating stem cells migrate to the synovium where they undergo their terminal differentiation in the microenvironment provided by other synovial lining cells (Fig. 5, frame C). These possibilities have very different therapeutic predictions. If differentiation to a presynoviocyte is "committed" within the bone marrow, then specific markers associated with this differentiation can be used to target therapy. On the other hand, if a pluripotential cell differentiates to a synoviocyte after arrival in the joint, then attempts to remove presynoviocytes from the bone marrow or circulation are likely to remove other important precursors (e.g., pre-Kupffer's cells).

Several indirect lines of evidence suggest that monocytic precursors may differentiate to presynoviocytes in the bone marrow and that this step in pathogenesis may be an important site of action of currently used therapies. Both gold and penicillamine inhibit the formation of granulocytes and

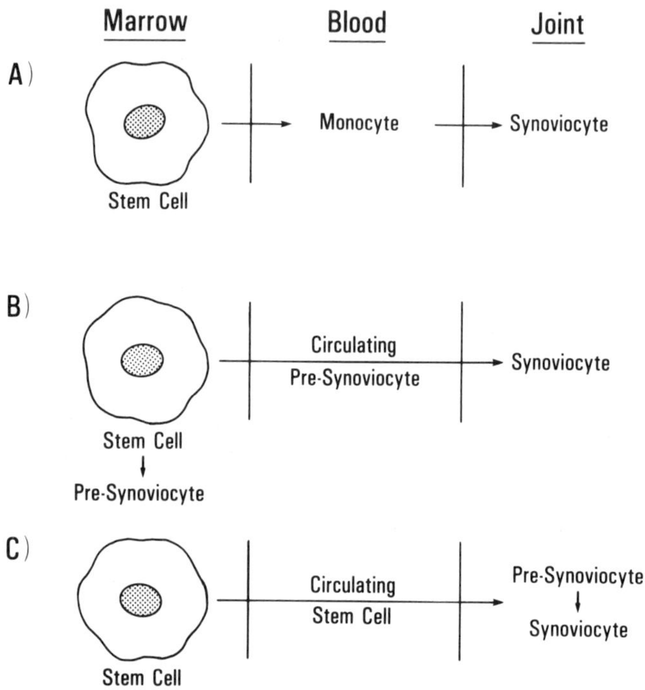

Figure 5 Sources of type A synoviocytes. The pattern of differentiation of presynoviocytes remains poorly understood. Several possibilities include (A) a stem cell precursor differentiates to yield a circulating monocyte; this cell undergoes terminal differentiation in the synovial microenvironment to become a type A synoviocyte; (B) A stem cell may undergo commitment to the synoviocyte lineage (i.e., become a presynoviocyte) within the bone marrow and this precommitted cell then enters the circulation and eventually arrives at the synovial tissue where it undergoes its terminal differentiation; and (C) pleuripotential stem cell are found in low frequency in the circulation of normal individuals; therefore, it is possible that such cells circulate in higher abundance in RA patients and migrate to the inflamed joint where they undergo terminal differentiation to synoviocytes.

marcrophage colonies from mouse and human bone marrow at doses that are in the therapeutic range (99-101). Littman et al. (102) found that gold inhibits the normal maturation-induced loss of peroxidase activity and the acquisition of spontaneous cytotoxicity. In comparison, the intra-articular administration of gold salts or penicillamine has little effect on synoviocytes (103). The therapeutic effects of gold may be relatively specific for presynoviocytes since RA patients do not suffer obvious generalized defects in their reticuloendothelial system (i.e., the occurrence of certain infections, such as pneumococcal septicemia, that occur in splenectomized patients) and significant granulocytopenias are relatively rare. This model would be consistent with the known slow onset of action of gold or penicillamine, since preexisting synovial type A cells in the joint would not be replaced and the delay in onset of therapeutic effects would represent the known slow half-life for replacement for these synoviocytes (34).

Allison (103) suggested that an important step in the differentiation of promonocytes into synoviocytes is the acquisition of the ability of the latter cells to produce high levels of IL-1 after stimulation. It is likely that this effect is important in RA, since patients with active disease have monocytes that spontaneously secrete large amounts of IL-1 in vitro, in comparison to patients with inactive disease (104,105). According to the paracrine model we have prooposed, the therapeutic benefit of gold would be due to decreasing the number of presynoviocytes (or activated monocytes) that reach the high endothelial venules of the inflamed arthritic joint. The decreased ability of IL-1 production would prevent these presynoviocytes from initiating paracrine interactions with resident type B synoviocytes or further influencing other adjacent cells (such as HEV) to perpetuate the cycle of synovitis.

C. Effect of Lymphocytes on Generation of Synoviocytes

Although our models of pathogenesis have not emphasized the role of lymphocytes as the primary agents of RA pathogenesis, these cells clearly play an important role. In addition to their secretion of lymphokines within the synovial tissues, lymphoid cells influence hematopoiesis (84). Anemia of chronic disease is frequent in patients with active RA, and the occurrence of severe neutropenia in these patients is termed Felty's syndrome (8). These associated conditions may occur as a result of an attempt by the RA patient's immune system to downregulate the production of presynoviocytes in the marrow. Certain effective treatments for RA, such as total nodal lymphoid irradiation (TLI), lead to markedly decreased synovitis but lymphoid activity (as measured by rheumatoid factor or proportion of activated T cells in the circulation) is increased (106). These studies make two important points:

first, it is possible to dissociate abnormalities in the lymphoid system from synovitis; and second, remission of synovitis is not necessarily associated with return to normality of the lymphoid system.

The strong association of RA with histocompatibility antigen HLA-DR4 suggests a role for T-lymphocytes in pathogenesis, since $CD4^+$ T-cells recognize antigens in the context of class II HLA-molecules. It has been proposed that T-cells directly "attack" $HLA\text{-}DR^+$ synovial lining cells. However, this seems unlikely since the synovial lymphocytes are not in direct contact with the DR^+ synoviocytes. An alternative model is that the critical influence of HLA-DR in RA pathogenesis occurs at the level of the bone marrow, where promonocytes differentiate into pre-synoviocytes. Since the monocytic precursors are $HLA\text{-}DR^+$, $CD4^+$ T-cells probably regulate production of type A synoviocytes. In particular, the ability of an individual to "downregulate" synoviocyte production may be deficient in individuals with HLA-DR4, thus conferring susceptibility to the disease RA. This hypothesis would be consistent with observations about the T-cell's role in regulating the differentiation of other hematopoetic lineages, observations about responses to current remittive therapies and provides testable hypotheses that may lead to new therapies.

D. Intra-articular Therapy

Although rheumatoid arthritis is a systemic disease, therapy can be specifically directed to particular joints. In this regard, it is important to remember that the RA synovium has invasive growth characteristics that have been compared to those of localized tumors (107,108). The frequent use of intra-articular glucocorticoid injections as well as surgical synovectomy provides examples of effective (but transient) "local treatments." Since the inflamed joint constitutes a localized space, a pharmacological synovectomy that can be administered by intra-articular injection and may be safely repeated at periodic intervals (if necessary) might prove cost-effective in disease management.

In view of the complex interactions of cytokines on particular cell types (i.e., either augmentation or inhibition depending on other factors present), it seems unlikely that simple intra-articular infusion of a single lymphokine will give a lasting therapeutic response. Likewise, it seems unlikely that a simple antagonist (i.e., a structure that blocks the receptor for lymphokine) will be able to block the very high affinity of cytokines for their receptors, particularly since these signals may be delivered by cell-to-cell contact. Therefore, an alternate approach for the future might be to conjugate the pharmacological agent to the specific ligand. This is shown schematically in Fig. 6, frame A. The infused drug-ligand would be directed to the appropriate cell by binding to the receptor for the cytokine, the drug-ligand would be internalized

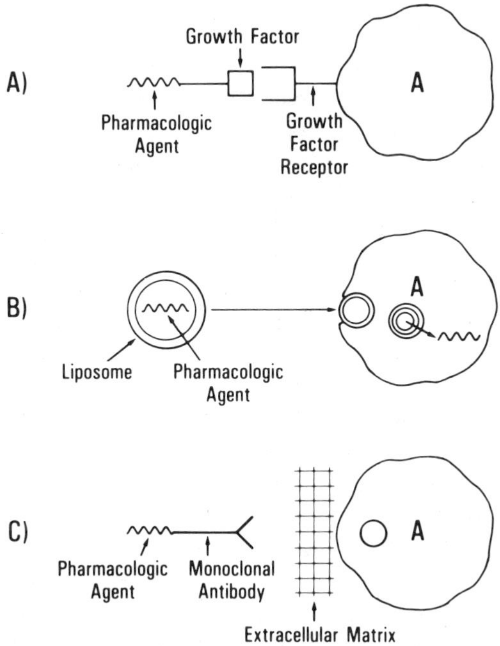

Figure 6 Possible methods for targeting intra-articular therapy in RA patients. (A) Therapeutic agents may be directly coupled to a specific ligand (i.e., a lymphokine or growth factor) that is expressed on the surface of a type A synoviocyte. The ligand is then internalized by binding to the receptor and the drug is delivered to the cell cytoplasm. (B) Therapeutic agents are encoated in liposomes. This might aid in protecting them from hydrolytic enzymes present in the synovial fluid. Since type A synoviocytes have phagocytic properties, it is likely that the lysosomes will selectively be taken up by these cells. (C) Therapeutic agents are coupled to specific monoclonal antibodies. The antibodies could be directed either at a specific cell surface molecule or at a component of the extracellular matrix (located at a critical region of the synovium such as the advancing margin of the pannus as it invades bone). After binding in the critical region, the chemical linkage between the antibody and pharmacological agent would dissolve, allowing the drug to diffuse into cells within a specific microenvironment.

by the "normal" receptor cycling process, and the drug would be delivered intracytoplasmically in certain receptor-mediated systems to the target cell. Another approach would be to encoat the therapeutic agent in a liposome (Fig. 6, frame B), since this structure would be phagocytosed by the type A synoviocyte. This mode of uptake would provide selectively in drug delivery. In rabbits with experimentally induced arthritis, intra-articularly injected corticosteroids encapsulated in liposomes were more effective than a threefold higher dose of microcyrstalline glucocorticoid (109). The phagocytosis of liposomes by synoviocytes might be further enhanced by the addition of specific proteins (i.e., ligands that bind to the synoviocyte cell surface receptors) into the lipids that form the liposome.

The above approaches are designed to target a pharmacological agent to a specific cell by virtue of a cell surface marker (e.g., a ligand receptor or antigen) or functional property (e.g., phagocytosis). Alternatively, therapy might be directed to a specific region of the RA joint, where it may kill all cells within that microenvironment. For example, a key goal for RA treatment is to prevent the synovial membrane from invading the adjacent bone. For example, fibronectins are located at particularly important sites such as the interface of the advancing pannus and the articular cartilage (43-45). Therefore, pharmacological agents could be coupled to specific antibodies to reactive with such extracellular matrix molecules or crosslinked combinations of matrix molecules. In this manner, the pharmacological agent would become localized in the pannus region after intra-articular infusion. After the drug conjugate had become localized, the linkage between drug and antibody would dissolve, liberate a high concentration of the drug within that microenvironment, and kill the cells within that region.

Other extracellular matrix proteins such as chondroitan sulfate, heparin sulfate, laminins, vitronectin, or particular collagen molecules might be studied by immunohistochemical methods to determine whether they would be important candidates for site-directed therapy. Also, connective tissue repair and remodeling at the cellular level in a chronic inflammatory site might provide novel epitopes in abnormal molecular combinations of these molecules that could provide sites for antibody-based site-directed therapy.

In order to deliver the therapeutic agent optimally to the target cell (and to minimize any extra-articular side effects due to leakage of the agent outside to joint cavity), particular linkers between the ligand and drug could be developed. For example, a releasable linker could be created that only dissociates within the type A synoviocyte or perhaps dissolved by an enzyme present in abundance only in the pannus. Alternatively, linker technology sensitive exposure to low-dose X ray or ultrasound might be employed; after intra-articular injection, the desired joint would be given a low-dose X-ray or ultrasound treatment to release the therapeutic agent. In this manner, a two-step approach to drug localization would be used. First, the drug would be targeted by ligand or monoclonal antibody to the specific cell type (i.e., bearing ligand receptor) or microenvironment (i.e., defined by monoclonal antibody to extracellular matrix) or other pannus-associated antigens. Then, the second signal (i.e., a specific enzyme in the microenvironment or an exogenous signal such as X ray) would cause the drug linkage to dissolve and allow local critical concentrations to be achieved.

The choice of therapeutic agents for intra-articular use remains unclear since relatively little is known about synoviocyte growth requirements. In view of their low growth fraction (i.e., low mitotic index), cell cycle agents such as vinca alkaloids are less likely to be effective. However, type A synoviocytes may express receptors for particular growth factors (26) and it remains possible that intra-articularly administered growth factor (in the form of a drug conjugates) may be able to stimulate a round of cell division and thus facilitate the action of a drug such as a vinca alkaloid. As an alternative, attention might be given to catalytically active protein toxins such as ricin, pokeweed antiviral protein, or gelonin. These agents generally act by interfering with ribosomal function and protein synthesis. It is predicted that they should be effective in view of the well-developed, active rough endoplasmic reticulum in synoviocytes (13). The polypeptide nature of these toxins, however, may limit their use in the synovial cavity that is filled with hydrolytic enzymes. Other drugs with nondegradable organic structures may be required, or the toxin may need to be protected from proteolysis by inclusion in liposome-like structures.

V. SUMMARY

The ideal treatment for rheumatoid arthritis would be recognition of the inciting agent and prevention of the disease (perhaps by vaccination) before symptom onset. However, we are currently faced with a spectrum of patients who differ in their disease severity, rapidity of disease progression, distribution of joint involvement, and response to currently existing therapeutic agents. At the present time, few rheumatoid patients achieve total remission and many progress to more erosive disease. Therefore, attention needs to be given to novel approaches to treatment. Since we may treat "too little, too late," we should carefully examine the synovial histology, immunogenetic characteristics, and autoantibody profiles of RA patients with the best response to our current medications. The aim is to allow selection of specific medications for patients based on their chance for therapeutic response and their decreased risk of serious side effects. In view of the significant expense of "blind" treatment regimens with gold or penicillamine, such diagnostic "profiles" may prove cost-effective. This approach is summarized in Table 4.

As more becomes known about the generation of presynoviocytes in the bone marrow, specific therapies can be directed toward blocking this differentiation. It is likely that drugs already in use (e.g., gold) may affect these

Table 4 Questions for Future Research

1. What are the genetic and environmental factors that interact to cause RA?
2. Can methods be developed to predict which medication will be most likely to induce a disease remission in a particular RA patient?
3. Can new models of RA pathogenesis be developed that will provide insights into pathogenesis or treatment?
   a. Does RA result from a paracrine interaction of type A and type B synoviocytes?
   b. Can RA be prevented by interrupting the generation of presynoviocytes in bone marrow or their "homing" to the joint tissue?
4. Can medications be used intra-articularly to effect a pharmacological synovectomy?
   a. By coupling drugs to specific cytokines or growth factors?
   b. By coupling drugs to specific monoclonal antibodies?
   c. By encoating the drugs in liposomes to facilitate their phagocytosis by type A synoviocytes?

stem cells and drug analogs have better efficacy with lower toxicity. The presynoviocytes migrate from the bone marrow through the circulation until they reach a high endothelial venule (HEV) at the inflamed joint. The interruption of this presynoviocyte traffic into the joint provides a site for therapeutic intervention.

Finally, "local" therapy may be administered intra-articularly to achieve a pharmacological synovectomy. Drugs might be conjugated to a specific monoclonal antibody or to a growth factor that binds to a specific synoviocyte cell surface receptor. Encoating drugs in liposomes may help facilitate their phagocytosis and thus destruction of the type A synoviocytes. In addition to cell surface antigens as targets, drug conjugates also may be directed to extracellular matrix molecules. In this case, releasable linkers with a defined kinetics of dissociation in vivo would hold the drug and antibody together long enough to permit localization; then the linkage would dissolve and release the drug in a form that could freely diffuse into cells within the relevant microenvironment.

ACKNOWLEDGMENTS

I thank Drs. A. C. Allison, George Fey, Jack Gauldie, Ed Amento, Martin Lotz, John Vaughan, Dennis Carson, Mark Totoritis, Mark Ginsberg, and

Frank Kozin for their stimulating discussions on the ontogeny of synoviocytes and the potential effects of long-acting drugs on bone marrow.

This work is supported in part by grant AR33983 and RR00833 from the National Institutes of Health, and a gift from the Henning Foundation. It is publication number 5367BCR of the Research Institute of Scripps Clinic, La Jolla, California.

REFERENCES

1. McDuffie FC. Morbidity impact of rheumatoid arthritis on society. Am J Med 1985; 78(Suppl aA):1-5.
2. Meenan RF, Yelin EH, Newitt M, et al. The impact of chronic disease. A sociomedical profile of rheumatoid arthritis. Arth Rheum. 1981; 24: 544-9.
3. Lightfoot RW. Treatment of rheumatic arthritis. In: McCarty DJ, ed. Arthritis and allied conditions. Philadelphia: Lea and Febiger, 1979:513.
4. Calin A. Diagnosis and management of rheumatoid arthritis. San Francisco: Addison-Wesley, 1983.
5. Iannuzzi L, Dawson N, Zein N, Kushner I. Does drug therapy slow radiographic deterioration in RA. N Engl J Med 1983; 309:1023.
6. McCarty DJ, Carrera GF. Intractable rheumatoid arthritis. Treatment with combined cyclophosphamide, azathioprine, and hydroxychloroquine. JAMA 1982; 248:1718-23.
7. Kinlen LJ. Incidence of cancer in rheumatoid arthritis patients and other disorders after immunosuppressive treatment. Am J Med 1985; 78(Suppl 1A):44-9.
8. Kelley WN, Harris ED, Rubby S, Sledge CB. (eds.). In: Textbook of rheumatology. Philadelphia: W.B. Saunders, 1981:785-95.
9. Sledge CB, Zuckerman JD, Zalutsky MR, Atcher RW, Shortkroff S, Lionberger DR, Rose HA, Hurson BJ, Lankenner PA Jr, Anderson RJ, et al. Treatment of rheumatoid synovitis of the knee with intraarticular injection of dysprosium 165-ferric hydroxide makcroaggregates. Arth Rheum. 1986; 29:153-9.
10. Sledge CB, Zuckerman JD, Shortkroff S, Zalutsky MR, Venkatesan P, Snyder MA, Barrett WP. Synovectomy of the rheumatoid knee using intra-articular injection of dysprosium-165-ferric hydroxide macroaggregates. J Bone Joint Surg [Am] 1987; 69:970-5.
11. Boerbooms AM, Buijs WC, Danen M, van de Putte LB, Vandenbroucke JP. Radio-synovectomy in chronic synovitis of the knee joint in patients with rheumatoid arthritis. Eur J Nucl Med 1985; 10:446-9.
12. Fox RI, Carson DA. Monoclonal antibodies and construction of antibody to specific determinants. In: Bennett JC, Cohen AS, eds.

Rheumatology and immunology. New York: Grune and Stratton, 1986: 438-43.

13. Fassbender H. Rheumatoid arthritis. In: Pathology of rheumatic diseases. New York: Springer-Verlag, 1980:26-106.
14. Cooper NS, Soren A, McEwen C, Rosenberger JL. Diagnostic specificity of synovial lesions. Hum Pathol 1981; 12:314-28.
15. Schumacher HR, Kitridou RC. Synovitis of recent onset: a clinicopathologic study during the first month of disease. Arth Rheum 1972; 15: 465-83.
16. Schumacher HR, Jr. Synovial membrane and fluid morphologic alterations in early rheumatoid arthritis: microvascular injury and virus-like particles. Ann NY Acad Sci 1975; 256:39-64.
17. Kulka JP, Bocking D, Ropes MW, Bauer W. Early joint lesions of rheumatoid arthritis. Arch Pathol 1955; 59:129-50.
18. Koch A, Polverini P, Leibovitch Stimulation of neovascularization by human rheumatoid synovial tissue macrophages. Arth Rheum 1986; 29: 471-9.
19. Leibovich. Macrophage induced angiogenesis is mediated by tumor necrosis factor-alpha. Nature 1987; 329:630-2.
20. Fudenberg HH. Molecular theology, immunophilosophy and autoimmune disease. Scand J Immunol 1980; 12:459-65.
21. Schiozawa S, Shiozawa K, Futita T. Morphologic observations in the early phase of the cartilage-pannus junction. Arth Rheum 1983; 26:472-7.
22. Norton W, Ziff M. Electron microscopic observations on rheumatoid synovial membranes. Arth Rheum 1966; 9:589.
23. Shiozawa S, Jasin H, Ziff M. Absence of immunoglobulins in rheumatoid cartilage-pannus junctions. Arth Rheum 1980; 23:816-21.
24. Hamilton J. In vitro evidence for the invasive and tumor-like properties of the rheumatoid pannus. J Rheumatol 1983; 10:845-51.
25. Canalis E, McCarthy T, Centrella M. Growth factors and the regulation of bone remodeling. J Clin Invest 1988; 81:277-81.
26. Young CL, Adamson III TC, Vaughan JH, Fox RI. Immunohistologic characterization of synovial membrane lymphocytes in rheumatoid arthritis. Arth Rheum 1984; 27:32-9.
27. Barland P, Novikoff AB, Hamerman D. Electron microscopy of the human synovial membrane. J Cell Biol 1962; 14:207-14.
28. Soren A, Waugh T. The giant cells in synovial membrane. Ann Rheum Dis 1981; 40:496-500.
29. Gadially FN. Fine structure of joints. In: Solokoff L. ed. The joints and synovial fluid. New York: Academic Press, 1978:110-20.
30. Graabaek PM. Ultrastructural evidence for two distinct types of synoviocytes in rat synovial membrane. J Ultrastruct Res 1982; 78:321-39.

31. Hermanns W, Schulz LC. Enzyme histochemical studies of the homogeneity of the mononuclear phagocyte system with special reference to the synovium. Agents Actions 1982; 11:117–29.
32. Henderson JA, et al The biochemistry of the human synovial lining with special reference to alterations in metabolism in rheumatoid arthritis. Pathol Res Pract 1981; 172:1–24.
33. Todd JA, Acha-Orbea H, Bell JI, Chao N, Fronek Z, Jacob CO, McDermott M, Sinha AA, Timmerman L, Steinman L, McDevitt HO. A molecular basis for MHC class II-associated autoimmunity. Science 1988; 240:1003–10.
34. Edwards JCW, Willoughby DA. Demonstration of bone marrow-derived cells in synovial lining by means of giant intracellular granules as genetic markers. Ann Rheum Dis 1982; 41:177–82.
35. Krawisz B, Florine D, Scott R. Differentiation of fibroblast-like cell into macrophages. Cancer Res 1981; 41:2891–9.
36. Thomas ED, Ramberg RE, Sale GE, Sparkes RS, Golde DW. Direct evidence for a bone marrow origin of the alveolar macrophage in man. Science 1976; 192:1016–8.
37. Gale RP, Sparkes RS, Golde DW. Bone marrow origin of hepatic macrophages (Kupffer cells) in humans. Science 1978; 201:937–8.
38. O'Rahilly R, Gardner E. The embryology of movable joints. In: Sokoloff L. ed. The joints and synovial fluid. New York: Academic Press, 1978:48–97.
39. Edwards JCW, Sedgwick AD, Willoughby DA. The formation of a structure with the essential features of synovial lining by subcutaneous injection of air. J Pathol 1981; 134:147–56.
40. Bevilacqua MP, Pober JS, Wheeler ME, Cotran RS, Gimbrone Jr MA. Interleukin 1 acts on cultured human vascular endothelium to increase the adhesion of polymorphonuclear leukocytes, monocytes, and related leukocyte cell lines. J Clin Invest 1985; 76:2003–11.
41. Freemont A, Jones C, Bromley P, Andrews P. Changes in vascular endothelium related to lymphocyte collections in diseased synovium. Arth Rheum 1983; 26:1427–33.
42. Jalkanen S, Steere AC, Fox RI, Butcher EC. A distinct endothelial cell recognition system controlling lymphocyte traffic into inflamed synovium. Science 1986; 233:556–8.
43. Scott CL, et al. Significance of fibronectin in rheumatoid arthritis and osteoarthritis. Ann Rheum Dis 1981; 40:142–53.
44. Scott DL, Walton W. The significance of fibronectin in rheumatoid arthritis. Sem Arth Rheum 1984; 13:244–54.
45. Scott D, Delamere J, Walton K. The distribution of fibronectin in the pannus of rheumatoid arthritis. Br J Exp Pathol 1981; 62:362–5.

46. Peterson GL. A simplification of the protein assay method of Lowry et al. which is more generally applicable. Anal Biochem 1977; 83:346-56.
47. Dayer J-M, Beutler B, Cerami A. Cachetin/tumor necrosis factor stimulates collagenase and prostaglandin E2 production by human synovial cells and dermal fibroblasts. J Exp Med 1985; 162:2163-8.
48. Dayer JM, Byrne MH, Krane SM. Effects of mononuclear cell factor (MCF), indomethacin, and prostaglandin E2 (PGE2) on collagen and fibronectin synthesis by cultured rheumatoid synovial cells. Clin Res 1980; 28:348A.
49. Allison AC. Immunopathogenetic mechanisms of arthritis and modes of action of anti-rheumatic therapies. In: *Immunopathogenetic Mechanisms in Arthritis*. Laster, England: MPP Press, 1988:213-30.
50. Seiff CA. Hematopoietic growth factors. J Clin Invest 1987; 79:1549-57.
51. Wong GG, Clark CC. Multiple actions of interleukin 6 within a cytokine network. Immunol Today 1988; 137-9.
52. Dayer J-M, Russell RGG, Krane SM. Collagenase production by rheumatoid synovial cells: stimulation by a human lymphocyte factor. Science 1977; 195:181-3.
53. Mizel SB, Dayer J-M, Krane SM, Mergenhagen SE. Stimulation of rheumatoid synovial cell collagenase and prostaglandin production by partially purified lymphocyte-activating factor (interleukin 1). Proc Natl Acad Sci USA 1981; 78:2474-7.
54. Stashenko P, Dewhirst FE, Peros WJ, Kent R, Ago JM. Synergistic interactions between interleukin-1, tumour necrosis factor, and lymphotoxin in bone resorption. J Immunol 1987; 138:1464-8.
55. Johnston Jr RB. Current concepts: immunology. Monocytes and macrophages. N Engl J Med 1988; 318:747-50.
56. Miyasaka N, Sato K, Makoto G, Minoru S, Natsuyama M, Inoue K, Nishioka K. Augmented interleukin-1 production and HLA-DR expression in the synovium of rheumatoid arthritis patients: possible involvement in joint destruction. Arth Rheum. 1988; 31:480-6.
57. Kaushansky K, Lin N, Adamson JW. Interleukin 1 stimulates fibroblasts to synthesize granulocyte-macrophage and granulocyte colony-stimulating factors. J Clin Invest 1988; 81:92-7.
58. Elias JA, Chein P, Gustilo KM, Schreiber AD. Differential interleukin-1 elaboration by density-defined human monocyte subpopulations. Blood 1985; 668:298-301.
59. Khansary N, Chou Y, Fudenberg H. Human monocyte heterogeneity: interleukin-1 and prostaglandin E2 production by separate subsets. Eur J Immunol 1985; 15:48-51.
60. Elias JA, Schreiber AD, Gustilo K, Chien P, Rossman MD, Lammie PJ, Daniele RP. Differential interleukin 1 elaboration by density

fractionated human alveolar macrophages and blood monocytes: relationship to cell maturity. J Immunol 1985; 135:3198-3204.

61. Burmester GR, Kalden JR, Peter HH, Schedel PI, Beck P, Wittenborg A. Immunological and functional characteristics of peripheral blood and synovial fluid lymphocytes from patients with rheumatoid arthritis. Scand J Immunol 1978; 7:405-17.
62. Burmester GR, Yu DTY, Irani A-M, Kunkel HG, Winchester RJ. Ia+ T cells in synovial fluid and tissues of patients with rheumatoid arthritis. Arth Rheum 1981; 24:1370-6.
63. Fox RI, Fong S, Sabharwal N, Carstens SA, Kung PC, Vaughan JH. Synovial fluid lymphocytes differ from peripheral blood lymphocytes in patients with rheumatoid arthritis. J Immunol 1982; 128: 351-4.
64. Egeland T, Lund H. Immunoregulating lymphokines in rheumatoid joints. I. Search for interleukin-2 in synovial fluid. Scand J Immunol 1987; 25:101-6.
65. Husby G, Williams Jr RC. Immunohistochemical studies of interleukin-2 and gamma-interferon in rheumatoid arthritis. Arth Rheum 1985; 28: 174-81.
66. Combe B, Pope RM, Fischbach M, Darnell B, Baron S, Talal N. Interleukin-2 in rheumatoid arthritis: production and response to interleukin-2 in rheumatoid synovial fluid, synovial tissue and peripheral blood. Clin Exp Immunol 1985; 59:520-8.
67. Malaise MG, Franchimont P. Defective in vitro gamma-interferon production in rheumatoid arthritis. Arth Rheum 1987; 30:230-1.
68. Paul WE. Interleukin 4/B cell stimulatory factor 1: one lymphokine, many functions. FASEB J 1987; 1:456-61.
69. McInnes A, Rennick DM. Interleukin 4 induces cultured monocytes/macrophages to form giant multinucleated cells. J Exp Med 1988; 167: 598-611.
70. Hirano T, Matsuda T, Turner M, Ohmoto Y, Tang B, Miyasaka N, Shimizu M, Feldmann M, Kishimoto T. Abnormal increase of B cell stimulatory factor-2 (BSF-2/IL-6) production in rheumatoid arthritis. Eur J Imm 1988; 18:1797-801.
71. Kishimoto T, Hirano T. Molecular regulation of B lymphocyte response. Ann Rev Immunol 1988; 6:485-512.
72. Gauldie J, Richards C, Harnish D, Lansdorp P, Baumann H. Interferon beta-2/B cell stimulatory factor type 2 shares identity with monocyte-derived hepatocyte-stimulating factor and regulates the major acute phase protein response in liver cells. Proc Natl Acad Sci USA 1987; 84: 7251-5.
73. Hirano T, Taga T, Nakano N, Yasukawa K, Kashiwamura S, Shimizu K, Nakajima K, Pyun KH, Kishimoto T. Purification to homogeneity and

characterization of human B-cell differentiation factor (BCDF or BSFp-2). Proc Natl Acad Sci USA 1985; 82:5490–4.
74. Sporn MB, Roberts AB. Peptide growth factors are multifunctional. Nature 1988; 332:217–9.
75. Ranges G, Figari I, Espevik T, Palladino M. The inhibition of CTL development by TGFβ and reversal by TGFα. J Exp Med 1987; 166:991–8.
76. Rennick D, Yang G, Takabe Y, Gemmell L. Interleukin-4 can enhance or antagonize the factor dependent growth of hematopoietic progenitor cells. Proc Natl Acad Sci USA 1987; 84:6889–93.
77. Sporn MB, Todaro GJ. Autocrine secretion and malignant transformation of cells. N Engl J Med 1980; 303:878–80.
78. Sherr C, Rettenmaier C, Socca R, Stanley E. The c-fms protooncogene is related to receptor for mononuclear growth factor CSF-1. Cell 1985; 41: 665–76.
79. Durum SK, Schmidt JA, Oppenheim JJ. Interleukin 1: an immunological perspective. Annu Rev Immunol 1985; 3:263–87.
80. Dinarello CA. Interleukin-1. Rev Infect Dis 1984; 6:51.
81. Dayer JM, Passwell JH, Schneeberger EE, Krane SM. Interactions among rheumatoid synovial cells and monocyte-macrophages: production of collagenase-stimulating factor by human monocyte exposed to concanavalin A or immunoglobulin Fc fragments J Immunol 1980; 124:1712–20.
82. Rupp EA, Cameron PM, Ranawat CS, Schmidt JA, Bayne EK. Specific bioactivities of monocyte-derived interleukin 1 alpha and interluekin 1 beta are similar to each other on cultured murine thymocytes and on cultured human connective tissue cells. J Clin Invest 1986; 78:836–9.
83. Kawasaki E, Ladner M, Wang A, Mark D. Molecular cloning of a cDNA encoding human macrophage specific colon stimulating factor (CSF-1). Science 1985; 230:291–4.
84. Cantrell M, Anderson D, Cerretti D, Gillis S, Cosman D. Cloning, sequence and expression of a human granulocyte/macrophage colony stimulating factor. Proc Natl Acad Sci USA 1985; 82:6250–4.
85. Wollheim F, Heinegard D, Palladino M, Saxne T, Talal N. TNF-alpha in synovial fluid. Differences between RA and reactive arthritis. Arth Rheum 1987; 30:S129.
86. Firestein GR, Xu WD, Townsend K, Glasebrook A, Broide DH, Zvaifler N. Cytokine profile of rheumatoid arthritis suggests a localized autologous mixed lymphocyte reaction. Arth Rheum Abstr 1988; 31:R16.
87. Wood D, Ihrie E, Hammerman T. Release of interleukin-1 from human synovial tissue in vitro. Arth Rheum 1985; 28:853–60.
88. Hirano T, Yasukawa K, Harada, H, Taga T, Watanabe Y, Matsuda T, Kashiwamura S, Nakajima K, Koyama K, Iwamatsu A, Tsunasawa S, Sakiyama F, Matsui H, Takahara Y, Taniguchi T, Kishimoto T.

Complementary DNA for a novel interleukin that induces B lymphocytes to produce immunoglobulin. Nature 1986; 324:73–6.

89. Amos R, Constable T, Crockson R, MacConkey B. Relation of serum CRP and ESR to radiographic changes. Br Med J 1977; 1:195.
90. Schooley JC, Kullgren B, Allison AC. Inhibition of interleukin-1 of the action of erythropoietin on erythroid precursors and its possible role in the pathogenesis of hypoplastic anaemias. Br J Haematol 1988; 67:11–17.
91. Gregerson PK, Silver J, Winchester RJ. The shared epitope hypothesis. Arth Rheum 1987; 30:1205–13.
92. Malone DG, Wahl SM, Tsokos M, Cattell H, Decker JL, Wilder RL. Immune function in severe, active rheumatoid arthritis. A relationship between peripheral blood mononuclear cell proliferation to soluble antigens and synovial tissue immunohistologic characteristics. J Clin Invest 1984; 74:1173–85.
93. Decker JL, Malone DG, Haraoui B, Wahl SM, Schrieber L, Klippel JH, Steinberg AD, Wilder RL. NIH conference. Rheumatoid arthritis: evolving concepts of pathogenesis and treatment. Ann Intern Med 1984; 101:810–24.
94. Stastny P. Rheumatoid arthritis: relationship with HLA-D. Am J Med 1983; 75:9–15.
95. Stastny P, Fink CW. Different HLA-D associations in adult and juvenile rheumatoid arthritis. J Clin Invest 1979; 63:124–130.
96. Gregersen PK, Shen M, Song Q-L, Merryman P, Degar S, Seki T, Maccari J, Goldberg D, Murphy H, Schwenzer J, Wang CY, Winchester RJ, Nepom GT, Silver J. Molecular diversity of HLA-DR4 haplotypes. Proc Natl Acad Sci USA 1986; 83:2642–6.
97. Erlich HA, Gelfand DH, Saiki RK. Specific DNA amplification. Nature 1988; 331:461–2.
98. Oste C. Polymerase chain reaction. Biotechniques 1988; 6:162–70.
99. Hamilton JA, Williams N. In vitro inhibition of myelopoiesis by gold salts and D-penicillamine. J Rheumatol 1985; 12:892–6.
100. Hamilton JA, Williams N. Effects of auranofin and other anti-rheumatic drugs on human myelopoiesis in vivo. J Rheumatol 1987; 14:216–20.
101. Waters RV, Allison AC. Gold salts inhibit proliferation of promonocytic cells and accelerate their differentiation. Unpublished. 1987.
102. Adinolfi M. Anti-I antibody in normal human newborn infants. Immunology 1965; 9:43–52.
103. Ikebuchi K, Wong GG, Clark SC, Ihle JN, Hirai Y, Ogawa M. Interleukin 6 enhancement of interleukin 3-dependent proliferation of multipotential hemopoietic progenitors. Proc Natl Acad Sci USA 1987; 84: 9035–9.

104. Shore A, Jaglal S, Keystone EC. Enhanced interleukin-1 generation by monocytes is temporally linked to an early event in the onset or exacerbation of rheumatoid arthritis. Clin Exp Immunol 1986; 65: 293–302.
105. Dani VA, March LM, Nelson DS, Brooks PM. Interleukin-1 secretion by peripheral blood monocytes and synovial macrophages from patients with rheumatoid arthritis. J Rheumatol 1987; 14:33–9.
106. Kotzin BL, Kansas GS, Engleman EG, Hoppe RT, Kaplan HS, Strober S. Changes in T cell subsets in patients with rheumatoid arthritis treated with total lymphoid irradiation. Clin Immunol Immunopathol 1983; 27:250.
107. Fassbender H, Annefled M. The potential aggressiveness of synovial tissue in RA. J. Pathol 1983; 139:399.
108. O'Sullivan F, Fassbender H, Gay S, Koopman W. Etcopathogenesis of RA-like disease in MRL/1 mice. Arth Rheum. 1985; 28:529.
109. Bonanomi M-H, Velvart M, Stimpel M, Roos KM, Fehr K, Weder HG. Studies of pharmacokinetics and therapeutic effects of glucocorticoids entrapped in liposomes after intraarticular application in healthy rabbits and in rabbits with antigen-induced arthritis. Rheumatol Int 1987; 7:203–12.

Index

About the Editors

DANIEL E. FURST is Professor of Medicine and Rheumatology, University of Medicine and Dentistry of New Jersey, New Brunswick, and Director of Anti-Inflammatory/Pulmonary Clinical Research, CIBA-GEIGY Corporation, Summit, New Jersey. The author or coauthor of numerous publications, Dr. Furst is the editor of the *Inflammatory Disease and Therapy* series and the coeditor with Alan J. Lewis of *Nonsteroidal Anti-Inflammatory Drugs: Mechanisms and Clinical Use* (both titles, Marcel Dekker, Inc.). A member of the American College of Rheumatology and American Society for Clinical Pharmacology and Therapeutics, he received the M.D. degree (1968) from The Johns Hopkins University, Baltimore, Maryland.

MICHAEL E. WEINBLATT is an Associate Physician in the Department of Rheumatology and Immunology, Brigham and Women's Hospital, and Associate Professor of Medicine, Harvard Medical School, Boston, Massachusetts. The author or coauthor of numerous journal articles and book chapters, Dr. Weinblatt is a member of the American College of Rheumatology and American College of Physicians. He received the M.D. degree (1975) from the University of Maryland School of Medicine, Baltimore.